Type 2 Diabetes: Diagnosis and Management

Type 2 Diabetes: Diagnosis and Management

Edited by Solomon Fleming

AMERICAN
MEDICAL PUBLISHERS
www.americanmedicalpublishers.com

American Medical Publishers,
41 Flatbush Avenue,
1st Floor, New York,
NY 11217, USA

Visit us on the World Wide Web at:
www.americanmedicalpublishers.com

ISBN: 978-1-63927-129-0

Cataloging-in-Publication Data

Type 2 diabetes : diagnosis and management / edited by Solomon Fleming.
p. cm.
Includes bibliographical references and index.
ISBN 978-1-63927-129-0
1. Non-insulin-dependent diabetes. 2. Non-insulin-dependent diabetes--Diagnosis.
3. Non-insulin-dependent diabetes--Treatment. 4. Diabetes. I. Fleming, Solomon.
RC662.18 .T96 2022
616.462--dc23

Table of Contents

Preface

Type 2 diabetes, also known as adult-onset diabetes, is a form of diabetes that causes high blood sugar, insulin resistance and lack of insulin. Its symptoms include increased thirst, frequent urination, and weight loss. The long term complications that may occur due to the type 2 diabetes include heart disease, strokes and diabetic retinopathy. One of the major risk factors of type 2 diabetes is obesity. It is often treated with anti-diabetic medications. Type 2 diabetes is managed by focusing on lifestyle interventions and lowering cardiovascular risk factors. It is also managed through maintaining blood glucose levels. This book brings forth some of the most innovative concepts and elucidates the unexplored aspects of type 2 diabetes. It presents researches and studies performed by experts across the globe. This book will serve as a valuable source of reference for graduate and post graduate students.

Significant researches are present in this book. Intensive efforts have been employed by authors to make this book an outstanding discourse. This book contains the enlightening chapters which have been written on the basis of significant researches done by the experts.

Finally, I would also like to thank all the members involved in this book for being a team and meeting all the deadlines for the submission of their respective works. I would also like to thank my friends and family for being supportive in my efforts.

Editor

1

Molecular Modulation of Osteoblasts and Osteoclasts in Type 2 Diabetes

Selvalakshmi Rathinavelu,[1] Crissy Guidry-Elizondo,[1] and Jameela Banu[1,2]

[1]*Department of Health and Biomedical Sciences, College of Health Affairs, University of Texas Rio Grande Valley, 1201, W University Dr, Edinburg, TX 78539, USA*
[2]*Department of Biology, College of Sciences, University of Texas Rio Grande Valley, 1201, W University Dr, Edinburg, TX 78539, USA*

Correspondence should be addressed to Jameela Banu; jameela.banu@utrgv.edu

Academic Editor: Hiroshi Okamoto

Diabetes is a common disease affecting majority of populations worldwide. Since 1980, there has been an increase in the number of people diagnosed as prediabetic and diabetic. Diabetes is characterized by high levels of circulating glucose and leads to most microvascular and macrovascular complications such as retinopathy, nephropathy, neuropathy, stroke, and myocardial infarction. Bone marrow vascular disruption and increased adiposity are also linked to various complications in type II diabetes mellitus. In addition to these complications, type 2 diabetic patients also have fragile bones caused by faulty mineralization mainly due to increased adiposity among diabetic patients that affects both osteoblast and osteoclast functions. Other factors that increase fracture risk in diabetic patients are increased oxidative stress, inflammation, and drugs administered to diabetic patients. This review reports the modulation of different pathways that affect bone metabolism in diabetic conditions.

1. Introduction

Diabetic patients are at high risk of developing osteoporosis. Normal to high bone mineral density (BMD) measurements recorded in type II diabetes mellitus (T2DM) patients are misleading [1]. In diabetic patients, an increase in the risk of hip (1.4–1.7-fold) and vertebral fractures have been reported [2]. As one ages, both genders are not only susceptible to increased risk of fragile bones but are also at high risk of developing diabetes, which augments the risk of bone fractures [3–6]. Bone fragility in T2DM patients is related to decreased bone strength and malformation of collagen fibers that can result in faulty mineralization and increased micro damages [7–9]. Using BMD measurements alone to diagnose bone condition in T2DM may not be reliable as the strength of the bone may be compromised in these patients. It is suggested that BMD with body mass index (BMI) adjustments may be a better indicator [10]. Supplemental data such as biochemical markers can be additional diagnostic tool. Bone biochemical markers such as C-terminal telopeptide (CTX) and N-terminal telopeptide (NTX) will reflect on the bone resorption process and breakdown of the collagen fibers. Interestingly, in T2DM patients, there is decreased CTX and increased NTX levels [11], and other reports did not find any difference between the two markers [12].

However, in T2DM patients, the quality of collagen fibers is compromised rather than increased breakdown of the collagen fibers. In T2DM patients, the trabecular bone network was shown to have large holes, decreased osteoblast recruitment, and mineral apposition rates combined with increased osteoclastogenesis [13].

The major pathophysiology in T2DM patients is insulin resistance (IR). This can be attributed to lack of or decreased insulin secretion and/or insulin receptors on the cell membranes. A close relationship between glucose and bone metabolism has been reported [14–18]. Yamaguchi and Sugimoto have described the link between glucose, fat, and bone metabolism [2]. They have suggested that osteocalcin, an important bone-forming marker, in the uncarboxylated form and the Wnt signalling pathway proteins, may be modulated to increase the fragility of bones in diabetic patients [19]. Other hormones secreted by adipocytes like adiponectin

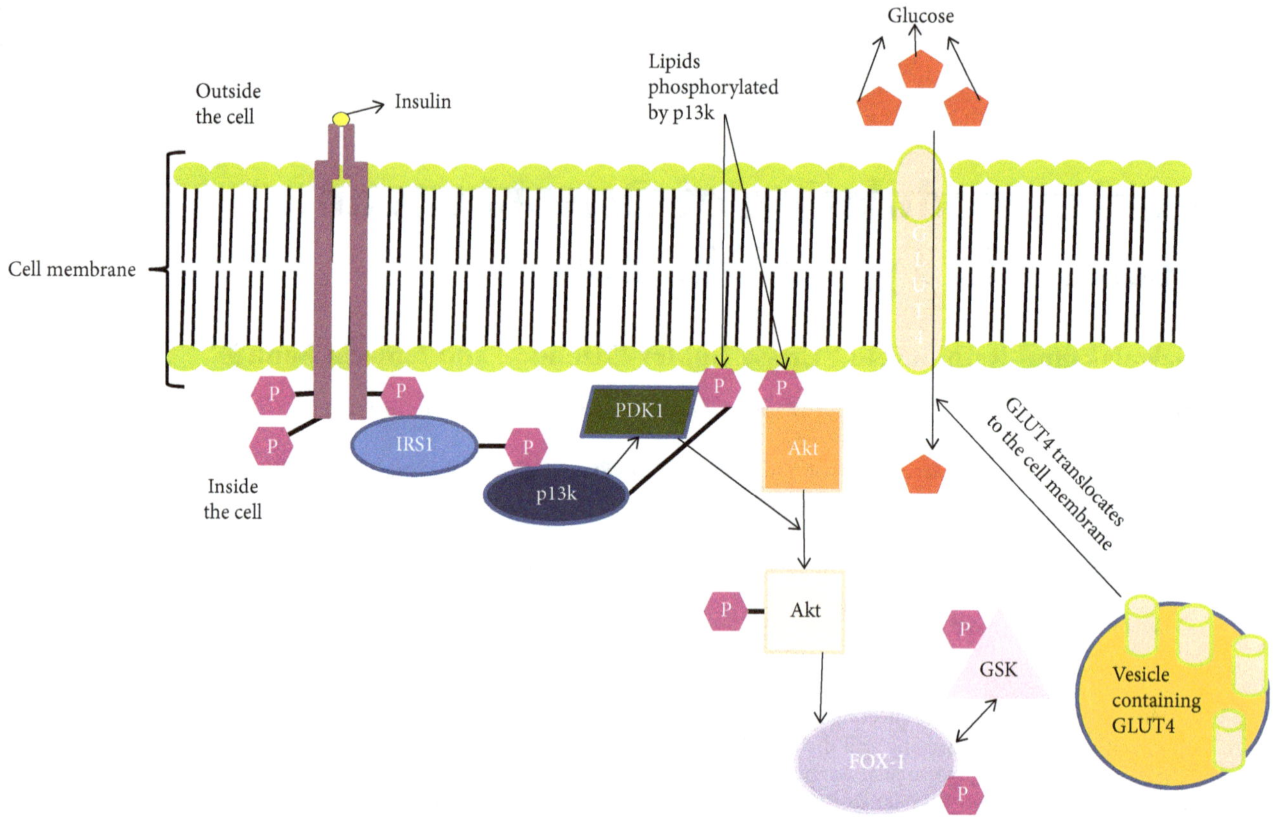

Figure 1: Insulin signalling pathway in normal cells.

decrease IR [20], while leptin increases IR [21, 22]; moreover, advanced glycation end products (AGEs) and insulin-like growth factor-I (IGF-1), which regulate bones, may be also modified in T2DM [1, 2]. AGE is formed by elevated blood glucose levels that cause nonenzymatic glycosylation and binds to its receptor (RAGE) which activates transcription factor nuclear factor-κB (NF-κB). This results in increased expression of receptor activator of nuclear factor kappa-B ligand- (RANKL-) mediated osteoclastogenesis [23, 24]. Accumulation of AGE may also stimulate interleukins (IL) such as IL-6, which reduces osteoblast proliferation and activity while increasing osteoclastic activity [1, 25–29]. In T2DM patients, there is hypersecretion of calcium and decreased calcium absorption due to decreased vitamin D levels and estrogenic levels, especially in females [30].

In addition, drugs used to treat diabetes can also have an effect on bone health. One such group of drugs is thiazolidiones (TZD), which increases the risk of osteoporosis in T2DM patients. TZDs are capable of influencing the mesenchymal cells to differentiate more into adipocytes rather than osteoblasts which results in increased cortical porosity [31]. Furthermore, insulin is administered to diabetic patients to help lower circulating glucose which directly acts on osteoclasts. A review of the drug effects on bone can be found in Montagnani et al. [1]. Although metformin has been shown to reduce bone loss, based on the severity of the side effects caused by this drug [32], absorption of nutrients essential for bone health may be compromised [30].

2. Materials and Methods

In this review, we are presenting information on the interaction of different pathways that influence bone, glucose utilization, and insulin signalling pathways. We collected literature using the following search engines: PubMed, Google Scholar, Cochrane Reviews, and Medline. The keywords used for the search were type II diabetes, insulin, bone, insulin and osteoclasts, insulin and osteoblasts, insulin and Wnt, insulin and inflammation, and insulin and oxidative stress.

3. Results and Discussion

3.1. Insulin Signalling Pathway under Normal and Diabetic Conditions. Normally, insulin activates several cascades of intracellular signalling pathways, which begins with phosphorylation of insulin receptor substrate 1 & 2 (IRS-1 & 2) and is followed by activation of phosphotidylinositide 3 kinase (PI3-K) and protein kinase B (AKT). This series of phosphorylation events, in turn, deactivates forkhead box proteins (FOX) and phosphorylates glycogen synthase (GSK), which plays an important role in controlling gluconeogenesis, glycogenolysis, and maintaining glucose homeostasis [33] (Figure 1). *In vitro* DNA-binding assays and transfection experiments showed that both mammalian FoxO and FoxA proteins can bind to IRS and mediate transcriptional activation [34].

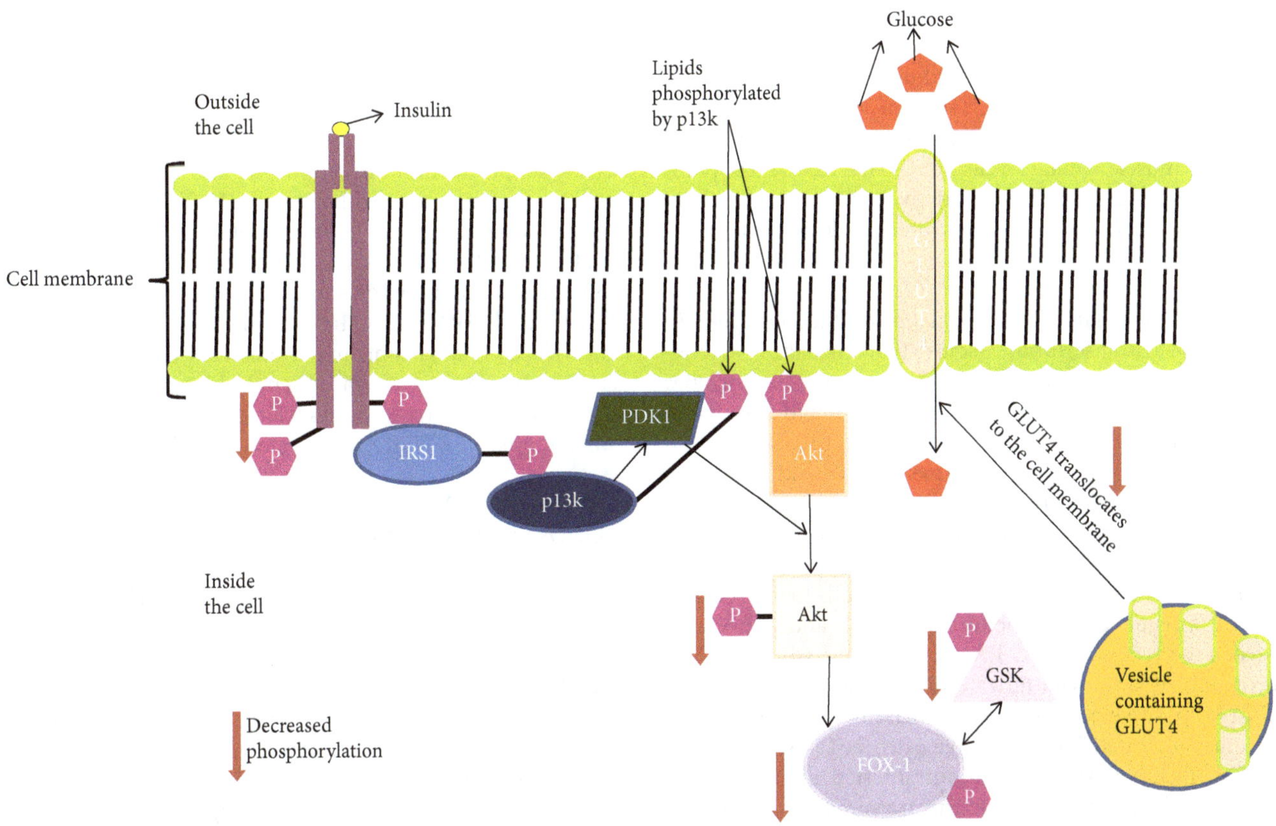

Figure 2: Insulin signalling pathway in cells of patients with type 2 diabetes mellitus.

Insulin regulates the transcriptional activity of hundreds of genes involved in glucose and lipid metabolism in the liver. Insulin along with growth hormone activates serine/threonine protein kinase (AKT), AKT phosphorylate FOXOs, and causes retention of FOXOs in the cytoplasm. In response to stress, decreased insulin, and growth hormone, FOXOs are activated and mediate bone cell functions [35, 36]. In T2DM, due to IR, there is decreased phosphorylation of IRS 1 & 2, decreasing PI3-K and increasing mitogen-activated protein kinase (MAPK) activation. This results in increased FOXO1 [33] (Figure 2). FOXO1 is activated in tissues associated with diabetic complications such as wound healing and bone fractures [33].

FOXOs play an important role in maintaining skeletal homeostasis by mediating both osteoclast and osteoblast function [35–41]. Other proteins like AGE, proinflammatory cytokines, and reactive oxygen species (ROS) are increased with high circulating blood glucose [33]. In T2DM, prolonged high levels of proinflammatory cytokines such as TNF-α, IL-1β, IL-6, and IL-18 enhance lipid peroxidation and dyslipidemia, resulting in increased osteoclastogenesis [42–44]. High levels of TNF-α increase the RANK/osteoprotegerin (OPG) ratio which enhances bone resorption [45].

Increased AGE, ROS, and proinflammatory cytokines increase bone loss. When AGE is formed, it bonds to its receptor RAGE and activates nuclear factor-κB (NF-κB) resulting in increased expression of RANKL-mediated osteoclastogenesis [23, 24, 46]. Prolonged inflammation also stimulates the expression of proapoptotic genes such as bcl-2-like protein (Bax). This reduces the expression of genes that stimulate osteoblast formation such as Fos-related antigen (FRA-1) and Runt-related transcription factor (RUNX2) [33] resulting in decreased bone formation. Oxidative stress reduces differentiation to osteoblasts and can directly degrade bone [47]. NF-κB responds to oxidative stress and increases osteoclast activity and decreases osteoblast differentiation [47].

3.2. Type 2 Diabetes Modulation of Bone Marrow Stem Cells. The microenvironment in bone marrow cells is affected by complications of diabetes. The mesenchymal stem cells (MSC) can differentiate into adipocytes or osteoblasts depending on the prevailing signalling molecules. Long-standing diabetes causes disruption of the bone marrow microenvironment by depleting and altering stem/progenitor cells resulting in enhanced adipogenesis and depressed osteogenesis [3, 48–56]. *In vitro* studies on RAW264.7 cells have demonstrated that high glucose decreases autophagy of osteoclasts thereby increasing osteoclastogenesis [57]. The multifactorial causes of enhanced adipogenesis are augmented insulin signalling, hyperlipidemia, and ROS. One of the major players is peroxisome proliferator-activated receptor gamma (PPARγ), an important regulator of lipid, glucose, and insulin metabolism. It consists of two isoforms—PPARγ1 and PPARγ2. PPARγ2 regulates the differentiation of MSC to either adipocytes or osteoblast [58]. Inside the cells, high levels of blood glucose activate phosphatidylinositol 4,5 bisphosphate 3 kinase (PI3k) and phosphorylate protein kinase B (PKB). This decreases peroxisome proliferator-activated receptor gamma (PPARγ) through FOXO1 and increases adipogenesis.

Activation of mechanistic target of rapamycin (mTOR) increases adipocyte specific factors in preadipocytes and increases muscle satellite cells [33]. The PI3K/PKB pathway is also stimulated by oxidative stress generated by ROS and enhances adipogenesis, thereby decreasing osteoclastogenesis [55].

3.3. FOXO1 Regulates RANKL-Mediated Osteoclastogenesis. FOX-1 is a transcription factor that mediates RANK-induced osteoclast formation. Osteoclast formation includes several steps such as differentiation of myeloid precursors to preosteoclasts, fusion of mononuclear preosteoclast to multinucleated osteoclasts, and maturation and activation of osteoclasts. Several proteins are involved in osteoclastogenesis such as RANKL, NK-κB, TNF, macrophage colony stimulating factor (M-CSF), and nuclear factor of activated T cells (NFATC1) [36]. Initially, M-CSF binds to its receptor, which upregulates and activates RANK and NF-κB in osteoclast precursor cells. RANK signalling stimulates the formation of single-cell tartrate-resistant acid phosphatase-(TRAP-) positive preosteoclasts, which fuse together to form the multinucleated TRAP-positive osteoclast [34].

Cell fusion is the most important step in osteoclastogenesis and dendritic cell-specific transmembrane protein (DC-STAMP), which induces NFATC1, the master gene in osteoclastogenesis [33]. Other NFATC1-mediated fusion molecules are TRAP, osteoclast-associated receptor (OSCAR), Cathepsin K, proto oncogene tyrosine protein kinase (C-SRC), and β3 integrin. Cell fusion can also be induced by other molecules independent of NFATc1 such as CD9, CD44, E-cadherin, merlin α, and macrophage fusion receptor [39]. When RANK stimulates NFATC1 through extracellular signal-regulated kinases (ERK)/c-Jun amino-terminal kinases (JNK)/MAP kinase p38 [33, 36], it also activates phospholipase C (PLC). This releases inositol triphosphate (IP_3) which causes extracellular calcium influx and intracellular calcium release inducing calcium oscillation.

These calcium oscillations activated by NFATc1 are regulated by Transmembrane 64 (Tmem 64) and interact with sarcoplasmic endoplasmic reticulum carbonic anhydrase (SERCA), causing osteoclast differentiation [59]. Tmem64 also interacts with SERCA2 through tyrosine-based activation motif (ITAM) that has a common Fc receptor gamma subunit (FCRγ) and DNAX-activating protein 12 (DAP12). This costimulation leads to activation of phospholipase gamma (PLCγ) and IP_3 causing calcium release from endoplasmic reticulum (ER), generating calcium oscillations. These oscillations activate Ca^{2+}/calmodulin-dependent protein kinase (CaMK) IV and cyclic AMP response element-binding protein (CREB), which plays an important role in the generation of mitochondrial ROS, induction of NFATc1 and C-FOS necessary for osteoclast production. NFATc1 induced by CREB is short acting but continuously spike cycling Ca^{2+} by activating SERCA2, which is necessary to sustain NFATc1 activity during osteoclastogenesis [38]. Later, osteoclasts are polarized by actin, integrin αV, and integrin β3, which activates vacuolar ATPase and release of cathepsin K (CTSK), lysosomal cysteine, and protease to degrade bone matrix, causing bone resorption.

FOX-1 which mediates the effect of RANK on osteoclastogenesis also modulates Toll-like receptor (TLR) and cytokine production in monocyte and dendritic cells as well as downstream regulation of NFATC1. This, in turn, regulates dendritic cell-derived protein (DC-STAMP) and ATP 6VOD2, which play an important role in cell fusion [33]. The differentiated osteoclast expresses NFATc1, OSCAR, CTSK, and PPARγc1b. In diabetic conditions, increased RANKL/OPG ratio contributes to increased osteoclastogenesis [35]. Interestingly, in the absence of RANK, NF-κB can be activated by TNF receptor-associated factor 6 (TRAF6) pathway, ectopic NFATC1, and activated RANKL promoters [41].

3.4. Role of FOXOs against Oxidative Stress in Osteoblasts. FOXOs protect osteoblasts from oxidative stress by interacting with transcription factor which regulates amino acid import, proliferation of osteoblasts, and generation of antioxidant enzymes such as catalase, superoxide dismutase (SOD), and glutathione [40]. In response to oxidative stress generated by reactive oxygen species (ROS), FOX 1, 3, and 4 are activated in the nucleus of the osteoblasts and produce antioxidants to decrease bone resorption. Oxidative stress is the critical step for osteoclast differentiation and function [35].

Both FOX1 and activating transcription factor 4 (ATF4) are located in the cytoplasm and respond to stress. Both are translocated to the nucleus which promotes protein and amino acid synthesis. ATF4 controls protein synthesis through a negative feedback mechanism that leads to accumulation of glutathione and collagen production. FOX1 also promotes osteoblast proliferation by increasing cell cycle cyclin D1 and D2 and suppressing cell cycle inhibitor p27Kip1. Decreased FOX1 suppresses osteoblastogenesis by decreasing osterix and type 1 collagen protein levels but does not affect levels of Runx2 and Bsp (bone sialoprotein) [40]. FOXOs are potent repressors of osteoblastogenesis by also decreasing PPAR-γ [37, 40]. This increase in bone resorption may be attributed to activation of antiosteoclastogenic factor osteoprotegerin (OPG) which promotes FOX-mediated transcription of β-catenin/T-cell specific transcription factor (TCF), thereby promoting RANK-mediated osteoclastogenesis by increasing PPAR-γ. This increases apoptosis of osteocytes and enhances adipogenesis as indicated by decreased bone markers such as calcitonin, TRAP, and cathepsin K [37]. Osteoblasts exposed to oxidative stress also have decreased expression of RUNX2 and osteocalcin and increased adipogenesis-related factors PPAR-γ and fatty acid binding protein-4 (FABP4) [55].

3.5. Wnt/β-Catenin Pathways in Metabolic Syndrome. Activation of Wnt (β-catenin) signalling promotes differentiation of progenitor stem cells into osteoblasts and prevents adipogenesis. Regulation of Wnt signalling is a balance between adipogenesis and myogenesis [60]. Wnt/(β-catenin) is activated when PPAR-γ binds with lymphoid enhancer factor/T cell factor (LEF/TCF), binding domain of β-catenin, and facilitates its phosphorylation by glycogen synthase kinase3b

(GSK3b), thereby resulting in increased differentiation within preadipocytes [61, 62]. The Wnt family has 19 ligands, 10 Wnt receptors, frizzled (Fz) coreceptors, and low-density lipoprotein receptor-related proteins (LRP-5 and LRP-6). The actions of Wnt include canonical and noncanonical pathways. Noncanonical Wnt signalling cascade also plays an important role in adipogenesis. Wnt binds to its receptor and activates phospholipase C (PLC), generating diacylglycerol (DAG) and inositol triphosphate (IP_3), which results in the release of intracellular calcium from the endoplasmic reticulum. Efflux of intracellular calcium activates protein kinase C (PKC). This leads to the phosphorylation of SET domain bifurcated-1 (SETB1) histone methyltransferase, inhibiting PPAR-γ through histone methylation H3-K9, and upregulates RUNX2 required for osteoblastogenesis [63, 64]. PKC has a dual role in adipogenesis. Its isoforms α, δ, and μ inhibit adipogenesis, while β1 and γ isoforms promote adipogenesis. Hyperglycemia-induced noncanonical Wnt pathway increased adipogenesis through activation of various PKC isoforms [55]. Wnt/β catenin pathway inhibitor, sclerostin, is increased in the serum of T2DM and is inversely related to levels of bone turnover markers [65, 66].

Regulation of Wnt signalling is a balance between adipogenesis and myogenesis. Insulin action and insulin resistance can be modulated by Wnt and lipoprotein receptor-related protein 5 (LRP5) activity [57]. Wnt canonical pathway acts on Fz/(LRP5/6), decreasing GSK-3β and increasing β-catenin, which translocates to the nucleus, conjuncts with lymphoid enhancer factor/T-cell factor (TCF), and regulates transcription of Wnt target genes. The *in vitro* study using human adipose-derived stem cells has shown that during the differentiation of insulin-producing cells (IPC), protein levels of Wnt 1, β-catenin, and GSK3β are increased [67]. At the same time, TCF-1 and cyclin-D increased from day 1 to day 9 and decreased from day 9 onwards and continued to decrease. Inhibition of Wnt signalling does not decrease differentiation from day 1 to day 9 but upregulates IPC specific markers such as insulin promoter 1 (PDX-1), insulin, and insulin receptor substrates 1 and 2 (IRS-1 and 2) from day 9 to day 12. Wnt signalling specific marker such as glucokinase decreased from day 9 to day 12. Activation of Wnt signalling on day 9 decreases IPC specific markers, and deactivation of Wnt signalling is necessary for IPC maturation [39, 67]. Overall, Wnt signalling may be more involved in IPC maturation [58]. In the pancreas and hepatocytes, β catenin/Wnt signalling pathways activate glucokinase promoter activities in the presence of PPAR-γ and cyclin-D promoter with transcription factor 7-like 2 (TCF7L2) binding sites [68] and play an important role in maintaining β-cell function [69].

IRS-2 and Akt are key signalling molecules in maintaining β-cell mass [70]. Akt prevents free fatty acid-induced β-cell apoptosis through inhibition of proapoptotic proteins like germinal center kinase 3α, β(GCK3α/β), FOX 1, and p53 [70]. The cross talk between insulin and Wnt signalling occurs at the level of coreceptor LRP 5, which has a profound positive effect on insulin signalling in preadipocytes [71].

The direct interaction between insulin receptors and LRP 5 occurs in an insulin/Wnt inducible manner. Insulin receptor/LRP 5 plays an important role in the pathogenesis of IR and obesity. Decreased Wnt canonical pathway receptor LRP5/6 increases the risk of diabetes mellitus and impaired glucose intolerance [33, 60].

Wnt signalling varies slightly in different cells. In preadipocytes, both insulin and Wnt3a lead to phosphorylation of LRP 6, GSK3b, Akt, and extracellular signal-regulated kinase (ERK1/2). If both IGF receptors and insulin receptors decrease, insulin-mediated Wnt3a phosphorylation decreases. Whereas, Wnt-mediated phosphorylation decreases not only when insulin receptors and IGF receptors are decreased but also in the absence of these receptors.

In skeletal muscles, Wnt/β-catenin signalling (1) increases muscle-specific myogenic transcription factor, (2) decreases PPAR-γ-related adipogenesis and C/EBP α expression, (3) converts type 2 skeletal muscle fibers into type 1 muscle fibers, (4) decreases c-myc-mediated activation of p27, which decreases myogenesis and increases adipogenesis, and (5) activates mitogenic factor 5 (Myf 5), which in turn activates myoblast determination protein D (myoD) [72, 73]. Risk of T2DM increases with decreased Wnt signalling in the skeletal muscle and increased adipogenesis [55, 74].

In hepatocytes, canonical Wnt3a stimulation decreases key enzymes of gluconeogenesis such as phosphoenolpyruvate carboxykinase (PEPCK) and glucose 6-phosphatase (G6Pase). Noncanonical Wnt 11 stimulation decreases glucose output by hepatocytes. Insulin increases TCF7L2, which increases cyclin D, a downstream target of the Wnt signalling pathway [75]. β-Catenin phosphorylation is positively correlated with transcriptional activity of β-cat/TCF. β-catenin phosphorylation occurs with (1) protein kinase A (PKA) activation; (2) PKA/cyclic adenosine monophosphate (cAMP) activator and glucagon stimulate cAMP responsive element-binding protein (CREB) phosphorylation, and (3) insulin is able to stimulate β-catenin phosphorylation [76].

In response to feeding, insulin mediates a repressor effect on gluconeogenesis through TCF7L2 and β-catenin phosphorylation. In the absence of TCF7L2, insulin also decreases gluconeogenesis by attenuating FOX [77]. Wnt and TCF7L2 are negative regulators of gluconeogenesis, while FOX is a positive regulator of gluconeogenesis [76]; insulin increases TCF7L2 in intestinal L-cells and stimulates the expression of proglucagon gene and incretin hormone glucagon-like peptide 1 (GLP-1) [77]; glucagon increases FOX through cAMP, and insulin decreases FOX through PI3K/Akt-mediated nuclear exclusion of FOXO1 [78], and TCF7L2 increases hepatic glucose production and the risk of T2DM [77].

3.6. Hormonal Balance in Skeletal Homeostasis and Metabolic Syndrome. Certain hormones associated with bone metabolism and energy balance such as osteocalcin, leptin, and adiponectin affect insulin signalling pathways and other hormones related to calcium homeostasis [70]. Osteocalcin is the marker of osteoblast activity [79] and is modulated in the osteoblast-specific gene esp, which encodes osteotesticular protein tyrosine phosphatase (OST-PTP) [80]. This OST-PTP dephosphorylates the insulin receptor [79]. Decreased OST-PTP increases insulin signalling through

Table 1: Effects of antidiabetic drugs on bone metabolism.

Antidiabetic drugs	Mode of action	References
Amylin	At low concentrations ↓ osteoclastogenesis	[90]
Incretin	↓ GLP-1 receptors; ↑ GIP influence on bone resorption and bone formation	[30, 71, 86]
Insulin	↑ Bone formation	[87–89]
Metformin	↓ Indigenous glucose production; ↑ insulin sensitivity; ↑ osteogenic markers	[31, 51, 78, 79, 80–82]
Sodium glucose cotransporter inhibitors	Interferes with calcium and phosphate homeostasis; ↑ CTX and ↓ BMD	[91, 92]
Sulfonylureas	↓ CTX, NTX; ↑ ALP, osteocalcin, bone strength	[30, 81, 83]
Thiazolidinediones	↑ Adipogenesis; ↓ BMD	[31]

↑ = increases; ↓ = decreases. GLP-1 = Glucogon like peptide 1, GIP = G;ucose-dependent insulinotropic polypeptide, CTX = C-terminal telopeptide, NTX = N-terminal telopeptide, BMD = bone mineral density, ALP = alkaline phosphatase.

the insulin receptor and promotes pancreatic β-cell proliferation, while increasing insulin and insulin-sensitizing adiponectin [79, 81].

Leptin produced by adipocytes acts on the hypothalamus, which regulates decreases and increases on appetite and satiety, as well as decrease in bone formation by inhibiting osteocalcin production in new bones [82, 83]. Adiponectin, also produced by adipocytes, acts on bones in an age-dependent manner and is inversely proportional to BMD [84]. Adiponectin is an antagonist to leptin, acts on the brain, and increases sympathetic output to peripheral osteoblast [85].

Other hormones like vitamin D and estrogen levels may be associated with developing T2DM and IR [65, 86]. Decreased levels of vitamin D decrease renal reabsorption of calcium and reduce osteocalcin production by osteoblasts [87], resulting in diminished bone formation. Estrogen, on the other hand, is implicated in IR. Of the two estrogen receptors, ERα is positively associated with glucose metabolism [88]. Both direct and indirect effects of ERα on IR have been reported. Directly, ERα can act on insulin signalling and increase GLUT4 expression, while indirectly, it can modulate oxidative stress and inflammation [89].

3.7. Influence of Drugs Used for Treating Diabetes and Bone. Different drugs commonly prescribed for treating diabetes like metformin, thiazolidinedione, and sulfonylurea do affect bone mass (Table 1). Most of them act on different pathways to influence bone status in the patients. One highly prescribed medication for T2DM patients is metformin. This drug has been associated with the most bone protective properties. Metformin can activate adenosine monophosphate kinase (AMPK) to reduce indigenous glucose production or may also act independent of the AMPK pathway by inhibiting glycolytic enzymes or adenylate cyclase and decreases gluconeogenesis [90, 91]. At the mesenchymal cellular level, metformin reduces adipocyte formation in the bone marrow by preventing endothelial nitric oxide synthase (eNOS) expression [14]. Metformin acts as an insulin sensitizer, increases GLP-1 secretion in L-cells of the intestines, stimulates nuclear translocation of β-catenin, and increases transcription of luciferase reporter gene. GLP-1 increases (1) pancreatic insulin secretion, (2) proinsulin gene expression, and (3) β-cell mass. GLP-1 also decreases gastric emptying and glucagon release. Inside the cells, metformin increases IRS-2, p-PI3K, p-PKB, calcium/calmodulin-dependent protein kinase 2 (CaMK2), CREB, p-GSKSβ (inactive form), enzymes of glycolysis like phosphofructokinase (PFK), and Kreb's cycle enzymes (isocitrate dehydrogenase, malate dehydrogenase). Glucose utilization mediated by metformin is through calcium-dependent protein kinase [55]. Metformin also increases the markers of osteogenic differentiation and function [33]. Although metformin has beneficial effects on bone, there is concern for patients who have moderate to severe digestive intolerance after consuming this medication, as nutrients necessary for bone health may not be absorbed properly.

Sulfonylureas are organic compounds that act on the pancreatic cells and increase the release of insulin. They act on membrane channels, first by blocking the potassium channels, causing depolarization in the cell which then opens the Ca^{2+} channels and this increases the release of insulin [92]. There are very few studies that show the interaction between the consumption of these drugs and bone. The few reports show that C-terminal telopeptide (CTX) and N-terminal telopeptide (NTX) levels are decreased in patients who take these drugs [32, 93]. Sulfonylureas can also activate the PI3K/ATK pathway which then increases the expression of alkaline phosphatase and osteocalcin mRNA expression [94]. It has been reported that sulfonylureas protect against ovariectomy-induced bone loss and also increase the mechanical strength by increasing bone formation [95]. Based on the limited evidence available, sulfonylureas are beneficial to the bone. In-depth, long-term studies are necessary to know the exact function of sulfonylureas on the bone in T2DM patients.

Recently, incretin-based therapies are being used. Incretins are inhibitors of glucagon-like peptide 1 receptors (GLP-1) and dipeptidyl peptidase 4 (DPP-4). GLP-1 receptors are expressed in the pancreatic β cells and other cells promoting metabolic activity [32]. It has been reported that GLP-1 can control bone resorption by interacting with GLP-2 and glucose-dependent insulinotropic polypeptide (GIP) [96]. In addition, it can also act on a calcitonin-dependent pathway [96]. GLP-2 may have antiresorptive function [97] while GIP can influence bone resorption and bone formation [80, 98].

Many clinical studies with patients who are on insulin treatment for T2DM have reported increased risk of fracture, especially in postmenopausal women [99–101]. Insulin is known to increase bone formation generally, and lack of detailed study on the reasons for insulin increasing fracture rates is not understood.

Amylin is a peptide that is reported to have some effects on bone metabolism [32]. Both *in vitro* and *in vivo* studies show this peptide, when present in lower levels, is associated with inhibited osteoclastic activity [102]. However, there is not much data on clinical studies regarding the effects of amylin on the bone.

Sodium glucose cotransporter inhibitors (SGCT) are drugs that reduce the reabsorption of glucose from the kidneys by inhibiting the sodium glucose cotransporters. They are capable of altering the calcium and phosphate homeostasis; therefore, they affect the bone and may be more deleterious to the bone. Several reports have shown that imbalance in the calcium and phosphate homeostasis triggers secretion of PTH which increases bone resorption [103]. Increased levels of CTX and decreased BMD values are also reported with the use of these drugs [104]. However, some reports have not shown any significant influence on the mineral levels or the levels of parathyroid hormone (PTH) and vitamin D [105, 106]. This may be due to any differences in the intake of vitamins and minerals. At this point, it may be safe to say that these drugs may be deleterious to the bone although more in-depth studies are required to determine the mechanism by which these drugs affect the bone [32].

TZDs are the most popular set of drugs that are proven to be harmful to the bone. The primary mechanism of action in TZDs is through direct induction of PPAR-γ leading to improved insulin sensitivity. The stimulation of differentiation of multipotent stem cells into adipocytes and increased adiposity in bone marrow are seen in patients treated with TZDs. The most common side effect of TZDs is weight gain through promotion of PPAR-γ, with increased adipogenesis leading to increased subcutaneous and bone marrow fat depots and decreased bone formation. These properties of TZDs make the patients' bones become very fragile, and their BMD is significantly decreased [33].

4. Conclusion

There is increasing evidence about the interaction between the glucose metabolic pathway, insulin signalling, and bone metabolic pathways. In 2015, it was reported that there was a rise in people aged 66 and older having T2DM [107]. Unfortunately, this is also the age when both men and women have decreased bone mass and are at high risk of having hip and spine fractures [65]. This may be because of the interaction of signalling pathways that modulate bone and glucose metabolism in T2DM patients. In order to assess the fracture risk, a combination of BMD, FRAX, and biochemical markers should be used. T2DM patients should be tested for their bone health regularly, and bone status in T2DM patients should be recognized as a complication of diabetes as recommended by Sanches et al. [58]. Another factor that influences the bone in T2DM is as a side effect of the drugs that are prescribed to treat diabetes. It is important to note that there is an intricate connection between the different pathways that are altered in T2DM patients and bone metabolism. Although there is evidence of the effects of metformin and TZDs on bones, more research need to be conducted with the newer antidiabetic drugs. Therefore, patients being treated for diabetes should be tested for several vitamin and mineral levels. This information should be used to advise patients on the nutrient intake of specific vitamin and mineral deficiencies. In addition, medications used for treating diabetes should be carefully chosen, and any micronutrient deficiency should be supplemented.

Conflicts of Interest

All the authors declare that there is no conflict of interest.

Authors' Contributions

The first two authors are equal contributors of the content of the manuscript. The last author designed the review and prepared the first draft of the paper. All authors revised the paper critically for intellectual content and approved the final version. All authors agree to be accountable for the work, and they ensure that any questions relating to the accuracy and integrity of the paper are investigated and properly resolved.

Acknowledgments

We acknowledge the Undergraduate Research Initiative, UTPA, for supporting Ms. Crissy Guidry Elizondo.

References

[1] A. Montagnani, S. Gonnelli, M. Alessandri, and R. Nuti, "Osteoporosis and risk of fracture in patients with diabetes: an update," *Aging Clinical and Experimental Research*, vol. 23, no. 2, pp. 84–90, 2011.

[2] T. Yamaguchi and T. Sugimoto, "Bone metabolism and fracture risk in type 2 diabetes mellitus [review]," *Endocrine Journal*, vol. 58, no. 8, pp. 613–624, 2011.

[3] M. Janghorbani, R. M. Van Dam, W. C. Willett, and F. B. Hu, "Systematic review of type 1 and type 2 diabetes mellitus and risk of fracture," *American Journal of Epidemiology*, vol. 166, no. 5, pp. 495–505, 2007.

[4] M. A. Petit, M. L. Paudel, B. C. Taylor et al., "Bone mass and strength in older men with type 2 diabetes: the Osteoporotic Fractures in Men Study," *Journal of Bone and Mineral Research*, vol. 25, no. 2, pp. 285–291, 2009.

[5] C. L. Khoo and M. Perera, "Diabetes and the menopause," *The Journal of the British Menopause Society*, vol. 11, no. 1, pp. 6–11, 2005.

[6] D. Merlotti, L. Gennari, F. Dotta, D. Lauro, and R. Nuti, "Mechanisms of impaired bone strength in type 1 and 2 diabetes," *Nutrition, Metabolism, and Cardiovascular Diseases*, vol. 20, no. 9, pp. 683–690, 2010.

[7] P. K. Dixit and R. A. Ekstrom, "Decreased breaking strength of diabetic rat bone and its improvement by insulin treatment," *Calcified Tissue International*, vol. 32, no. 1, pp. 195–199, 1980.

[8] M. Saito and K. Marumo, "Collagen cross-links as a determinant of bone quality: a possible explanation for bone fragility in aging, osteoporosis, and diabetes mellitus," *Osteoporosis International*, vol. 21, no. 2, pp. 195–214, 2009.

[9] G. K. Reddy, L. Stehno-Bittel, S. Hamade, and C. S. Enwemeka, "The biomechanical integrity of bone in experimental diabetes," *Diabetes Research and Clinical Practice*, vol. 54, no. 1, pp. 1–8, 2001.

[10] D. W. Bowden, A. J. Cox, B. I. Freedman et al., "Review of the Diabetes Heart Study (DHS) family of studies: a comprehensively examined sample for genetic and epidemiological studies of type 2 diabetes and its complications," *The Review of Diabetic Studies*, vol. 7, no. 3, pp. 188–201, 2010.

[11] J. Starup-Linde, S. A. Eriksen, S. Lykkeboe, A. Handberg, and P. Vestergaard, "Biochemical markers of bone turnover in diabetes patients–a meta-analysis, and a methodological study on the effects of glucose on bone markers," *Osteoporosis International*, vol. 25, no. 6, pp. 1697–1708, 2014.

[12] M. Herrmann and M. J. Seibel, "The amino- and carboxyterminal cross-linked telopeptides of collagen type I, NTX-I and CTX-I: a comparative review," *Clinica Chimica Acta*, vol. 393, no. 2, pp. 57–75, 2008.

[13] J. M. Pritchard, L. M. Giangregorio, S. A. Atkinson et al., "Association of larger holes in the trabecular bone at the distal radius in postmenopausal women with type 2 diabetes mellitus compared to controls," *Arthritis Care & Research*, vol. 64, no. 1, pp. 83–91, 2011.

[14] Q. Gu, Y. Gu, H. Yang, and Q. Shi, "Metformin enhances osteogenesis and suppresses adipogenesis of human chorionic villous mesenchymal stem cells," *The Tohoku Journal of Experimental Medicine*, vol. 241, no. 1, pp. 13–19, 2017.

[15] J. Starup-Linde and P. Vestergaard, "Biochemical bone turnover markers in diabetes mellitus - a systematic review," *Bone*, vol. 82, pp. 69–78, 2016.

[16] J. Starup-Linde, M. Frost, P. Vestergaard, and B. Abrahamsen, "Epidemiology of fractures in diabetes," *Calcified Tissue International*, vol. 100, no. 2, pp. 109–121, 2016.

[17] J. Starup-Linde, S. Gregersen, and P. Vestergaard, "Associations with fracture in patients with diabetes: a nested case-control study," *BMJ Open*, vol. 6, no. 2, article e009686, 2016.

[18] J. Starup-Linde, S. Lykkeboe, S. Gregersen et al., "Differences in biochemical bone markers by diabetes type and the impact of glucose," *Bone*, vol. 83, pp. 149–155, 2016.

[19] K. J. Motyl, L. R. McCabe, and A. V. Schwartz, "Bone and glucose metabolism: a two-way street," *Archives of Biochemistry and Biophysics*, vol. 503, no. 1, pp. 2–10, 2010.

[20] C. B. Confavreux, R. L. Levine, and G. Karsenty, "A paradigm of integrative physiology, the crosstalk between bone and energy metabolisms," *Molecular and Cellular Endocrinology*, vol. 310, no. 1-2, pp. 21–29, 2009.

[21] F. J. A. de Paula, M. C. Horowitz, and C. J. Rosen, "Novel insights into the relationship between diabetes and osteoporosis," *Diabetes/Metabolism Research and Reviews*, vol. 26, no. 8, pp. 622–630, 2010.

[22] G. Wolf, "Energy regulation by the skeleton," *Nutrition Reviews*, vol. 66, no. 4, pp. 229–233, 2008.

[23] K. H. Ding, Z. Z. Wang, M. W. Hamrick et al., "Disordered osteoclast formation in RAGE-deficient mouse establishes an essential role for RAGE in diabetes related bone loss," *Biochemical and Biophysical Research Communications*, vol. 340, no. 4, pp. 1091–1097, 2006.

[24] J. Xie, J. D. Mendez, V. Mendez-Valenzuela, and M. M. Aguilar-Hernandez, "Cellular signalling of the receptor for advanced glycation end products (RAGE)," *Cellular Signalling*, vol. 25, no. 11, pp. 2185–2197, 2013.

[25] C. J. Hernandez, S. Y. Tang, B. M. Baumbach et al., "Trabecular microfracture and the influence of pyridinium and non-enzymatic glycation-mediated collagen cross-links," *Bone*, vol. 37, no. 6, pp. 825–832, 2005.

[26] Y. Katayama, T. Akatsu, M. Yamamoto, N. Kugai, and N. Nagata, "Role of nonenzymatic glycosylation of type I collagen in diabetic osteopenia," *Journal of Bone and Mineral Research*, vol. 11, no. 7, pp. 931–937, 1996.

[27] T. Miyata, K. Notoya, K. Yoshida et al., "Advanced glycation end products enhance osteoclast-induced bone resorption in cultured mouse unfractionated bone cells and in rats implanted subcutaneously with devitalized bone particles," *Journal of the American Society of Nephrology*, vol. 8, no. 2, pp. 260–270, 1997.

[28] M. Takagi, S. Kasayama, T. Yamamoto et al., "Advanced glycation endproducts stimulate interleukin-6 production by human bone-derived cells," *Journal of Bone and Mineral Research*, vol. 12, no. 3, pp. 439–446, 1997.

[29] X. Wang, X. Shen, X. Li, and C. Mauli Agrawal, "Age-related changes in the collagen network and toughness of bone," *Bone*, vol. 31, no. 1, pp. 1–7, 2002.

[30] G. Isaia, L. Bodrato, V. Carlevatto, M. Mussetta, G. Salamano, and G. M. Molinatti, "Osteoporosis in type II diabetes," *Acta Diabetologica Latina*, vol. 24, no. 4, pp. 305–310, 1987.

[31] L. D. Sardone, R. Renlund, T. L. Willett, I. G. Fantus, and M. D. Grynpas, "Effect of rosiglitazone on bone quality in a rat model of insulin resistance and osteoporosis," *Diabetes*, vol. 60, no. 12, pp. 3271–3278, 2011.

[32] M. Chandran, "Diabetes drug effects on the skeleton," *Calcified Tissue International*, vol. 100, no. 2, pp. 133–149, 2017.

[33] H. Jiao, E. Xiao, and D. T. Graves, "Diabetes and its effect on bone and fracture healing," *Current Osteoporosis Reports*, vol. 13, no. 5, pp. 327–335, 2015.

[34] S. Hannenhalli and K. H. Kaestner, "The evolution of Fox genes and their role in development and disease," *Nature Reviews. Genetics*, vol. 10, no. 4, pp. 233–240, 2009.

[35] S. M. Bartell, H. N. Kim, E. Ambrogini et al., "FoxO proteins restrain osteoclastogenesis and bone resorption by attenuating H_2O_2 accumulation," *Nature Communications*, vol. 5, no. 1, p. 3773, 2014.

[36] Y. Wang, G. Dong, H. H. Jeon et al., "FOXO1 mediates RANKL-induced osteoclast formation and activity," *Journal of Immunology*, vol. 194, no. 6, pp. 2878–2887, 2015.

[37] E. Ambrogini, M. Almeida, M. Martin-Millan et al., "FoxO-mediated defense against oxidative stress in osteoblasts is indispensable for skeletal homeostasis in mice," *Cell Metabolism*, vol. 11, no. 2, pp. 136–146, 2010.

[38] H. Kim, T. Kim, B. C. Jeong et al., "Tmem64 modulates calcium signaling during RANKL-mediated osteoclast differentiation," *Cell Metabolism*, vol. 17, no. 2, pp. 249–260, 2013.

[39] K. Kim, S. H. Lee, J. Ha Kim, Y. Choi, and N. Kim, "NFATc1 induces osteoclast fusion via up-regulation of Atp6v0d2 and the dendritic cell-specific transmembrane protein (DC-STAMP)," *Molecular Endocrinology*, vol. 22, no. 1, pp. 176–185, 2008.

[40] M. T. Rached, A. Kode, L. Xu et al., "FoxO1 is a positive regulator of bone formation by favoring protein synthesis and

resistance to oxidative stress in osteoblasts," *Cell Metabolism*, vol. 11, no. 2, pp. 147–160, 2010.

[41] H. Takayanagi, S. Kim, T. Koga et al., "Induction and activation of the transcription factor NFATc1 (NFAT2) integrate RANKL signaling in terminal differentiation of osteoclasts," *Developmental Cell*, vol. 3, no. 6, pp. 889–901, 2002.

[42] D. T. Graves and R. A. Kayal, "Diabetic complications and dysregulated innate immunity," *Frontiers in Bioscience*, vol. 13, no. 13, pp. 1227–1239, 2008.

[43] K. F. Moseley, "Type 2 diabetes and bone fractures," *Current Opinion in Endocrinology, Diabetes, and Obesity*, vol. 19, no. 2, pp. 128–135, 2012.

[44] S. Yamagishi, "Role of advanced glycation end products (AGEs) in osteoporosis in diabetes," *Current Drug Targets*, vol. 12, no. 14, pp. 2096–2102, 2011.

[45] S. Pacios, J. Kang, J. Galicia et al., "Diabetes aggravates periodontitis by limiting repair through enhanced inflammation," *The FASEB Journal*, vol. 26, no. 4, pp. 1423–1430, 2012.

[46] Z. Makita, S. Radoff, E. J. Rayfield et al., "Advanced glycosylation end products in patients with diabetic nephropathy," *The New England Journal of Medicine*, vol. 325, no. 12, pp. 836–842, 1991.

[47] M. Abdollahi, B. Larijani, R. Rahimi, and P. Salari, "Role of oxidative stress in osteoporosis," *Therapy*, vol. 2, no. 5, pp. 787–796, 2005.

[48] S. Botolin, M. C. Faugere, H. Malluche, M. Orth, R. Meyer, and L. R. McCabe, "Increased bone adiposity and peroxisomal proliferator-activated receptor-gamma2 expression in type I diabetic mice," *Endocrinology*, vol. 146, no. 8, pp. 3622–3631, 2005.

[49] S. Botolin and L. R. McCabe, "Bone loss and increased bone adiposity in spontaneous and pharmacologically induced diabetic mice," *Endocrinology*, vol. 148, no. 1, pp. 198–205, 2007.

[50] I. I. de Liefde, M. van der Klift, C. E. D. H. de Laet, P. L. A. van Daele, A. Hofman, and H. A. P. Pols, "Bone mineral density and fracture risk in type-2 diabetes mellitus: the Rotterdam Study," *Osteoporosis International*, vol. 16, no. 12, pp. 1713–1720, 2005.

[51] R. Dhaliwal, D. Cibula, C. Ghosh, R. S. Weinstock, and A. M. Moses, "Bone quality assessment in type 2 diabetes mellitus," *Osteoporosis International*, vol. 25, no. 7, pp. 1969–1973, 2014.

[52] M. Janghorbani, D. Feskanich, W. C. Willett, and F. Hu, "Prospective study of diabetes and risk of hip fracture: the Nurses' Health Study," *Diabetes Care*, vol. 29, no. 7, pp. 1573–1578, 2006.

[53] G. Leidig-Bruckner and R. Ziegler, "Diabetes mellitus a risk for osteoporosis?," *Experimental and Clinical Endocrinology & Diabetes*, vol. 109, Supplement 2, pp. S493–S514, 2001.

[54] A. Oikawa, M. Siragusa, F. Quaini et al., "Diabetes mellitus induces bone marrow microangiopathy," *Arteriosclerosis, Thrombosis, and Vascular Biology*, vol. 30, no. 3, pp. 498–508, 2010.

[55] M. A. Piccinin and Z. A. Khan, "Pathophysiological role of enhanced bone marrow adipogenesis in diabetic complications," *Adipocytes*, vol. 3, no. 4, pp. 263–272, 2014.

[56] S. Yaturu, B. Bryant, and S. K. Jain, "Thiazolidinedione treatment decreases bone mineral density in type 2 diabetic men," *Diabetes Care*, vol. 30, no. 6, pp. 1574–1576, 2007.

[57] Z. Y. Cai, B. Yang, Y. X. Shi et al., "High glucose downregulates the effects of autophagy on osteoclastogenesis via the AMPK/mTOR/ULK1 pathway," *Biochemical and Biophysical Research Communications*, vol. 503, no. 2, pp. 428–435, 2018.

[58] C. P. Sanches, A. G. D. Vianna, and F. d. C. Barreto, "The impact of type 2 diabetes on bone metabolism," *Diabetology and Metabolic Syndrome*, vol. 9, no. 1, p. 85, 2017.

[59] D. A. Arvanitis, E. Vafiadaki, G. C. Fan et al., "Histidine-rich Ca-binding protein interacts with sarcoplasmic reticulum Ca-ATPase," *American Journal of Physiology. Heart and Circulatory Physiology*, vol. 293, no. 3, pp. H1581–H1589, 2007.

[60] J. Palsgaard, B. Emanuelli, J. N. Winnay, G. Sumara, G. Karsenty, and C. R. Kahn, "Cross-talk between insulin and Wnt signaling in preadipocytes: role of Wnt co-receptor low density lipoprotein receptor-related protein-5 (LRP5)," *The Journal of Biological Chemistry*, vol. 287, no. 15, pp. 12016–12026, 2012.

[61] S. R. Farmer, "Regulation of PPARγ activity during adipogenesis," *International Journal of Obesity*, vol. 29, Supplement 1, pp. S13–S16, 2005.

[62] J. R. Miller, "The Wnts," *Genome Biology*, vol. 3, no. 1, 2002.

[63] I. Fleming, S. J. MacKenzie, R. G. Vernon, N. G. Anderson, M. D. Houslay, and E. Kilgour, "Protein kinase C isoforms play differential roles in the regulation of adipocyte differentiation," *The Biochemical Journal*, vol. 333, no. 3, pp. 719–727, 1998.

[64] Y. Zhou, D. Wang, F. Li, J. Shi, and J. Song, "Different roles of protein kinase C-βI and -δ in the regulation of adipocyte differentiation," *The International Journal of Biochemistry & Cell Biology*, vol. 38, no. 12, pp. 2151–2163, 2006.

[65] M. R. Rubin, "Bone cells and bone turnover in diabetes mellitus," *Current Osteoporosis Reports*, vol. 13, no. 3, pp. 186–191, 2015.

[66] E. Canalis, "Wnt signalling in osteoporosis: mechanisms and novel therapeutic approaches," *Nature Reviews Endocrinology*, vol. 9, no. 10, pp. 575–583, 2013.

[67] Q. Shi, S. Luo, H. Jia et al., "Wnt/β-catenin signaling may be involved with the maturation, but not the differentiation, of insulin-producing cells," *Biomedicine & Pharmacotherapy*, vol. 67, no. 8, pp. 745–750, 2013.

[68] H. J. Welters and R. N. Kulkarni, "Wnt signaling: relevance to β-cell biology and diabetes," *Trends in Endocrinology and Metabolism*, vol. 19, no. 10, pp. 349–355, 2008.

[69] J. Mei, L. S. Holst, T. R. Landstrom et al., "C_2-ceramide influences the expression and insulin-mediated regulation of cyclic nucleotide phosphodiesterase 3B and lipolysis in 3T3-L1 adipocytes," *Diabetes*, vol. 51, no. 3, pp. 631–637, 2002.

[70] M. H. Kim, S. H. Hong, and M. K. Lee, "Insulin receptor-overexpressing β-cells ameliorate hyperglycemia in diabetic rats through Wnt signaling activation," *PLoS One*, vol. 8, no. 7, article e67802, 2013.

[71] C. S. Cselenyi, K. K. Jernigan, E. Tahinci, C. A. Thorne, L. A. Lee, and E. Lee, "LRP6 transduces a canonical Wnt signal independently of Axin degradation by inhibiting GSK3's phosphorylation of β-catenin," *Proceedings of the National Academy of Sciences of the United States of America*, vol. 105, no. 23, pp. 8032–8037, 2008.

[72] D. D. Armstrong and K. A. Esser, "Wnt/β-catenin signaling activates growth-control genes during overload-induced skeletal muscle hypertrophy," *American Journal of Physiology. Cell Physiology*, vol. 289, no. 4, pp. C853–C859, 2005.

[73] S. Tajbakhsh, U. Borello, E. Vivarelli et al., "Differential activation of Myf5 and MyoD by different Wnts in explants of mouse paraxial mesoderm and the later activation of myogenesis in the absence of Myf5," *Development*, vol. 125, no. 21, pp. 4155–4162, 1998.

[74] D. Zhou, R. S. Strakovsky, X. Zhang, and Y. X. Pan, "The skeletal muscle Wnt pathway may modulate insulin resistance and muscle development in a diet-induced obese rat model," *Obesity*, vol. 20, no. 8, pp. 1577–1584, 2012.

[75] V. Lyssenko, R. Lupi, P. Marchetti et al., "Mechanisms by which common variants in the *TCF7L2* gene increase risk of type 2 diabetes," *The Journal of Clinical Investigation*, vol. 117, no. 8, pp. 2155–2163, 2007.

[76] P. W. Smith and P. G. Rusnak, "APIC guideline for infection prevention and control in the long-term care facility," *American Journal of Infection Control*, vol. 19, no. 4, pp. 198–215, 1991.

[77] W. Ip, W. Shao, Y. T. A. Chiang, and T. Jin, "The Wnt signaling pathway effector TCF7L2 is upregulated by insulin and represses hepatic gluconeogenesis," *American Journal of Physiology. Endocrinology and Metabolism*, vol. 303, no. 9, pp. E1166–E1176, 2012.

[78] L. Wegner, M. S. Hussain, K. Pilgaard et al., "Impact of *TCF7L2* rs7903146 on insulin secretion and action in young and elderly Danish twins," *The Journal of Clinical Endocrinology and Metabolism*, vol. 93, no. 10, pp. 4013–4019, 2008.

[79] Q. Zhang, R. C. Riddle, and T. L. Clemens, "Bone and the regulation of global energy balance," *Journal of Internal Medicine*, vol. 277, no. 6, pp. 681–689, 2015.

[80] Q. Zhong, T. Itokawa, S. Sridhar et al., "Effects of glucose-dependent insulinotropic peptide on osteoclast function," *American Journal of Physiology. Endocrinology and Metabolism*, vol. 292, no. 2, pp. E543–E548, 2007.

[81] M. Ferron, J. Wei, T. Yoshizawa et al., "Insulin signaling in osteoblasts integrates bone remodeling and energy metabolism," *Cell*, vol. 142, no. 2, pp. 296–308, 2010.

[82] P. Ducy, M. Amling, S. Takeda et al., "Leptin inhibits bone formation through a hypothalamic relay: a central control of bone mass," *Cell*, vol. 100, no. 2, pp. 197–207, 2000.

[83] S. Takeda, F. Elefteriou, R. Levasseur et al., "Leptin regulates bone formation via the sympathetic nervous system," *Cell*, vol. 111, no. 3, pp. 305–317, 2002.

[84] P. K. Wiklund, L. Xu, Q. Wang et al., "Lactation is associated with greater maternal bone size and bone strength later in life," *Osteoporosis International*, vol. 23, no. 7, pp. 1939–1945, 2012.

[85] J. B. Richards, A. M. Valdes, K. Burling, U. C. Perks, and T. D. Spector, "Serum adiponectin and bone mineral density in women," *The Journal of Clinical Endocrinology and Metabolism*, vol. 92, no. 4, pp. 1517–1523, 2007.

[86] C. Mathieu, C. Gysemans, A. Giulietti, and R. Bouillon, "Vitamin D and diabetes," *Diabetologia*, vol. 48, no. 7, pp. 1247–1257, 2005.

[87] J. T. Chaiban and K. G. Nicolas, "Diabetes and bone still a lot to learn," *Clinical Reviews in Bone and Mineral Metabolism*, vol. 13, no. 1, pp. 20–35, 2015.

[88] L. Zirilli, V. Rochira, C. Diazzi, G. Caffagni, and C. Carani, "Human models of aromatase deficiency," *The Journal of Steroid Biochemistry and Molecular Biology*, vol. 109, no. 3-5, pp. 212–218, 2008.

[89] A. A. Gupte, H. J. Pownall, and D. J. Hamilton, "Estrogen: an emerging regulator of insulin action and mitochondrial function," *Journal of Diabetes Research*, vol. 2015, Article ID 916585, 9 pages, 2015.

[90] A. K. Madiraju, D. M. Erion, Y. Rahimi et al., "Metformin suppresses gluconeogenesis by inhibiting mitochondrial glycerophosphate dehydrogenase," *Nature*, vol. 510, no. 7506, pp. 542–546, 2014.

[91] Z.'e. Zhou, Y. Tang, X. Jin et al., "Metformin inhibits advanced glycation end products-induced inflammatory response in murine macrophages partly through AMPK activation and RAGE/NFκB pathway suppression," *Journal of Diabetes Research*, vol. 2016, Article ID 4847812, 10 pages, 2016.

[92] P. Proks, F. Reimann, N. Green, F. Gribble, and F. Ashcroft, "Sulfonylurea stimulation of insulin secretion," *Diabetes*, vol. 51, Supplement 3, pp. S368–S376, 2002.

[93] K. Kanazawa and A. Kudo, "Self-assembled RANK induces osteoclastogenesis ligand-independently," *Journal of Bone and Mineral Research*, vol. 20, no. 11, pp. 2053–2060, 2005.

[94] P. Ma, B. Gu, J. Ma et al., "Glimepiride induces proliferation and differentiation of rat osteoblasts via the PI3-kinase/Akt pathway," *Metabolism*, vol. 59, no. 3, pp. 359–366, 2010.

[95] J. Fronczek-Sokol and M. Pytlik, "Effect of glimepiride on the skeletal system of ovariectomized and non-ovariectomized rats," *Pharmacological Reports*, vol. 66, no. 3, pp. 412–417, 2014.

[96] C. Yamada, Y. Yamada, K. Tsukiyama et al., "The murine glucagon-like peptide-1 receptor is essential for control of bone resorption," *Endocrinology*, vol. 149, no. 2, pp. 574–579, 2008.

[97] D. B. Henriksen, P. Alexandersen, B. Hartmann et al., "Disassociation of bone resorption and formation by GLP-2: a 14-day study in healthy postmenopausal women," *Bone*, vol. 40, no. 3, pp. 723–729, 2007.

[98] D. Xie, Q. Zhong, K. H. Ding et al., "Glucose-dependent insulinotropic peptide-overexpressing transgenic mice have increased bone mass," *Bone*, vol. 40, no. 5, pp. 1352–1360, 2007.

[99] A. V. Schwartz, D. E. Sellmeyer, K. E. Ensrud et al., "Older women with diabetes have an increased risk of fracture: a prospective study," *The Journal of Clinical Endocrinology and Metabolism*, vol. 86, no. 1, pp. 32–38, 2001.

[100] R. Q. Ivers, R. G. Cumming, P. Mitchell, A. J. Peduto, and Blue Mountains Eye Study, "Diabetes and risk of fracture: the Blue Mountains Eye Study," *Diabetes Care*, vol. 24, no. 7, pp. 1198–1203, 2001.

[101] K. K. Nicodemus, A. R. Folsom, and Iowa Women's Health Study, "Type 1 and type 2 diabetes and incident hip fractures in postmenopausal women," *Diabetes Care*, vol. 24, no. 7, pp. 1192–1197, 2001.

[102] J. Cornish, K. E. Callon, U. Bava, S. A. Kamona, G. J. S. Cooper, and I. R. Reid, "Effects of calcitonin, amylin, and calcitonin gene-related peptide on osteoclast development," *Bone*, vol. 29, no. 2, pp. 162–168, 2001.

[103] S. I. Taylor, J. E. Blau, and K. I. Rother, "Possible adverse effects of SGLT2 inhibitors on bone," *The Lancet Diabetes and Endocrinology*, vol. 3, no. 1, pp. 8–10, 2015.

[104] J. P. Bilezikian, N. B. Watts, K. Usiskin et al., "Evaluation of bone mineral density and bone biomarkers in patients with type 2 diabetes treated with canagliflozin," *The Journal of Clinical Endocrinology and Metabolism*, vol. 101, no. 1, pp. 44–51, 2016.

[105] H. E. Bays, R. Weinstein, G. Law, and W. Canovatchel, "Canagliflozin: effects in overweight and obese subjects without diabetes mellitus," *Obesity*, vol. 22, no. 4, pp. 1042–1049, 2014.

[106] K. Ways, M. D. Johnson, R. N. V. S. Mamidi, J. Proctor, S. de Jonghe, and C. Louden, "Successful integration of nonclinical and clinical findings in interpreting the clinical relevance of rodent neoplasia with a new chemical entity," *Toxicologic Pathology*, vol. 43, no. 1, pp. 48–56, 2014.

[107] CDC, "National diabetes statistics report. Estimates of diabetes and its burden in the United States," 2017, https://www.cdc.gov/diabetes/pdfs/data/statistics/national-diabetes-statistics-report.pdf.

2

Effects of Newer Antidiabetic Drugs on Endothelial Function and Arterial Stiffness

Konstantinos Batzias,[1] Alexios S. Antonopoulos,[1] Evangelos Oikonomou,[1] Gerasimos Siasos,[1] Evanthia Bletsa,[1] Panagiota K. Stampouloglou,[1] Chara-Vasiliki Mistakidi,[1] Marina Noutsou,[2] Niki Katsiki,[3] Periklis Karopoulos,[1] Georgios Charalambous,[1] Anastasia Thanopoulou,[2] Nicholas Tentolouris,[4] and Dimitris Tousoulis[1]

[1] *1st Department of Cardiology, Hippokration Hospital, National and Kapodistrian University of Athens Medical School, Athens, Greece*

[2] *Diabetes Center, 2nd Department of Internal Medicine, Medical School, National and Kapodistrian University of Athens, Hippokration General Hospital of Athens, Athens, Greece*

[3] *Second Department of Internal Medicine, Hippokration University Hospital, Aristotle University of Thessaloniki, Thessaloniki, Greece*

[4] *First Department of Propaedeutic and Internal Medicine, Division of Diabetes, Laiko University Hospital, National and Kapodistrian University of Athens Medical School, Athens, Greece*

Correspondence should be addressed to Evangelos Oikonomou; boikono@gmail.com

Academic Editor: Yoshifumi Saisho

Background. Newer antidiabetic drugs, i.e., dipeptidyl peptidase-4 (DPP-4) inhibitors, sodium-glucose cotransporter-2 (SGLT-2) inhibitors, and glucagon-like peptide-1 receptor agonists (GLP-1 RAs) may exert distinct cardiovascular effects. We sought to explore their impact on vascular function. *Methods.* Published literature was systematically searched up to January 2018 for clinical studies assessing the effects of DPP-4 inhibitors, GLP-1 RAs, and SGLT-2 inhibitors on endothelial function and arterial stiffness, assessed by flow-mediated dilation (FMD) of the brachial artery and pulse wave velocity (PWV), respectively. For each eligible study, we used the mean difference (MD) with 95% confidence intervals (CIs) for FMD and PWV. The pooled MD for FMD and PWV were calculated by using a random-effect model. The presence of heterogeneity among studies was evaluated by the I^2 statistic. *Results.* A total of 26 eligible studies ($n = 668$ patients) were included in the present meta-analysis. Among newer antidiabetic drugs, only SGLT-2 inhibitors significantly improved FMD (pooled MD 1.14%, 95% CI: 0.18 to 1.73, $p = 0.016$), but not DPP-4 inhibitors (pooled MD = 0.86%, 95% CI: -0.15 to 1.86, $p = 0.095$) or GLP-1 RA (pooled MD = 2.37%, 95% CI: -0.51 to 5.25, $p = 0.107$). Both GLP-1 RA (pooled MD = −1.97, 95% CI: -2.65 to -1.30, $p < 0.001$) and, to a lesser extent, DPP-4 inhibitors (pooled MD = -0.18, 95% CI: -0.30 to -0.07, $p = 0.002$) significantly decreased PWV. *Conclusions.* Newer antidiabetic drugs differentially affect endothelial function and arterial stiffness, as assessed by FMD and PWV, respectively. These findings could explain the distinct effects of these drugs on cardiovascular risk of patients with type 2 diabetes.

1. Introduction

Type 2 diabetes (T2D) is a chronic disease affecting 8.3% of the adult population worldwide, with a rising prevalence that renders its tackling a global challenge [1]. Patients with T2D are at high cardiovascular disease (CVD) risk [2, 3] and are characterized by micro- and macrovascular dysfunction which is of multifactorial origin [4, 5].

The safety and effects of newly licensed antidiabetic drugs on the cardiovascular system represent important clinical issues [6, 7]. Recent evidence from clinical trials suggests that newer antidiabetic drugs can not only exert glycemic-lowering properties but also decrease CVD risk [8, 9]. In this context, sodium-glucose cotransporter-2 (SGLT-2) inhibitors, i.e., empagliflozin in the Empagliflozin Cardiovascular Outcome Event Trial in Type 2 Diabetes Mellitus Patients-Removing Excess Glucose (EMPA-REG OUTCOME) study [8] and canagliflozin in the Canagliflozin Cardiovascular Assessment Study [10], significantly reduced the rates of CVD events, hospitalization for heart failure (HF), CVD, and total mortality, as well as improved kidney function in T2D patients with established CVD. Similar beneficial effects were reported for liraglutide, an once-daily glucagon-like peptide-1 receptor agonist (GLP-1 RA), and for semaglutide, an once-weekly GLP-1 RA, both of which reduced CVD morbidity and mortality (but not hospitalization for HF) in T2D patients with established CVD, in the Liraglutide Effect and Action in Diabetes: Evaluation of Cardiovascular Outcome Results (LEADER) trial [9] and the Trial to Evaluate Cardiovascular and Other Long-term Outcomes with Semaglutide in Subjects with Type 2 Diabetes (SUSTAIN-6) [11], respectively. In contrast, lixisenatide once daily and exenatide once weekly did not affect CVD risk in the Evaluation of Lixisenatide in Acute Coronary Syndrome (ELIXA) trial [12] and the Exenatide Study of Cardiovascular Event Lowering (EXSCEL) [13], respectively. Furthermore, dipeptidyl peptidase-4 (DPP-4) inhibitors seem to exert neutral effects on CVD risk as shown for alogliptin in the Examination of Cardiovascular Outcomes with Alogliptin versus Standard of Care (EXAMINE) trial [14] and for sitagliptin in the Trial Evaluating Cardiovascular Outcomes with Sitagliptin (TECOS) [15]. Saxagliptin was reported to increase the rate of hospitalization for HF [16] in the Saxagliptin Assessment of Vascular Outcomes Recorded in Patients with Diabetes Mellitus (SAVOR)–Thrombolysis in Myocardial Infarction (TIMI) 53 trial. Despite this evidence provided by large randomized clinical trials, the mechanisms by which antidiabetic drugs can affect CVD risk remain not entirely clear.

Vascular dysfunction is one of the initial steps in the atherosclerotic process [17, 18]. Endothelial function and arterial stiffness [17, 19] are two widely used indices of vascular function, which both offer prognostic information on the risk of CVD events in T2D patients [19]. Improvement of these indices represents one of the mechanisms by which drugs with established CVD benefits, such as statins, exert their effects [20, 21]. Currently, it remains unknown how newer antidiabetic drugs may affect vascular function as studies have yielded conflicting results.

We conducted a systematic review of the literature, followed by a meta-analysis, to investigate the effects of newer antidiabetic drugs, i.e., DPP-4 inhibitors, GLP-1 RAs, and SGLT-2 inhibitors, on vascular function as assessed by flow-mediated dilation (FMD) of the brachial artery and pulse wave velocity (PWV).

2. Patients and Methods

2.1. Literature Search. Eligible studies evaluating the effects of DPP-4 inhibitors, GLP-1 RAs, and SGLT-2 inhibitors on FMD and PWV were drawn from a systematic review of the English literature in the MEDLINE and Web of Science databases up to 31 January 2018. The medical terms (MeSH) used were the following: sodium-glucose cotransporter-2 OR SGLT2 OR empagliflozin OR canagliflozin OR dapagliflozin OR DPP-4 OR dipeptidyl peptidase-4 inhibitors OR sitagliptin OR saxagliptin OR vildagliptin OR linagliptin OR gemigliptin OR canagliptin OR teneligliptin OR alogliptin OR trelagliptin OR omarigliptin OR evogliptin OR dutogliptin OR GLP-1 OR glucagon-like peptide-1 OR exenatide OR lixisenatide OR dulaglutide OR liraglutide OR semaglutide AND endothelial function OR arterial stiffness OR flow-mediated dilation OR pulse wave velocity. Studies were also identified from searching the references of published articles. The PRISMA flow chart for the study is presented in Figure 1.

2.2. Study Eligibility. Studies were eligible if they were full-length publications in peer-reviewed journals reporting on (a) endothelium-dependent vasodilatory response by FMD and/or (b) arterial stiffness assessed by carotid-femoral, carotid-radial, or brachial-ankle PWV. Studies need also to be either double-blind, placebo-controlled, randomized clinical trials or observational studies assessing the outcomes of interest before and after treatment with a newer antidiabetic drug. No restriction criteria were imposed with regard to the size of the population studied. Analysis did not include studies assessing endothelial function or arterial stiffness by other markers. Only human studies were included in the analysis, whereas review articles were excluded.

2.3. Extraction of Data. Literature search, selection of studies, and extraction of data were performed independently by two investigators (KB and AA). Means and standard deviations (SD) of FMD and PWV as well as their changes following drug treatment were recorded from cumulative published data. In studies reporting standard error, SD was calculated using the equation $SD = \text{standard error} * \sqrt{n}$. In studies reporting median and interquartile range, mean and SD were calculated and used in further analyses [22]. In those studies where extraction of cumulative statistics could not be reliably performed based on the full-length publication, a communication with the corresponding author was attempted to provide summary statistics [23–27].

2.4. Statistical Analysis. For each eligible study, we used the mean difference (MD) with 95% confidence intervals (CIs) for endothelium-dependent vasodilation and arterial stiffness as summary statistics (MD pre- and posttreatment). The difference in mean $\pm$ SD for FMD and PWV was included in the quantitative synthesis to explore the pooled MD after treatment with any of the studied antidiabetic drugs; the results were presented in respective forest plots. Subgroup analysis was performed for different drug classes. The presence of heterogeneity was evaluated by the I^2 statistic. A random-effect model was used to obtain pooled MD and 95% CIs. Results were considered statistically significant at two-tailed p value < 0.05. The findings of the meta-analysis were also confirmed in leave-one-out sensitivity analysis. The quality of published studies was assessed by the modified version of

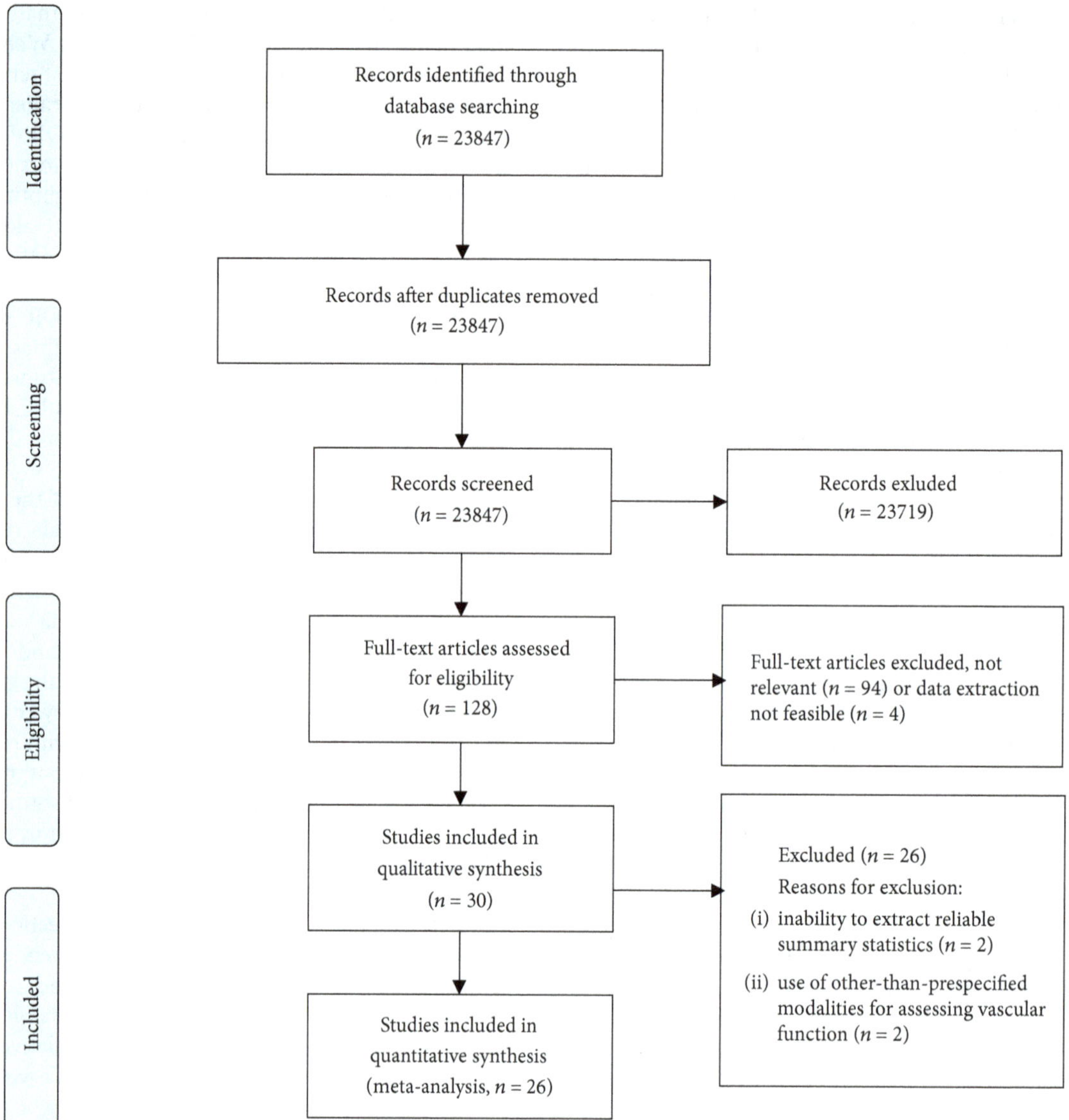

Figure 1: Study flow chart.

the Downs and Black questionnaire [28]. The effect of publication bias on pooled estimates was explored by the Duval and Tweedie nonparametric "trim and fill" method and the construction of relevant funnel plots. All statistical analyses were performed by STATA software version 13.0 (StataCorp LLC, College Station, Texas, US).

3. Results

3.1. Qualitative Summary. The literature search identified 30 studies for potential inclusion in the present meta-analysis. Certain identified studies that were originally included in the qualitative synthesis had to be excluded from the quantitative synthesis due to not fulfilling the eligibility criteria. One study was excluded because it assessed endothelial function by reactive hyperemia peripheral arterial tonometry [29] and one because it used a 24 h approach to measure PWV [30]. Also, two studies had to be excluded due to inability to extract reliable summary statistics for the outcomes of interest [26, 27] (Figure 1). Therefore, a total of 26 studies ($n = 668$ patients) were finally included in the quantitative synthesis. The details of the individual studies included in the meta-analysis are summarized in Table 1.

All studies were published since 2012. The sample sizes of the studies ranged from 10 to 51 patients. The mean follow-up time was 152 days after initiation of treatment. The majority of studies were randomized controlled trials [23–25, 31–48], but some of them were uncontrolled or single-arm observational studies [49–53]. All studies performed the ultrasound-based technique to assess brachial artery FMD and PWV to assess arterial stiffness.

3.2. Quantitative Synthesis

3.2.1. Effects of Newer Antidiabetic Drugs on Endothelial Function. The effects of newer antidiabetic drugs on FMD

Table 1: Summary characteristics of studies included in the analysis.

Author	Class	Agent	Study design	N	Duration (days)	FMD (%) Baseline	FMD (%) Post	PWV (m/s) Baseline	PWV (m/s) Post
Ayaori et al. [31]	DPP-4i	Sitagliptin	RCT	42	42	7.2 ± 5.9	4.4 ± 5.9		
		Alogliptin				6.9 ± 6.3	4.4 ± 6.2		
Baltzis et al. [32]	DPP-4i	Linagliptin	RCT	19	84	6.5 ± 2.1	7.2 ± 2.5		
de Boer et al. [33]	DPP-4i	Linagliptin	RCT	22	182			8.7 ± 1.6	8.3 ± 1.3
Dell'Oro et al. [34]	DPP-4i	Saxagliptin	RCT	16	360	3.6 ± 0.3	7.4 ± 0.8		
Duvnjak et al. [49]	DPP-4i	Sitagliptin/vildagliptin	Open label (NR)	51	90			8.6 ± 0.3	8.4 ± 0.3
Gurkan et al. [35]	GLP-1 RA	Exenatide	RCT	17	182	6.4 ± 5.7	8.6 ± 4.7		
Hong et al. [50]	GLP-1 RA	Exenatide	Single arm (NR)	32	90			7.2 ± 2.2	5.1 ± 0.1
Hopkins et al. [51]	GLP-1 RA	Exenatide/liraglutide	Single arm (NR)	11	180	6.2 ± 2.3	5.1 ± 2.7		
Ida et al. [52]	DPP-4i	Trelagliptin	Single arm (NR)	27	84	2.4 ± 2.7	2.7 ± 3.8	16.3 ± 2.4	15.6 ± 2.2*
Irace et al. [36]	GLP-1 RA	Exenatide	RCT	10	112	1.6 ± 2.9	9.1 ± 3.6		
Nakamura et al. [24]	DPP-4i	Sitagliptin	RCT	24	90	5.4 ± 2.3	6.2 ± 2.0		
Kim et al. [37]	DPP-4i	Vildagliptin	RCT	17	84	9.4 ± 5.0	7.9 ± 4.3		
Kitao et al. [38]	DPP-4i	Vildagliptin	RCT	48	84	5.5 ± 2.0	5.1 ± 2.3		
Kubota et al. [53]	DPP-4i	Sitagliptin	Single arm (NR)	40	90	4.1 ± 1.5	5.1 ± 1.6		
Lambadiari et al. [39]	GLP-1 RA	Liraglutide	RCT	30	180	8.9 ± 3.0	13.2 ± 6.0	11.8 ± 2.5	10.3 ± 3.3
Leung et al. [40]	DPP-4i	Sitagliptin/vildagliptin	RCT	25	365	2.4 ± 1.6	7.3 ± 1.6		
Li et al. [41]	DPP-4i	Saxagliptin	RCT	14	84	9.3 ± 4.7	14.3 ± 4.3		
Nomoto et al. [42]	DPP-4i	Sitagliptin	RCT	48	182	5.6 ± 2.8	5.6 ± 2.8		
Nomoto et al. [43]	GLP-1 RA	Liraglutide	RCT	16	98	6.0 ± 2.6	5.6 ± 1.6		
Shigiyama et al. [44]	SGLT-2i	Dapagliflozin	RCT	37	112	4.8 ± 1.9	5.7 ± 2.1		
Shigiyama et al. [45]	DPP-4i	Linagliptin	RCT	29	112	4.9 ± 2.7	6.3 ± 2.7		
Solini et al. [46]	SGLT-2i	Dapagliflozin	RCT	16	2	2.8 ± 2.3	4.0 ± 2.1	10.1 ± 1.6	8.9 ± 1.6
Suzuki et al. [25]	DPP-4i	Sitagliptin	RCT	12	90	3.7 ± 2.3	5.4 ± 2.2		
Maruhashi et al. [23]	DPP-4i	Sitagliptin	RCT	17	720	4.3 ± 2.6	4.4 ± 2.3		
Widlansky et al. [47]	DPP-4i	Saxagliptin	RCT	16	56	5.6 ± 2.3	5.8 ± 2.3		
Zografou et al. [48]	DPP-4i	Vildagliptin	RCT	32	180			8.6 ± 2.1	8.3 ± 1.5

DPP-4i: dipeptidyl peptidase-4 inhibitor; FMD: flow-mediated dilation; GLP-1 RA: glucagon-like peptide-1 receptor agonist; NR: nonrandomized; RCT: randomized clinical trial; SGLT-2i: sodium-glucose cotransporter-2 inhibitor; PWV: pulse wave velocity. *N* refers to the active treatment group. The full list of references of the studies included in the table is provided in the supplementary material. *Measured as brachial-ankle PWV.

are summarized in Figure 2. Overall, 16 studies investigated the effects of DPP-4 inhibitors on FMD. In the pooled meta-analysis, the effects of DPP-4 inhibitors on FMD was not statistically significant (pooled MD = 0.86%, 95% CI: -0.15 to 1.86, $p = 0.095$). But there was significant heterogeneity between studies ($I^2 = 87.8\%$, $p < 0.0001$). In leave-one-out sensitivity analysis, the results were unchanged (Table 2); only by excluding the study of Ayaori et al. [31] was a significant effect of DPP-4 on FMD observed (pooled MD = 1.25%, 95% CI: 0.24 to 2.27, $p = 0.015$), but heterogeneity among studies remained significant. Even within the group of DPP-4 inhibitors, no specific agent was associated with significant improvements in FMD.

For the effect of GLP-1 RAs (liraglutide and exenatide) on FMD (5 studies; $n = 84$ patients), the pooled estimate effect was not significant (pooled MD = 2.38%, 95% CI: -0.51 to 5.25, $p = 0.107$). Heterogeneity among studies was significant ($I^2 = 88.4\%$, $p < 0.001$). In leave-one-out sensitivity analysis, the results were unchanged and the heterogeneity among studies remained significant.

Only 2 eligible studies ($n = 53$ patients) evaluated the effects of SGLT-2 inhibitors on FMD. Dapagliflozin was the only SGLT-2 inhibitor used in these studies. SGLT-2 inhibitors increased FMD significantly (pooled MD = 0.95%, 95% CI: 0.18 to 1.73, $p = 0.016$).

In metaregression analysis, the mean difference in FMD was not associated with the size of the study ($b = -0.033$, $p = 0.489$), the duration of intervention ($b = 0.002$, $p = 0.460$), the age ($b = -0.162$, $p = 0.163$) or the sex (for males: $b = 0.004$, $p = 0.931$) of participants enrolled.

3.2.2. Effects of Newer Antidiabetic Drugs on Arterial Stiffness. The effects of newer antidiabetic drugs on PWV are summarized in Figure 3. Marked heterogeneity was observed among analyzed studies ($I^2 = 80.7\%$, $p < 0.001$). A total of 4 studies ($n = 132$ patients) investigated the effects of DPP-4 inhibitors on arterial stiffness, which were associated with a significant reduction in PWV (pooled MD = −0.18, 95% CI: -0.30 to -0.07, $p = 0.002$). A similar effect was identified for GLP-1 RAs (2 studies; $n = 62$ patients), which were associated with

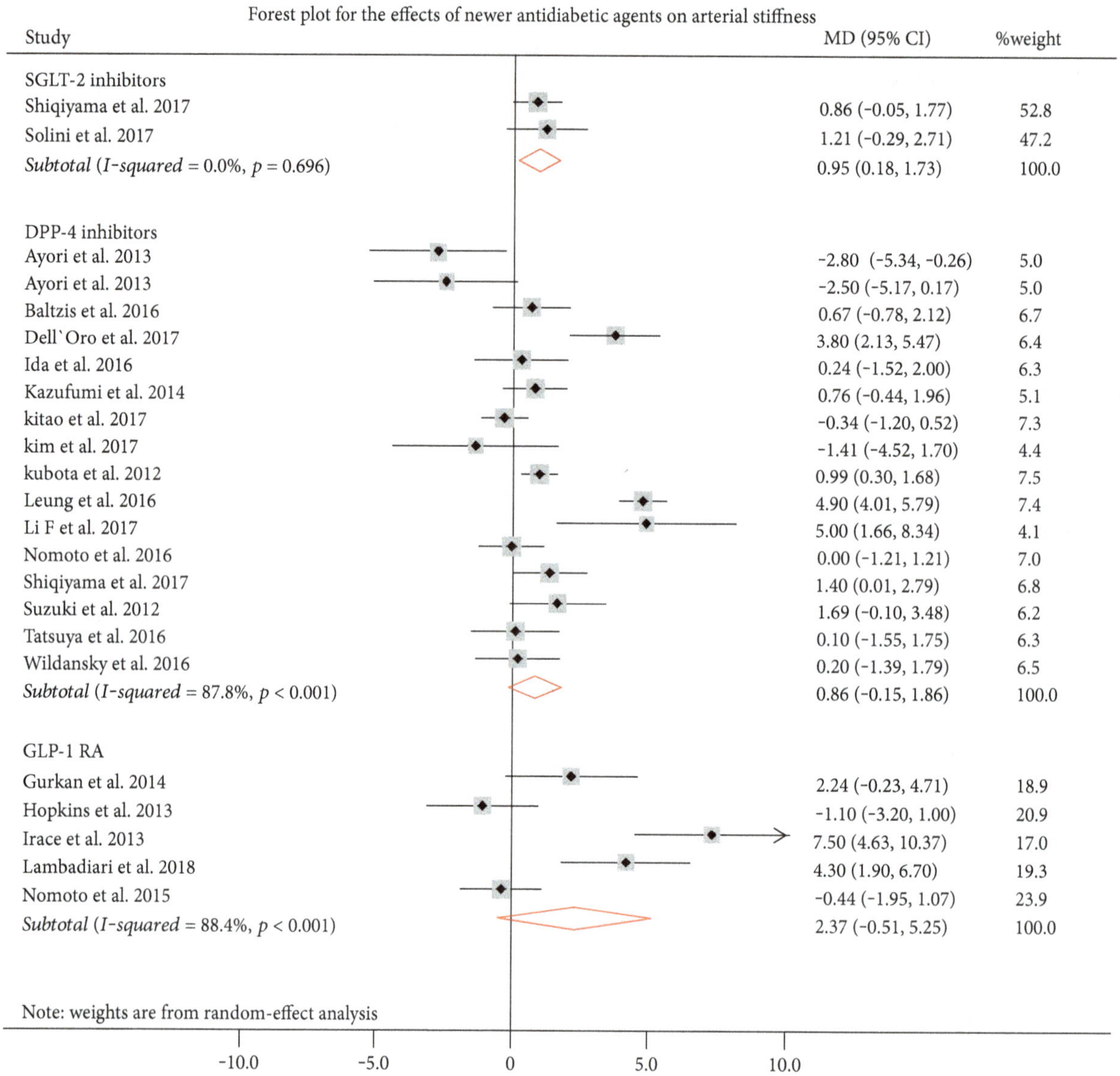

Figure 2: Effects of newer antidiabetic drugs on endothelial function. Squares indicate the mean difference (MD) and the respective 95% confidence intervals in flow-mediated dilatation (FMD) before/after treatment from eligible studies. The size of the squares corresponds to the weight of each study. The diamonds and their width represent the pooled MD and the 95% CI, respectively. DPP-4 = DPP-4 inhibitors, SGLT-2 inhibitors, and GLP-1 RAs and defines them under the figure. DPP-4: dipeptidyl peptidase-4; GLP-1 RAs: glucagon-like peptide-1 receptor agonists; SGLT-2: sodium-glucose cotransporter-2.

a significant reduction in PWV (pooled MD = −1.97, 95% CI: -2.65 to -1.30, $p < 0.001$). For SGLT-2 inhibitors, only one study reported a reduction in PWV, and therefore, no safe conclusions can be drawn.

3.3. Quality Assessment of Included Studies and Publication Bias. The quality of published studies was assessed by the modified Downs and Black checklist [28]. The quality of published studies is considered moderate with a mean modified Downs and Black score of 23.1. To explore publication bias, we constructed a funnel plot of published studies for the effect size of antidiabetic drugs on the primary endpoint of our study, i.e., endothelial function assessed by FMD. The funnel plot was symmetric, suggesting the absence of publication bias (Figure 4).

4. Discussion

In the present systematic review, we sought to explore the effects of newer antidiabetic drugs, namely, SGLT-2 inhibitors, DPP-4 inhibitors, and GLP-1 RAs, on vascular function. We hypothesized that the distinct profile of each antidiabetic drug class could be also associated with differences in their vascular effects. The systematic review of the published literature showed that evidence in this field is modest, based mainly on small randomized clinical trials with significant heterogeneity. In this context, published studies supported a beneficial effect of SGLT-2 on FMD, which seems to not be shared by GLP-1 RAs or DPP-4 inhibitors. Accordingly, evidence suggested a reduction in PWV by both DPP-4 inhibitors and GLP-1 RAs. These findings are potentially

Table 2: Leave-one-out sensitivity analysis for the effects of newer antidiabetics on endothelial function.

Study excluded	MD (95% CI)	p value	Heterogeneity (I^2)
DPP-4 inhibitors			
Ayaori et al. [31]	1.253 (0.242 to 2.265)	$p = 0.015$	87.7%, $p < 0.001$
Baltzis et al. [32]	0.866 (-0.205 to 1.936)	$p = 0.113$	88.6%, $p < 0.001$
Dell'Oro et al. [34]	0.658 (-0.365 to 1.682)	$p = 0.207$	87.8%, $p < 0.001$
Ida et al. [52]	0.897 (-0.151 to 1.945)	$p = 0.095$	88.5%, $p < 0.001$
Nakamura et al. [24]	0.858 (-0.226 to 1.943)	$p = 0.121$	88.6%, $p < 0.001$
Kim et al. [37]	0.962 (-0.066 to 1.990)	$p = 0.067$	88.3%, $p < 0.001$
Kitao et al. [38]	0.948 (-0.115 to 2.011)	$p = 0.080$	87.1%, $p < 0.001$
Kubota et al. [53]	0.832 (-0.329 to 1.993)	$p = 0.160$	88.6%, $p < 0.001$
Leung et al. [40]	0.566 (-0.130 to 1.261)	$p = 0.111$	68.6%, $p < 0.001$
Li et al. [41]	0.679 (-0.337 to 1.695)	$p = 0.190$	88.1%, $p < 0.001$
Nomoto et al. [42]	0.917 (-0.153 to 1.986)	$p = 0.093$	88.2%, $p < 0.001$
Shigiyama et al. [44]	0.813 (-0.262 to 1.888)	$p = 0.138$	88.6%, $p < 0.001$
Suzuki et al. [25]	0.798 (-0.261 to 1.858)	$p = 0.140$	88.6%, $p < 0.001$
Maruhashi et al. [23]	0.906 (-0.152 to 1.964)	$p = 0.093$	88.4%, $p < 0.001$
Widlansky et al. [47]	0.899 (-0.161 to 1.960)	$p = 0.097$	88.5%, $p < 0.001$
GLP-1 RA			
Gurkan et al. [35]	2.435 (-1.177 to 6.047)	$p = 0.186$	91.2%, $p < 0.001$
Hopkins et al. [51]	3.275 (-0.132 to 6.682)	$p = 0.060$	89.2%, $p < 0.001$
Irace et al. [36]	1.141 (-1.194 to 3.476)	$p = 0.338$	80.2%, $p = 0.001$
Lambadiari et al. [39]	1.902 (-1.399 to 5.203)	$p = 0.259$	89.3%, $p < 0.001$
Nomoto et al. [42]	3.155 (-0.376 to 6.687)	$p = 0.080$	88.1%, $p < 0.001$

DPP-4: dipeptidyl peptidase-4 inhibitors; GLP-1 RA: glucagon-like peptide-1 receptor agonists.

important as they suggest a different impact of newer antidiabetic drugs on vascular function, which could be linked with their distinct effects on CVD risk. However, these results should be interpreted with caution given the modest quality of evidence in the published literature and the significant heterogeneity between studies.

DPP-4 inhibitors are an antidiabetic drug class on which there is abundant clinical experience, since they have been marketed for over a decade (since 2006). Large randomized clinical trials in the field are consistent in their findings and support a neutral effect of DPP-4 inhibitors on CVD outcomes. However, there is evidence that saxagliptin may increase the risk for HF hospitalization [16]. Recent meta-analyses have also found that DPP-4 inhibitors do not affect the risk for CVD mortality and stroke [54]. Data from the small clinical studies included in the present meta-analysis indicate a marginal effect of DPP-4 drugs on FMD and a significant reduction in PWV. These small effects could be related to the glucose-lowering properties of DPP-4 inhibition but may not be commonly shared by all agents of the DPP-4 drug class. This is an interest finding which (a) confirms the safety profile of this drug class and (b) may explain the neutral effect of certain DPP-4 drugs on CVD outcomes.

For SGLT-2 inhibitors, evidence suggests a beneficial effect of these agents on CVD risk and mortality in T2D patients with established CVD. Evidence from randomized clinical trials suggests that empagliflozin and canagliflozin significantly reduce the CVD morbidity, all-cause mortality, and CVD mortality as well as HF hospitalization and nephropathy development or progression [8]. Similar effects have also been reported for canagliflozin [10]. These benefits could be related to glucose-lowering as well as to reductions in blood pressure, weight, and serum uric acid and to improvements in oxidative stress, glomerular hyperfiltration, albuminuria, arterial stiffness, plasma lipids, sympathetic nervous system activity, myocardial oxygen consumption, and cardiac workload [55]. Our findings complement these SGLT-2 inhibitor actions, suggesting also a significant improvement in FMD. Concerning the impact of SGLT-2 inhibitors on arterial wave velocity, it should be noted that despite the ample evidence on the impact of this class of drugs on natriuresis and blood pressure [8, 10], more data are required to assess the effects of these drugs on PWV, as there are only few published data on this topic [46].

Our findings also agree with the published evidence from large randomized clinical trials on the effects of liraglutide [9] and semaglutide [11] on CVD outcomes in T2D patients. In the present meta-analysis, GLP-1 RAs significantly decreased PWV in T2D patients, although they did not affect FMD. Since the effects of these drugs on CVD risk is still debatable [12, 56], it remains to be seen whether their impact on vascular function may play a role in determining their CVD effects.

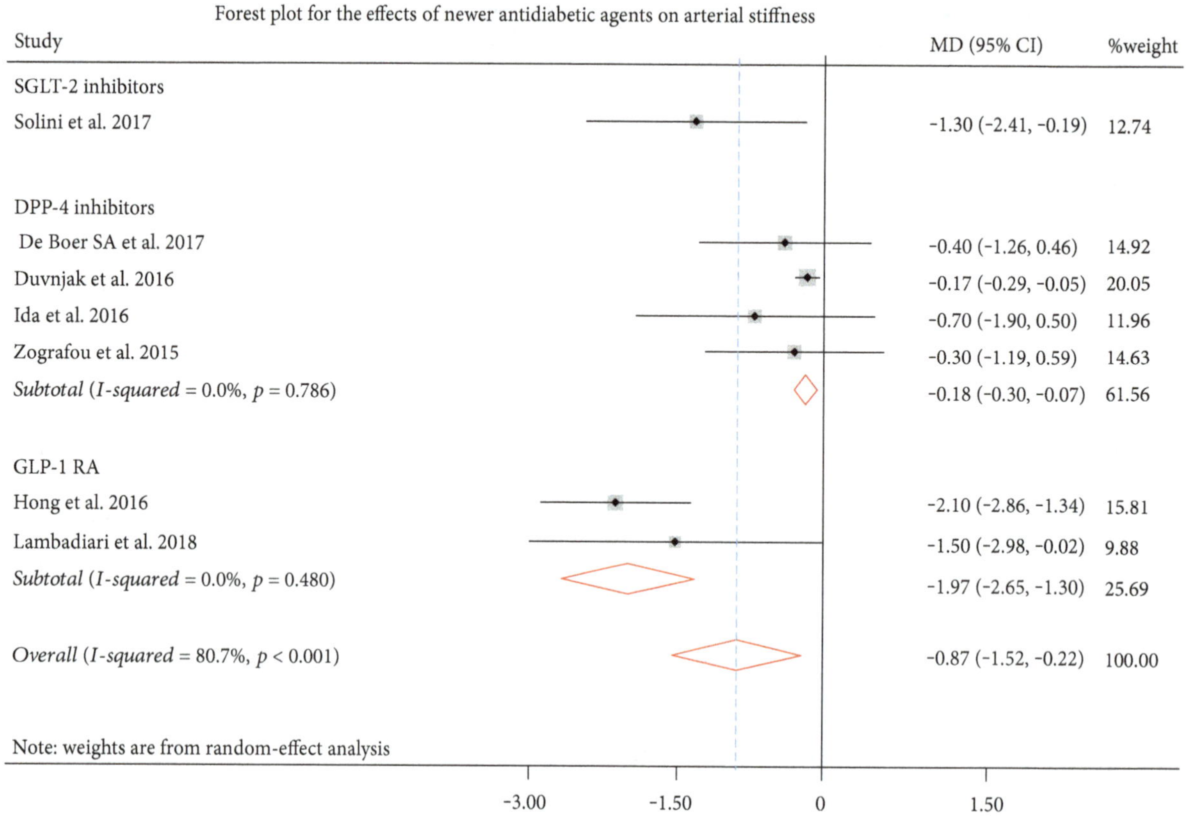

FIGURE 3: Effects of newer antidiabetic drugs on arterial stiffness. Squares indicate the mean difference (MD) and the respective 95% confidence intervals in pulse wave velocity (PWV) before/after treatment from eligible studies. The size of the squares corresponds to the weight of each study. The diamonds and their width represent the pooled weighted MD and the 95% CI, respectively. DPP-4: dipeptidyl peptidase-4; GLP-1 RAs: glucagon-like peptide-1 receptor agonists; SGLT-2: sodium-glucose cotransporter-2.

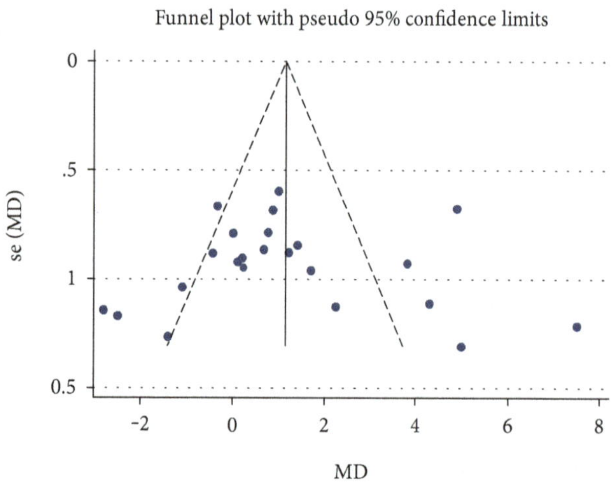

FIGURE 4: Funnel plot and assessment of publication bias. Funnel plot with 95% pseudoconfidence intervals of the effect size and its standard error for studies assessing the effects of newer antidiabetic drugs on the primary endpoint endothelial function. Large studies appear toward the top of the graph and tend to cluster near the mean effect size. Smaller studies appear toward the bottom of the graph and (since there is more sampling variation in effect size estimates in the smaller studies) will be dispersed across a range of values. The symmetric distribution of studies about the combined effect size indicates the absence of publication bias.

The limitations of the existing studies in the field should be noted. The published evidence is modest and mainly based on small-sized randomized clinical studies, some of which were uncontrolled. Furthermore, studies were significantly heterogeneous, and therefore, the results of the present meta-analysis should be interpreted cautiously. The number of the published studies in this field did not allow for subgroup analysis per drug class or for between-agent comparisons within the same drug class. Furthermore, based on the published literature, we cannot conclude whether beneficial effects of SGLT-2 inhibitors, DDP-4 inhibitors, and GLP-1 RAs are due to direct glucose-lowering effects or to indirect effects driven by the modulation of other cardiovascular risk factors such as body weight loss and arterial blood pressure modification [8–11, 57]. More data is also warranted for the effect of SGLT-2 inhibitors on arterial stiffness as well as endothelial function as there are limited published studies reporting on their effects.

5. Conclusion

In conclusion, the present meta-analysis suggests that the published literature in the field of newer antidiabetic drugs and vascular function is of modest quality and characterized by significant heterogeneity among studies. Overall, both DPP-4 inhibitors and GLP-1 RAs were shown to significantly decrease PWV without affecting FMD. In contrast, SGLT-2 inhibitors significantly improved FMD, but concrete data on their effects on PWV is still missing. Whether these distinct properties of newer antidiabetic drugs, in relation to their effects on endothelial function and arterial stiffness, may explain their differential effects on CVD risk remains to be elucidated in future studies.

Conflicts of Interest

The authors declare that they have no conflicts of interest.

References

[1] J. E. Shaw, R. A. Sicree, and P. Z. Zimmet, "Global estimates of the prevalence of diabetes for 2010 and 2030," *Diabetes Research and Clinical Practice*, vol. 87, no. 1, pp. 4–14, 2010.

[2] The Emerging Risk Factors Collaboration, "Diabetes mellitus, fasting blood glucose concentration, and risk of vascular disease: a collaborative meta-analysis of 102 prospective studies," *The Lancet*, vol. 375, no. 9733, pp. 2215–2222, 2010.

[3] C. C. Low Wang, C. N. Hess, W. R. Hiatt, and A. B. Goldfine, "Clinical update: cardiovascular disease in diabetes mellitus. Atherosclerotic cardiovascular disease and heart failure in type 2 diabetes mellitus - mechanisms, management and clinical considerations," *Circulation*, vol. 133, no. 24, pp. 2459–2502, 2016.

[4] A. S. Antonopoulos, G. Siasos, and D. Tousoulis, "Microangiopathy, arterial stiffness, and risk stratification in patients with type 2 diabetes," *JAMA Cardiology*, vol. 2, no. 7, pp. 820-821, 2017.

[5] A. S. Antonopoulos, M. Margaritis, P. Coutinho et al., "Adiponectin as a link between type 2 diabetes and vascular NADPH oxidase activity in the human arterial wall: the regulatory role of perivascular adipose tissue," *Diabetes*, vol. 64, no. 6, pp. 2207–2219, 2015.

[6] S. E. Nissen and K. Wolski, "Effect of rosiglitazone on the risk of myocardial infarction and death from cardiovascular causes," *The New England Journal of Medicine*, vol. 356, no. 24, pp. 2457–2471, 2007.

[7] R. R. Holman, H. Sourij, and R. M. Califf, "Cardiovascular outcome trials of glucose-lowering drugs or strategies in type 2 diabetes," *Lancet*, vol. 383, no. 9933, pp. 2008–2017, 2014.

[8] B. Zinman, C. Wanner, J. M. Lachin et al., "Empagliflozin, cardiovascular outcomes, and mortality in type 2 diabetes," *New England Journal of Medicine*, vol. 373, no. 22, pp. 2117–2128, 2015.

[9] S. P. Marso, G. H. Daniels, K. Brown-Frandsen et al., "Liraglutide and cardiovascular outcomes in type 2 diabetes," *New England Journal of Medicine*, vol. 375, no. 4, pp. 311–322, 2016.

[10] B. Neal, V. Perkovic, K. W. Mahaffey et al., "Canagliflozin and cardiovascular and renal events in type 2 diabetes," *New England Journal of Medicine*, vol. 377, no. 7, pp. 644–657, 2017.

[11] S. P. Marso, S. C. Bain, A. Consoli et al., "Semaglutide and cardiovascular outcomes in patients with type 2 diabetes," *The New England Journal of Medicine*, vol. 375, no. 19, pp. 1834–1844, 2016.

[12] M. A. Pfeffer, B. Claggett, R. Diaz et al., "Lixisenatide in patients with type 2 diabetes and acute coronary syndrome," *The New England Journal of Medicine*, vol. 373, no. 23, pp. 2247–2257, 2015.

[13] R. R. Holman, M. A. Bethel, R. J. Mentz et al., "Effects of once-weekly exenatide on cardiovascular outcomes in type 2 diabetes," *The New England Journal of Medicine*, vol. 377, no. 13, pp. 1228–1239, 2017.

[14] W. B. White, C. P. Cannon, S. R. Heller et al., "Alogliptin after acute coronary syndrome in patients with type 2 diabetes," *The New England Journal of Medicine*, vol. 369, no. 14, pp. 1327–1335, 2013.

[15] J. B. Green, M. A. Bethel, P. W. Armstrong et al., "Effect of sitagliptin on cardiovascular outcomes in type 2 diabetes," *New England Journal of Medicine*, vol. 373, no. 3, pp. 232–242, 2015.

[16] B. M. Scirica, D. L. Bhatt, E. Braunwald et al., "Saxagliptin and cardiovascular outcomes in patients with type 2 diabetes mellitus," *New England Journal of Medicine*, vol. 369, no. 14, pp. 1317–1326, 2013.

[17] A. S. Antonopoulos, F. Sanna, N. Sabharwal et al., "Detecting human coronary inflammation by imaging perivascular fat," *Science Translational Medicine*, vol. 9, no. 398, article eaal2658, 2017.

[18] A. S. Antonopoulos and D. Tousoulis, "The molecular mechanisms of obesity paradox," *Cardiovascular Research*, vol. 113, no. 9, pp. 1074–1086, 2017.

[19] A. S. Antonopoulos, G. Siasos, T. Konsola et al., "Arterial wall elastic properties and endothelial dysfunction in the diabetic foot syndrome in patients with type 2 diabetes," *Diabetes Care*, vol. 38, no. 11, pp. e180–e181, 2015.

[20] C. Antoniades, C. Bakogiannis, P. Leeson et al., "Rapid, direct effects of statin treatment on arterial redox state and nitric oxide bioavailability in human atherosclerosis via tetrahydrobiopterin-mediated endothelial nitric oxide synthase coupling," *Circulation*, vol. 124, no. 3, pp. 335–345, 2011.

[21] C. Antoniades, C. Bakogiannis, D. Tousoulis et al., "Preoperative atorvastatin treatment in CABG patients rapidly improves vein graft redox state by inhibition of Rac1 and NADPH-oxidase activity," *Circulation*, vol. 122, no. 11, Supplement 1, pp. S66–S73, 2010.

[22] S. P. Hozo, B. Djulbegovic, and I. Hozo, "Estimating the mean and variance from the median, range, and the size of a sample," *BMC Medical Research Methodology*, vol. 5, no. 1, p. 13, 2005.

[23] for the PROLOGUE Study Investigators, T. Maruhashi, Y. Higashi et al., "Long-term effect of sitagliptin on endothelial function in type 2 diabetes: a sub-analysis of the PROLOGUE study," *Cardiovascular Diabetology*, vol. 15, no. 1, 2016.

[24] K. Nakamura, H. Oe, H. Kihara et al., "DPP-4 inhibitor and alpha-glucosidase inhibitor equally improve endothelial function in patients with type 2 diabetes: EDGE study," *Cardiovascular Diabetology*, vol. 13, no. 1, p. 110, 2014.

[25] K. Suzuki, K. Watanabe, T. Suzuki et al., "Sitagliptin improves vascular endothelial function in Japanese type 2 diabetes patients without cardiovascular disease," *Journal of Diabetes Mellitus*, vol. 2, no. 3, pp. 338–345, 2012.

[26] T. Jax, A. Stirban, A. Terjung et al., "A randomised, active- and placebo-controlled, three-period crossover trial to investigate short-term effects of the dipeptidyl peptidase-4 inhibitor linagliptin on macro- and microvascular endothelial function in type 2 diabetes," *Cardiovascular Diabetology*, vol. 16, no. 1, p. 13, 2017.

[27] X. H. Wang, L. N. Han, Y. R. Yu et al., "Effects of GLP-1 agonist exenatide on cardiac diastolic function and vascular endothelial function in diabetic patients," *Sichuan Da Xue Xue Bao. Yi Xue Ban*, vol. 46, no. 4, pp. 586–590, 2015.

[28] S. H. Downs and N. Black, "The feasibility of creating a checklist for the assessment of the methodological quality both of randomised and non-randomised studies of health care interventions," *Journal of Epidemiology and Community Health*, vol. 52, no. 6, pp. 377–384, 1998.

[29] J. Matsubara, S. Sugiyama, E. Akiyama et al., "Dipeptidyl peptidase-4 inhibitor, sitagliptin, improves endothelial dysfunction in association with its anti-inflammatory effects in patients with coronary artery disease and uncontrolled diabetes," *Circulation Journal*, vol. 77, no. 5, pp. 1337–1344, 2013.

[30] K. Striepe, A. Jumar, C. Ott et al., "Effects of the selective sodium-glucose cotransporter 2 inhibitor empagliflozin on vascular function and central hemodynamics in patients with type 2 diabetes mellitus," *Circulation*, vol. 136, no. 12, pp. 1167–1169, 2017.

[31] M. Ayaori, N. Iwakami, H. Uto-Kondo et al., "Dipeptidyl peptidase-4 inhibitors attenuate endothelial function as evaluated by flow-mediated vasodilatation in type 2 diabetic patients," *Journal of the American Heart Association*, vol. 2, no. 1, article e003277, 2013.

[32] D. Baltzis, J. R. Dushay, J. Loader et al., "Effect of linagliptin on vascular function: a randomized, placebo-controlled study," *The Journal of Clinical Endocrinology and Metabolism*, vol. 101, no. 11, pp. 4205–4213, 2016.

[33] S. A. de Boer, H. J. L. Heerspink, L. E. Juárez Orozco et al., "Effect of linagliptin on pulse wave velocity in early type 2 diabetes: a randomized, double-blind, controlled 26-week trial (RELEASE)," *Diabetes, Obesity and Metabolism*, vol. 19, no. 8, pp. 1147–1154, 2017.

[34] R. Dell'Oro, A. Maloberti, F. Nicoli et al., "Long-term saxagliptin treatment improves endothelial function but not pulse wave velocity and intima-media thickness in type 2 diabetic patients," *High Blood Pressure & Cardiovascular Prevention*, vol. 24, no. 4, pp. 393–400, 2017.

[35] E. Gurkan, I. Tarkun, T. Sahin, B. Cetinarslan, and Z. Canturk, "Evaluation of exenatide versus insulin glargine for the impact on endothelial functions and cardiovascular risk markers," *Diabetes Research and Clinical Practice*, vol. 106, no. 3, pp. 567–575, 2014.

[36] C. Irace, S. de Luca, E. Shehaj et al., "Exenatide improves endothelial function assessed by flow mediated dilation technique in subjects with type 2 diabetes: results from an observational research," *Diabetes & Vascular Disease Research*, vol. 10, no. 1, pp. 72–77, 2012.

[37] G. Kim, S. Oh, S. M. Jin, K. Y. Hur, J. H. Kim, and M. K. Lee, "The efficacy and safety of adding either vildagliptin or glimepiride to ongoing metformin therapy in patients with type 2 diabetes mellitus," *Expert Opinion on Pharmacotherapy*, vol. 18, no. 12, pp. 1179–1186, 2017.

[38] N. Kitao, H. Miyoshi, T. Furumoto et al., "The effects of vildagliptin compared with metformin on vascular endothelial function and metabolic parameters: a randomized, controlled trial (Sapporo Athero-Incretin Study 3)," *Cardiovascular Diabetology*, vol. 16, no. 1, p. 125, 2017.

[39] V. Lambadiari, G. Pavlidis, F. Kousathana et al., "Effects of 6-month treatment with the glucagon like peptide-1 analogue liraglutide on arterial stiffness, left ventricular myocardial deformation and oxidative stress in subjects with newly diagnosed type 2 diabetes," *Cardiovascular Diabetology*, vol. 17, no. 1, p. 8, 2018.

[40] M. Leung, D. Y. Leung, and V. W. Wong, "Effects of dipeptidyl peptidase-4 inhibitors on cardiac and endothelial function in type 2 diabetes mellitus: a pilot study," *Diabetes & Vascular Disease Research*, vol. 13, no. 3, pp. 236–243, 2016.

[41] F. Li, J. Chen, F. Leng, Z. Lu, and Y. Ling, "Effect of saxagliptin on circulating endothelial progenitor cells and endothelial function in newly diagnosed type 2 diabetic patients," *Experimental and Clinical Endocrinology & Diabetes*, vol. 125, no. 6, pp. 400–407, 2017.

[42] H. Nomoto, H. Miyoshi, T. Furumoto et al., "A randomized controlled trial comparing the effects of sitagliptin and glimepiride on endothelial function and metabolic parameters: Sapporo Athero-Incretin Study 1 (SAIS1)," *PLoS One*, vol. 11, no. 10, p. e0164255, 2016.

[43] H. Nomoto, H. Miyoshi, T. Furumoto et al., "A comparison of the effects of the GLP-1 analogue liraglutide and insulin glargine on endothelial function and metabolic parameters: a randomized, controlled trial Sapporo Athero-Incretin Study 2 (SAIS2)," *PLoS One*, vol. 10, no. 8, p. e0135854, 2015.

[44] F. Shigiyama, N. Kumashiro, M. Miyagi et al., "Effectiveness of dapagliflozin on vascular endothelial function and glycemic control in patients with early-stage type 2 diabetes mellitus: DEFENCE study," *Cardiovascular Diabetology*, vol. 16, no. 1, p. 84, 2017.

[45] F. Shigiyama, N. Kumashiro, M. Miyagi et al., "Linagliptin improves endothelial function in patients with type 2 diabetes: a randomized study of linagliptin effectiveness on endothelial function," *Journal of Diabetes Investigation*, vol. 8, no. 3, pp. 330–340, 2017.

[46] A. Solini, L. Giannini, M. Seghieri et al., "Dapagliflozin acutely improves endothelial dysfunction, reduces aortic stiffness and renal resistive index in type 2 diabetic patients: a pilot study," *Cardiovascular Diabetology*, vol. 16, no. 1, p. 138, 2017.

[47] M. E. Widlansky, V. K. Puppala, T. M. Suboc et al., "Impact of DPP-4 inhibition on acute and chronic endothelial function in humans with type 2 diabetes on background metformin therapy," *Vascular Medicine*, vol. 22, no. 3, pp. 189–196, 2017.

[48] I. Zografou, C. Sampanis, E. Gkaliagkousi et al., "Effect of vildagliptin on hsCRP and arterial stiffness in patients with type 2 diabetes mellitus," *Hormones*, vol. 14, no. 1, pp. 118–125, 2015.

[49] L. Duvnjak and K. Blaslov, "Dipeptidyl peptidase-4 inhibitors improve arterial stiffness, blood pressure, lipid profile and inflammation parameters in patients with type 2 diabetes mellitus," *Diabetology and Metabolic Syndrome*, vol. 8, no. 1, p. 26, 2016.

[50] J. Y. Hong, K. Y. Park, B. J. Kim, W. M. Hwang, D. H. Kim, and D. M. Lim, "Effects of short-term exenatide treatment on regional fat distribution, glycated hemoglobin levels, and aortic pulse wave velocity of obese type 2 diabetes mellitus patients," *Endocrinology and Metabolism*, vol. 31, no. 1, pp. 80–85, 2016.

[51] N. D. Hopkins, D. J. Cuthbertson, G. J. Kemp et al., "Effects of 6 months glucagon-like peptide-1 receptor agonist treatment on endothelial function in type 2 diabetes mellitus patients," *Diabetes, Obesity & Metabolism*, vol. 15, no. 8, pp. 770–773, 2013.

[52] S. Ida, K. Murata, K. Betou et al., "Effect of trelagliptin on vascular endothelial functions and serum adiponectin level in patients with type 2 diabetes: a preliminary single-arm prospective pilot study," *Cardiovascular Diabetology*, vol. 15, no. 1, p. 153, 2016.

[53] Y. Kubota, M. Miyamoto, G. Takagi et al., "The dipeptidyl peptidase-4 inhibitor sitagliptin improves vascular endothelial function in type 2 diabetes," *Journal of Korean Medical Science*, vol. 27, no. 11, pp. 1364–1370, 2012.

[54] G. Savarese, C. D'Amore, M. Federici et al., "Effects of dipeptidyl peptidase 4 inhibitors and sodium-glucose linked cotransporter-2 inhibitors on cardiovascular events in patients with type 2 diabetes mellitus: a meta-analysis," *International Journal of Cardiology*, vol. 220, pp. 595–601, 2016.

[55] N. Katsiki, D. P. Mikhailidis, and M. J. Theodorakis, "Sodium-glucose cotransporter 2 inhibitors (SGLT2i): their role in cardiometabolic risk management," *Current Pharmaceutical Design*, vol. 23, no. 10, pp. 1522–1532, 2017.

[56] K. B. Margulies, K. J. Anstrom, A. F. Hernandez et al., "GLP-1 agonist therapy for advanced heart failure with reduced ejection fraction: design and rationale for the functional impact of GLP-1 for heart failure treatment study," *Circulation. Heart Failure*, vol. 7, no. 4, pp. 673–679, 2014.

[57] X. Zhang and Q. Zhao, "Effects of dipeptidyl peptidase-4 inhibitors on blood pressure in patients with type 2 diabetes: a systematic review and meta-analysis," *Journal of Hypertension*, vol. 34, no. 2, pp. 167–175, 2016.

3

Advanced Glycation End Products Increase MDM2 Expression via Transcription Factor KLF5

Pu Wang[1] **Yu Cheng Lu,**[1] **Yuan Fei Li,**[2] **Lan Wang,**[1] **and Shao Chin Lee**[1,3]

[1]*School of Life Sciences, Shanxi University, Taiyuan, Shanxi 030006, China*
[2]*Department of Oncology, The First Clinical Hospital of Shanxi Medical University, Taiyuan, Shanxi 030006, China*
[3]*Department of Bological Science, School of Life Sciences, Jiangsu Normal University, Xuzhou, Jiangsu 221000, China*

Correspondence should be addressed to Shao Chin Lee; lee_shao@hotmail.com

Academic Editor: Julia M. dos Santos

Type 2 diabetes increases the risk for all-site cancers including colon cancer. Diabetic patients present typical pathophysiological features including an increased level of advanced glycation end products (AGEs), which comes from a series of nonenzymatic reactions between sugars and biological macromolecules, positively associated with the occurrence of diabetic complications. MDM2 is an oncogene implicated in cancer development. The present study investigated whether diabetes promoted MDM2 expression in colon cells and the underlying mechanisms. Our results showed that AGE increased the protein level of MDM2 in a cell model and promoted binding between MDM2 and Rb as well as p53, which led to degradation of Rb and p53. KLF5 was able to bind to the regulatory sequence of the MDM2 gene, and knockdown of the KLF5 protein level inhibited the AGE-triggered MDM2 overexpression, which indicated that KLF5 was the transcription factor for MDM2. In a mouse model of diabetes, we found that AGE level was increased in serum. The protein levels of both KLF5 and MDM2 were increased. KLF5 was able to bind to the regulatory sequence of the MDM2 gene. In conclusion, our results suggest that diabetes increases the level of AGE which enhances the expression of MDM2 via transcription factor KLF5 in colon cells. MDM2 overexpression is a candidate biological link between type 2 diabetes and colon cancer development.

1. Introduction

Type 2 diabetes is a prevalent endocrine disease worldwide, which causes tremendous economic and health burden [1]. Epidemiologic research suggests that people who suffered from this diabetes have a significantly increased risk for many types of cancer such as colon cancer, endometrial cancer, and breast cancer [2]. For colon cancer, in particular, a 1.5- to 3.0-fold increase in cancer risk is observed [3–5]. Nevertheless, the biological links between type 2 diabetes and cancer remain unknown. Common pathophysiological factors in diabetes, hyperinsulinemia, hyperglycemia, increased level of saturated fatty acids, and advanced glycation end-products (AGEs) [2], are associated with increased cancer risk. However, the underlying molecular mechanisms are to be explored.

AGEs are a complex and heterogeneous group of compounds which comes from a series of nonenzymatic reactions between sugars and biological macromolecules (proteins, lipids, and nucleic acid) [6]. AGEs have been shown to accumulate in various tissues under diabetic conditions, and they participate in the development of diabetic vascular complications (nephropathy, retinopathy, and atherosclerosis) and nondiabetic disease such as senescence and tumours [7]. Glycosylated hemoglobin A1 has been used as an important indicator for diabetes diagnosis and treatment outcome. There is evidence of an association between AGEs and cancer development; epidemiological data demonstrate that the serum concentration of glyceraldehyde-derived AGEs in patients with colorectal cancer is increased and is closely related to an increased risk of rectal cancer [8]. Experiments *in vitro* show that AGEs can promote migration and invasion of breast and colon cancers through the ERK-MMP pathway; moreover, AGEs can enhance colon formation, as observed in soft agar colon formation assay [9, 10]. When BSA drove AGEs are administered ip, they are able to promote the liver metastasis of human colorectal cancer [11].

MDM2 is an oncogene, the amplification and overexpression of which are linked to progression and poor prognosis of different cancers. It can bind directly to cancer suppressors p53 and Rb to promote their inactivation and/or degradation [12].

In clinical samples, increase in MDM2 gene amplification and cytoplasmic expression are observed in colon cancer, which is associated with advanced cancer staging [13]. However, many tumours exhibit high MDM2 and MDMX protein levels without increased copy number [14]. Thus, transcriptional regulation of MDM2 expression in different tissues appears to be the mechanism for increased MDM2 expression [14]. Several transcription factors have been found in MDM2 transcriptional regulation, which include SP1, p53, NF-κB, and KLF6 [15–19]. MDM2 is expressed at different levels in different tissues without known reasons and mechanisms; trigger- or tissue-specific transcriptional factors have not been documented [14].

Kruppel-like factor 5 (KLF5) belongs to the family of Kruppel-like transcription factors, of which 17 members have been identified to date. Members of this family have been implicated in an extensive array of biological processes including embryonic development, control of cellular proliferation and differentiation, and stress response [20]. KLF5 is expressed in the reproductive organs, pancreas, prostate, skeletal muscle, and lung [21]. However, the highest level of its expression is found in intestinal epithelial cells [22]. Studies *in vivo* have demonstrated essential roles of this protein in various biological processes. KLF5 can function as a transcriptional activator or repressor, a promoter or inhibitor of cell growth and survival, and either an oncogene or tumor suppressor, depending on the cellular and genetic context in which it operates [23]. More importantly, evidence suggests that KLF5 plays an important role in intestinal tumorigenesis. In $LGR5^+$ stem cells, which contain an oncogenic mutant β-catenin, the production of lethal adenomas and carcinomas is completely inhibited by KLF5 deletion [24].

KLF family members are closely related to Sp1 transcription factors but are distinguished by a unique pattern of three cysteine-2/histidine-2 zinc finger motifs separated by seven conserved amino acids at the carboxy terminal of the proteins [25]. Both KLF5 and SP1 bind to similar elements within GC-rich promoter sequences of target genes. Existing data show that SP1 targets at the MDM2 gene basally or under different stimuli [26]. Differential transcriptional activities between SP1 and KLF5 have not been well documented.

From the above, we have a hypothesis that AGEs could promote colon cancer development through active KLF5.

2. Materials and Methods

2.1. Cell Culture. HCT116 (human colon cancer cell) cells were kindly provided by Dr. B. Vogelstein of the Johns Hopkins University School of Medicine, which were maintained in DMEM (low glucose, 5 mM) supplemented with 50 U/ml penicillin, 50 μg/ml streptomycin, and 10% (v/v) fetal calf serum. The culture medium and reagents for the colon cancer cells were purchased from Gibco (Beijing, China).

2.2. Chemicals and Antibodies. Chemicals were purchased from Sigma (St. Louis, MO, USA). Anti-KLF5 antibody (sc-398470, mice, 1 : 1000) was purchased from Santa Cruz (California, USA). Rabbit antibodies against p53 (D120082, 1 : 500), Rb (D221069, 1 : 500), p-Rb (D151284, 1 : 500), MDM2 (D155246, 1 : 500), SP1 (D161137, 1 : 500), actin (D110001,1 : 1000), anti-histone 2A antibody (D151717, 1 : 1000), and anti-BSA (D120272, 1 : 200) were purchased from Sangon (Shanghai, China). Anti-rabbit fluorescent antibody flux 488 (number 4412, Goat, 1 : 1000) was purchased from Cell Signaling. CHIP Kit (P2078) and Cell Cycle Detection kit (C1052) were purchased from Beyotime (Shanghai, China).

2.3. Preparation of AGEs. 50 mg/ml BSA (Sigma, USA) was incubated with 0.5 mmol/l D-glucose (Sigma, USA) for 8 weeks at 37°C. The unincorporated sugar was removed by dialysis against 0.2 mmol/l PBS (pH 7.4). 50 mg/ml nonglycated BSA was incubated without D-glucose as a negative control. The AGEs preparations were scanned for fluorescent intensity using a fluorospectrophotometer (SpectraMax M5, USA). AGEs had fluorescent peak at excitation wavelength of 370 nm and slit 2 nm. Data were processed using GraphPad Prism 6.

2.4. Flow Cytometric Analysis of AGEs Cell-Binding Assay. HCT116 cells seeded on 6-well plates were treated with 50 μg/ml AGEs at 37°C for 4 hours. Cells were collected by centrifugation at 1000g for 5 min, washed with ice-cold PBS, and then fixed with 70% cold ethanol and stored at 4°C for 24 h. Cells were centrifuged again, washed with cold PBS twice, and incubated with anti-BSA antibody for 1 hour at room temperature, and then cells were washed three times with ice-cold PBS followed by FITC-conjugated secondary antibody in 1x PBS for 1 hour at room temperature in the dark, then cells were washed again and measured by flow cytometry. Data were analyzed by FlowJo 7.6.

2.5. Western Blot Analysis. The cultured HCT116 cells and mouse colon tissues were lysed in RIPA buffer. Proteins were separated by polyacrylamide gel electrophoresis and transferred onto PVDF membrane. After blocking for 1 hour at room temperature with TBST containing 0.05% (v/v), Tween-20, and 5% (w/v) nonfat milk, the membranes were incubated with primary antibodies overnight at 4°C, followed by washes with TBST containing 0.05% Tween-20. The membranes were then incubated with a horseradish peroxidase-conjugated secondary antibody for 1 hour at room temperature. ECL reagents (number 32106, Thermo Biosciences) were used to visualize the protein bands, which were captured on an X-ray film.

2.6. Knockdown of Protein Level. The predesigned siRNA oligonucleotides (Sangon Technology, Shanghai, China) were as follows:

(1) KLF5, 5′-AAAGUAUAGACGAGACAGUGC-3′ (sense) and GCCTGTCTCGTCTTCTTT (antisense)

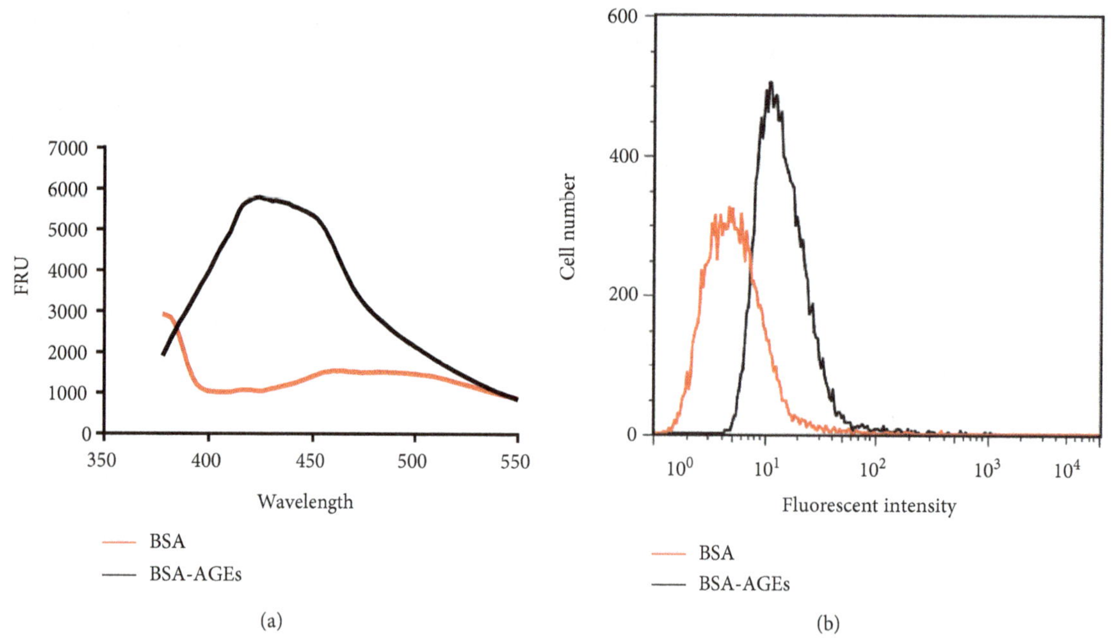

Figure 1: Quanlity assessment of BSA-AGEs and their binding to cells. (a) Full-wavelength scanning was performed to analyze the fluorescent density of quanlity of the prepared AGEs, which indicated the aunlity of the preparation. Excitation wavelength was 370 nm. (b) Cells were treated with AGEs for 4 hours and stained with indirect immunofluorescence staining against BSA and then measured by flow cytometry, which indicated the cell binding of AGE. Every experiment was repeated at least three times.

(2) SP1, 5′AACAGCGTTTCTGCAGCTACC-3′(sense) and GGTAGCTGCAGAAACGCTGTT (antisense)

(3) RAGE, 5′-GCCGGAAAUUGUGAAUCCUTT-3′ (sense) and AAGGTTCCTTTCCGGC (antisense)

HCT116 cells (5×10^4 cells per well) were seeded in 6-well plates and cultured for 24 hours and then were transfected with 200 nM SiRNA oligonucleotides using Lipofectamine 2000 transfection reagent (11668-019, Invitrogen), according to the manufacturer's instructions. Transfection efficiency was evaluated by Western blot analysis 24 hours after transfection.

2.7. Immunoprecipitation. Cultured HCT116 cells were harvested under nondenaturing conditions, washed by ice-cold PBS for 3 times, lysed in 0.5 ml ice-cold cell lysis buffer, and centrifuged. The supernatant was collected to a new tube and incubated with 20 μl Protein G Plus/Protein A agarose (IP05 Millipore) with gentle shaking for 2 hours at 4°C. Protein G Plus/Protein A agarose was then removed by centrifuge for 10 min at 4°C, and the supernatant was incubated with primary antibody overnight at 4°C with gentle shaking. Afterwards, 30 μl Protein G Plus/Protein A agarose were added and incubated under gentle shaking for 4 hours at 4°C. Finally, Protein G Plus/Protein A agarose was collected by centrifuge followed by 2x loading buffer resuspension and heating at 100°C and microcentrifuge for 1 minute at 14000*g*.

2.8. Chromatin Immunoprecipitation. Cultured HCT116 cells were washed and cross-linked using 1% formaldehyde for 20 min, and mouse colon tissues were cross-linked using 1% formaldehyde for 30 min and homogenized. After stopping cross-linking by addition of 0.1 mol/l glycine, cell lysates were sonicated and centrifuged. Immunoprecipitations were performed using the KLF5 antibody in the presence of BSA/salmon sperm DNA and a 50% slurry of protein A agarose beads. Input and immunoprecipitates were washed and eluted and then incubated for 2 h at 42°C in the presence of proteinase K followed by 6 h at 65°C to reverse the formaldehyde cross-linking. DNA fragments were recovered by phenol/chloroform extraction and ethanol precipitation. The related fragments on promoters of MDM2 were amplified by reverse transcription PCR. DNA bands on agarose gels were detected on a UV transilluminator, and graphs were reverse treated by FluorChem HD2 (Alpha Innotech 1.3.0.7). Primers used were as follows:

(i) Human primer 1 GGAGTGTCACAGCGCCAAA (forward) and CAATTGGGTCCGGGGCTC (reverse)

(ii) Human primer 2 TAAAAGCGCAGAGTAACCG CT (forward) and CGCTGGAGTTGTACCCAAA TG (reverse)

(iii) Human primer 3 GTGGACACTGAGTCATACT GCT (forward) and AAAAGAAGGGTCAGAA ATGAAGGC (reverse)

(iv) Mouse primer 1 ATTGCGGTTTCGAGCGGTAA (forward) and GCCGCCTCCTGGACCAATA (reverse)

(v) Mouse primer 2 TGTGGCGTGAGTGACTGAAA (forward) and AAGACTTTAAAAATAGGCAAG GTGA (reverse)

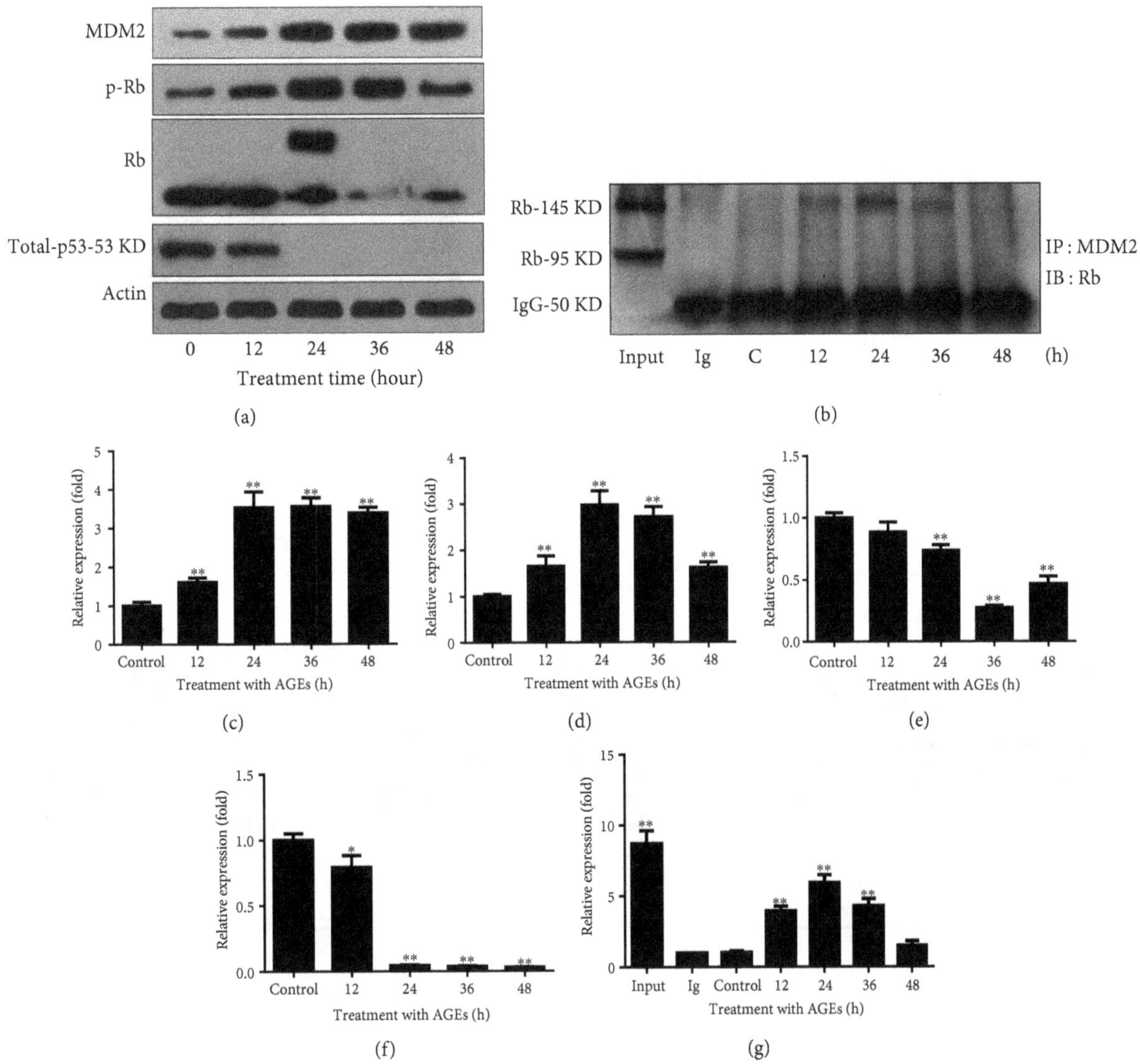

FIGURE 2: AGEs promote expression of MDM2, degradation of p53 and Rb degradation, and phosphorylation of Rb. (a) Cells were treated with AGEs (50 μg/ml) for indicated times; MDM2, p-Rb, Rb, and p53 were quantified by Western blot analysis, which showed that the expression level of MDM2 was increased and the level of RB as well as p53 was decreased. Phosphorylation of Rb was increased. (b) Cells were treated with BSA-AGEs (50 μg/ml) for indicated times, anti-MDM2 antibody was used for immunoprecipitation, and anti-Rb antibody was used for Western blot analysis, which showed the binding between MDM2 and Rb. Every experiment was repeated at least three times. (c–f) The bands of MDM2 (c), pRb (d), Rb (e), and total p53 (f) in Figure 2(a) were quantified using ImageJ. (g) The band of Rb in Figure 2(b) was quantified using ImageJ. Every experiment was repeated at least three times. Asterisks denote significant difference amongst experimental groups. $^{*}p < 0.05$ and $^{**}p < 0.01$.

2.9. Diabetic Mouse Model. Diabetes was induced in ICR mice by consecutive injection of 50 mg/kg streptozotocin (STZ) (0.05 mol/l sodium citrate, pH 5.5) for 5 days after an 8 h fast. Animals with fasting blood glucose >14 mg/dl were considered to be diabetic. After 8 weeks of injections, blood samples were collected by removing the eyeball; latter, mice were killed by dislocation of the cervical spine. Blood routine examinations were analyzed at the Hospital of Shanxi University by flow cytometry. All *in vivo* procedures were performed according to the National Institutes of Health Guide for the Care and Use of Laboratory animals. Animals were maintained at a barrier area of the laboratory animal center, and padding was changed every day. Blood AGEs were detected by fluorescence quantification at excitation wavelength 370 nm and emission wavelength was 440 nm. The fluorescent intensity was aligned by serum protein concentration.

2.10. Statistical Analysis. All of the experiments were performed in triplicate. The data in figures were expressed as mean ± SD, the data of quantified blot bands were expressed as mean (fold) ± SD, and nonparametric test was performed to compare the difference between two groups. One-way ANOVA was performed to show the time-dependent effects observed in the study. The statistical analysis software package SPSS21 was employed for statistical comparisons. A p value < 0.05 was considered as statistically significant.

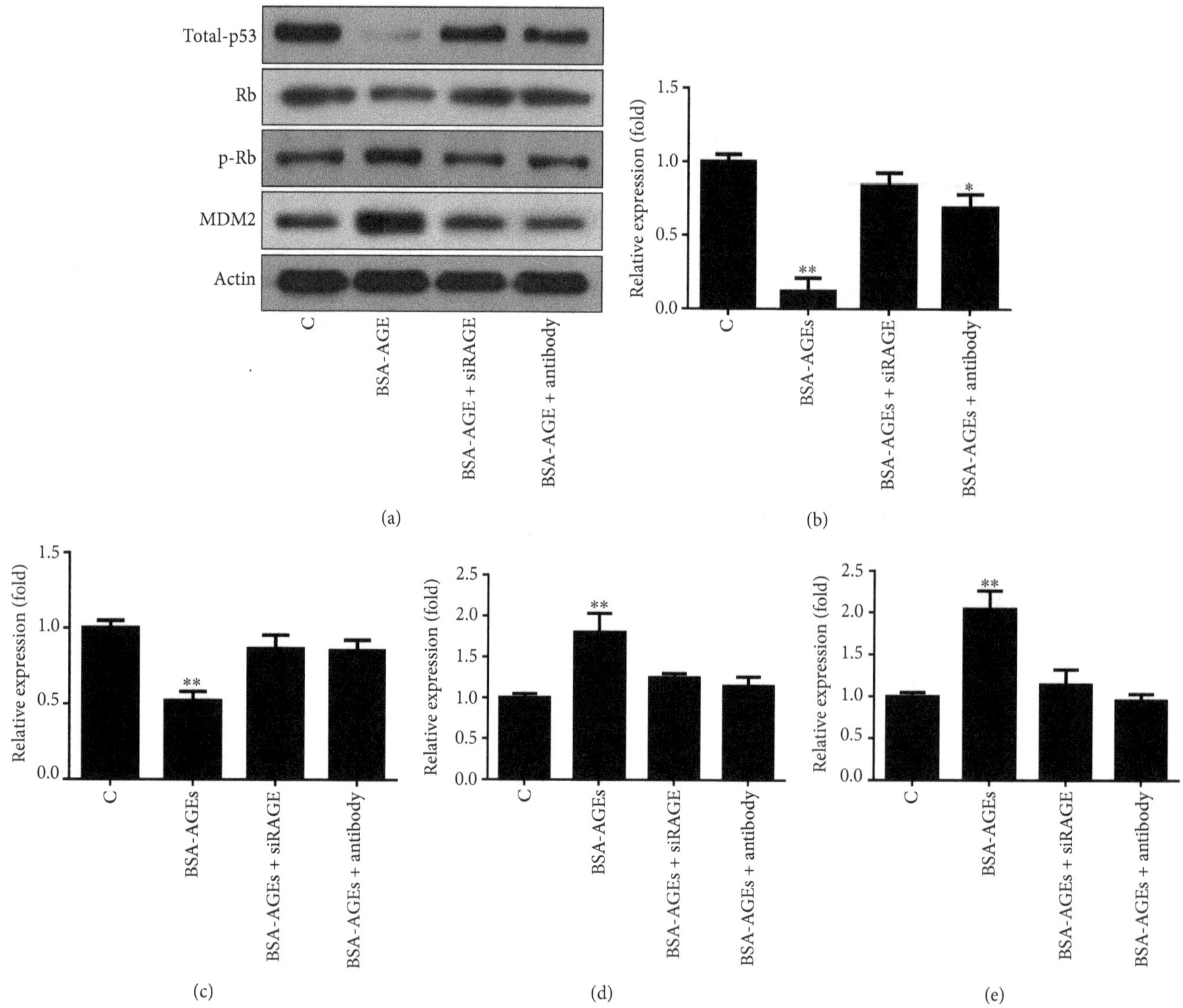

FIGURE 3: AGEs trigger signaling via their receptor RAGE. Cells were pretreated with RAGE siRNA or anti-RAGE antibody followed by treatment with BSA-AGEs (50 μg/ml) for 24 hours. Both siRNA and anti-RAGE inhibited the effects of AGEs on the levels of MDM2, Rb, and p53. (b–e) The bands of p53 (b), Rb (c), p-Rb (d), and MDM2 (e) in Figure 3(a) were quantified using ImageJ. Every experiment was repeated at least three times. Asterisks denote significant difference amongst experimental groups. $^{*}p < 0.05$ and $^{**}p < 0.01$.

2.11. Experimental Design. Firstly, we prepared the AGEs using the BSA-glucose incubation method. Flow cytometry was performed to verify its ability of binding the HCT116 cancer cell line. Then, we analyzed the protein levels of p53, Rb, p-Rb, and MDM2 by Western blot. Finally, we examined whether KLF5 was the transcription for MDM2. Candidate sequences of KLF5 binding to the human MDM2 gene regulatory sequence were predicted in the JASPAR database. Its binding ability was also verified by chromatin immunoprecipitation in the HCT116 cell line. We also quantified the protein level of klf5 and MDM2 and their binding in the colon tissues of healthy and diabetic mice, to show that their expressions and binding were also elevated in colon tissues in diabetes.

3. Results

3.1. BSA-AGEs Quality and Its Cell Binding. Wavelength spectrum scanning showed that the prepared BSA-AGEs had an obvious absorption peak at the wavelength between 400 and 450 nm (Figure 1(a)). There was a significant increase (6.1 ± 0.8, $p < 0.01$) in the area under the curve. Next, we investigated the cell-binding ability of the prepared BAS-AGEs using flow cytometry analysis. The results showed that after treatment with BSA-AGEs, cell fluorescence intensity was significantly increased, compared with that in the cells treated with BSA alone (23.1 ± 3.1 versus 7.81 ± 0.65; $p < 0.01$) (Figure 1(b)). Results from MTT assay showed that AGEs did not inhibit cell viability from the concentrations from 50 to 300 μg/ml (figure not shown). We used the concentration of 50 μg/ml in all the experimental treatments, since the cell appeared to psroliferate well at this concentration of BSA-AGEs.

3.2. BSA-AGEs Enhances the Expression of MDM2 and Phosphorylation of Rb and Decreases the Protein Levels of Rb and p53. Results from the Western blot analyses showed

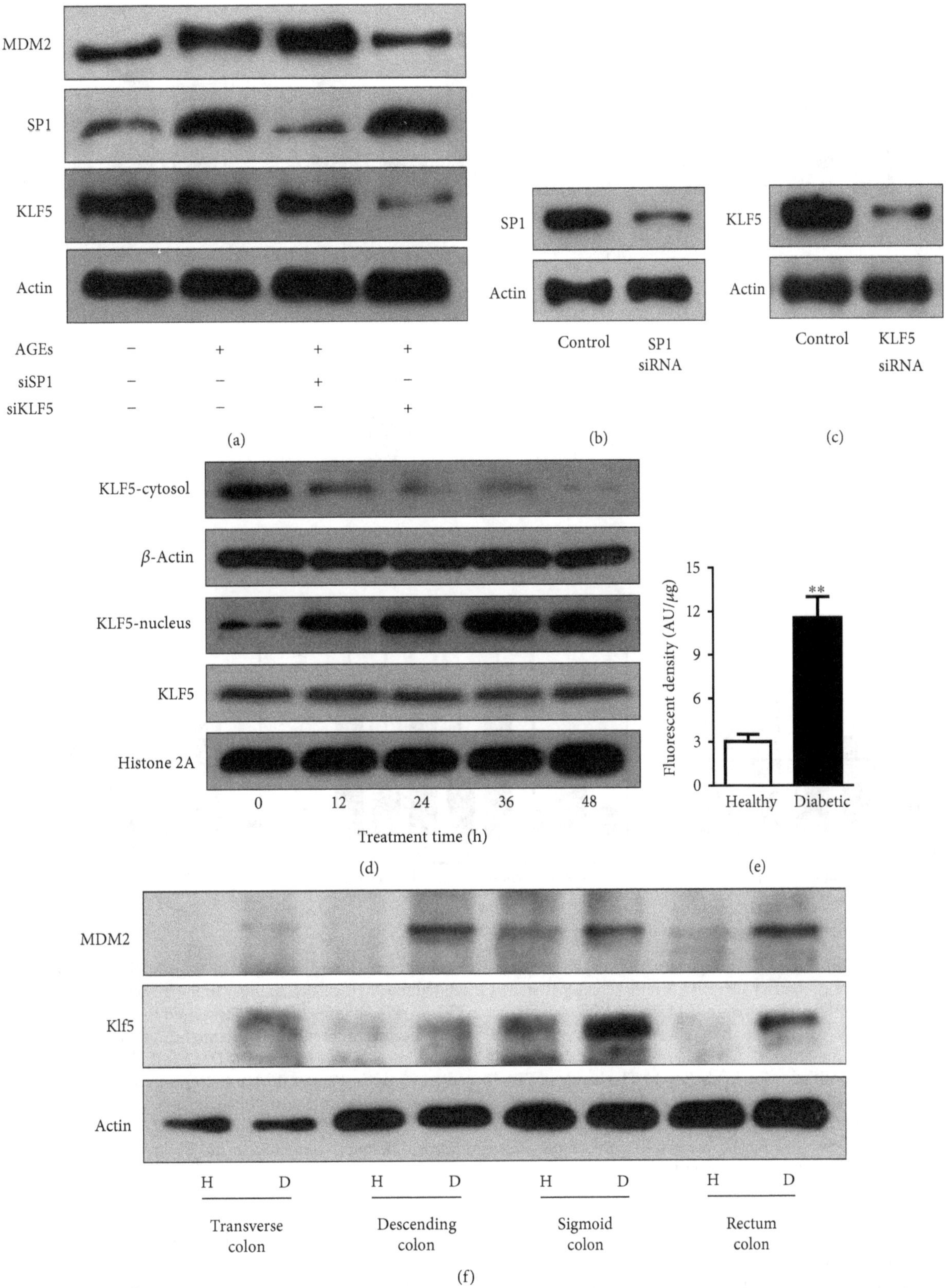

Figure 4: Continued.

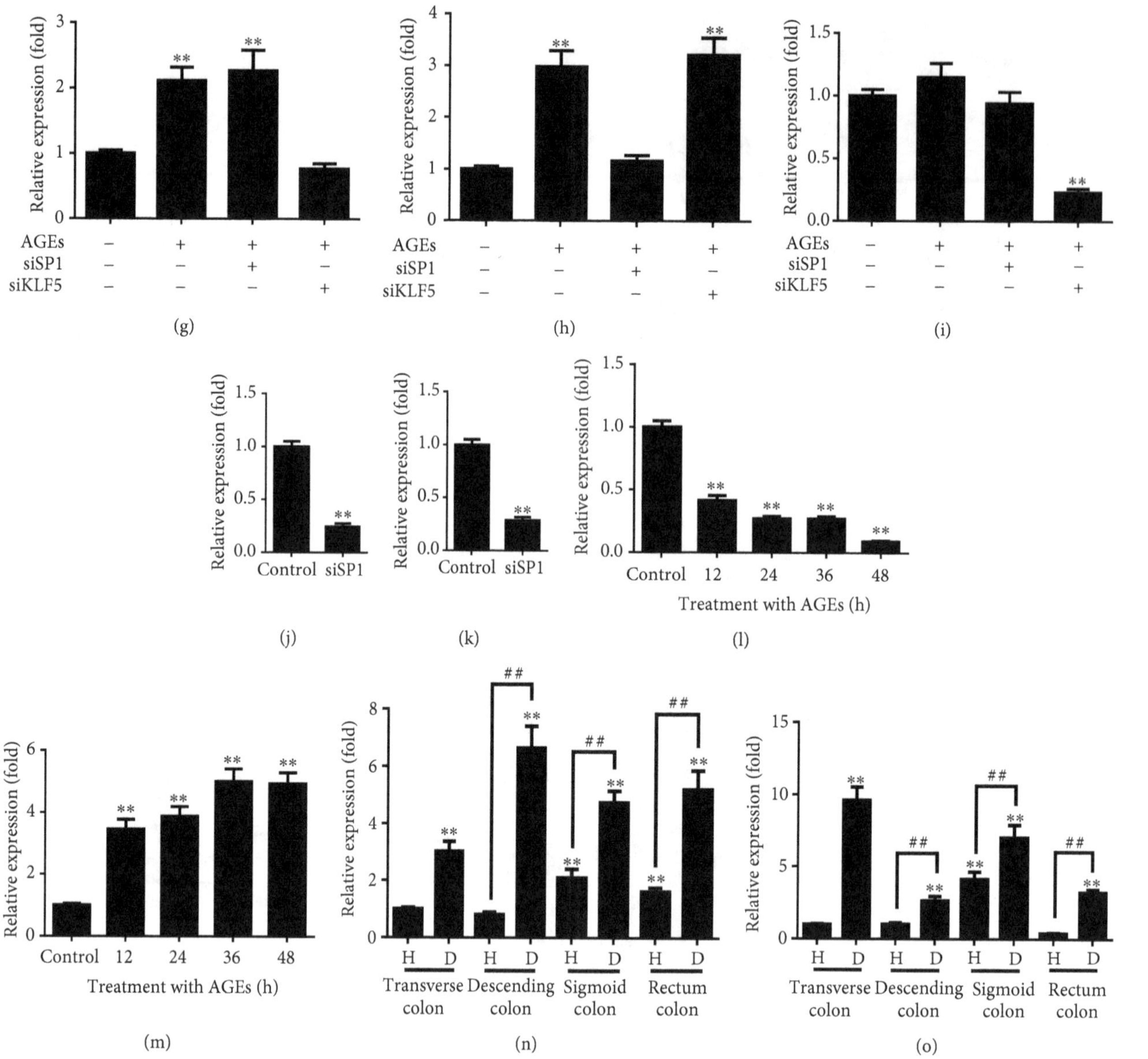

Figure 4: Transcription factor KLF5 regulates MDM2 gene expression. (a) Cells were treated with siRNA target of SP1 or KLF5 to test their effects on the levels of proteins. KLF5 siRNA rather than SP1 siRNA inhibited the AGE-caused changes in the protein levels. (b) SP1 siRNA knocked down the SP1 protein level; (c) KLF5 siRNA knocked down the KLF5 protein level; (d) AGEs triggered the nuclear translocation of KLF5; (e) the level of AGEs in serum of diabetic mice was increased. Serum fluorescent intensity represented the AGE level. (f) The protein levels of both KLF5 and MDM2 were increased in the colon of diabetic mice; (g–i) The bands of MDM2 (g), SP1 (h), and KLF5 (i) in Figure 4(a) were quantified using ImageJ. (j–k) The bands of SP1 (j) and KLF5 (k) in Figures 4(b) and 4(c) were quantified using ImageJ. (l–m) The bands of KLF5 in the cytosol (l) and nucleus (m) in Figure 4(d) were quantified using ImageJ. (n–o) The bands of MDM2 (n) and KLF5 (o) in Figure 4(f) were quantified using ImageJ. Every experiment was repeated at least three times. Asterisks denote significant difference compared to the control group; well number denotes significant difference compared to the healthy group within the same section of colons. $^{\#\#}p < 0.01$ and $^{**}p < 0.01$.

that AGEs upregulated the expression of MDM2 (control (1 ± 0.10): 12 h (1.6 ± 0.12): 24 h (3.5 ± 0.41): 36 h (3.6 ± 0.22): 48 h (3.4 ± 0.15), $p < 0.01$) and downregulated the protein levels of Rb (control (1 ± 0.04): 12 h (0.88 ± 0.08): 24 h (0.74 ± 0.04): 36 h (0.27 ± 0.016): 48 h (0.46 ± 0.06), $p < 0.01$) and p53 (control (1 ± 0.05): 12 h (0.79 ± 0.09): 24 h (0.04 ± 0.004): 36 h (0.038 ± 0.006): 48 h (0.029 ± 0.002), $p < 0.01$) as well as phosphorylation of Rb (control (1 ± 0.05): 12 h (1.6 ± 0.22): 24 h (2.9 ± 0.35): 36 h (2.7 ± 0.22): 48 h (1.6 ± 0.11), $p < 0.01$), which leads to its inactivation, in a time-dependent manner (Figure 2(a)). Moreover, MDM2 directly bound to Rb after 12 (3.9 ± 0.33), 24 (5.9 ± 0.55), and 36 (4.3 ± 0.51) hours of treatment ($p < 0.01$); the maximum binding occurred at 24 hours (Figure 2(b)).

3.3. AGE Signals through Its Receptor. To investigate whether the AGEs bound to its receptor (receptor of advanced glycation end product (RAGE)) to regulate the levels of Rb and

Table 1: Demographic data of experimental animals.

	Healthy subjects	Diabetic subjects
n	6	6
Weight (g)	29.4 ± 2.57	20.8 ± 1.48**
Blood glucose (mmol/l)	8.04 ± 1.34	28.7 ± 1.99**
HbA1c (mmol/l)	6.55 ± 1.04	17.38 ± 4.64**
LDL (mmol/l)	0.12 ± 0.05	0.44 ± 0.27*
HDL (mmol/l)	2.59 ± 0.64	3.536 ± 0.76*
TC (mmol/l)	3.1 ± 1.2	5.12 ± 1.08*
TG (mmol/l)	0.33 ± 0.25	4.58 ± 1.39**

Data are means ± SD or medians (range). $^{*}p < 0.05$ and $^{**}p < 0.01$.

p53, we treated the cells with RAGE siRNA that knocked down the RAGE level (Figure 3(a)) or RAGE antibody, which is aimed at inhibiting RAGE signaling, and found that both treatments were able to inhibit the AGEs-caused decrease in protein levels of p53 (control (1.0 ± 0.05): BSA-AGEs (0.12 ± 0.09): BSA-AGEs + siRAGE (0.85 ± 0.08): BSA-AGEs + antibody (0.69 ± 0.09), $p < 0.01$) and Rb (control (1.0 ± 0.05): BSA-AGEs (0.52 ± 0.06): BSA-AGEs + siRAGE (0.87 ± 0.09): BSA-AGEs + antibody (0.85 ± 0.07), $p < 0.01$) as well as the AGE-caused increase in Rb phosphorylation (control (1.0 ± 0.05): BSA-AGEs (1.80 ± 0.23): BSA-AGEs + siRAGE (1.25 ± 0.05): BSA-AGEs + antibody (1.15 ± 0.11), $p < 0.01$) (Figure 3(a)).

3.4. KLF5 Transcribes MDM2 in the Cell Model. We next examined the responsible transcription factor that enhanced the MDM2 expression by targeting at SP1 and KLF5. We found that the treatment increased the protein level of SP1 (1.0 ± 0.05 versus 2.98 ± 0.31, $p < 0.01$) (Figure 4(a)). However, knockdown of SP1 (1.0 ± 0.05 versus 0.28 ± 0.03, $p < 0.01$) (Figure 4(b)) had no effect on the AGEs-enhanced MDM2 expression (Figure 4(a)). Although the protein level of KLF5 was not significantly increased in the AGEs-treated cells (Figure 4(a)), KLF5 siRNA which decreased its protein level (1.0 ± 0.05 versus 0.24 ± 0.03, $p < 0.01$) (Figure 4(c)) was able to abolish the upregulation of MDM2 expression by AGEs (Figure 4(a)). Since the activity of transcription factors is often dependent on subcellular localizations, we investigated the level of KLF5 in the cytosol and nucleus fractions to test whether AGEs increased the nuclear translocation. The results showed that the concentration of KLF5 started to decrease in the cytosol fraction and to translocate to the nucleus from 12 hours (1.0 ± 0.05 versus 0.41 ± 0.04, $p < 0.01$) of the AGEs treatment, which continued to 48 hours (1.0 ± 0.05 versus 0.09 ± 0.007, $p < 0.01$) (Figure 4(d)). We investigated whether KLF5 transcribed the MDM2 animal model of diabetes. Mice were treated with STZ to induce diabetes. Table 1 shows that the mice became diabetic after 8 weeks of STZ treatment, in particular the AGEs level, as indicated by the increase in fluorescent intensity of serum from diabetic mice (3.0 ± 0.2 versus 11.5 ± 0.7; $p < 0.01$) (Figure 4(e)). The fluorescent intensity was measured at a wavelength of 350 nm which indicated the level of AGEs. The protein level of KLF5 was both increased in the transverse colon (1.0 ± 0.05 versus 3.0 ± 0.35, $p < 0.01$), descending colon (0.8 ± 0.09 versus 6.6 ± 0.77, $p < 0.01$), sigmoid colon (2.1 ± 0.3 versus 4.7 ± 0.41, $p < 0.01$), and rectum colon (1.6 ± 0.14 versus 5.2 ± 0.66, $p < 0.01$) of diabetic mice (Figure 4(f)) as well as the protein level of MDM2 in the transverse colon (1.0 ± 0.05 versus 9.6 ± 0.9, $p < 0.01$), descending colon (1.0 ± 0.1 versus 2.6 ± 0.3, $p < 0.01$), sigmoid colon (4.1 ± 0.5 versus 7.0 ± 0.6, $p < 0.01$), and rectum colon (0.39 ± 0.04 versus 3.2 ± 0.2, $p < 0.01$) of diabetic mice.

3.5. Evidence that KLF5 Transcribes MDM2 in an Animal Model of Diabetes. To obtain further evidence that KLF5 transcribed MDM2, we performed chromatin immunoprecipitation to pull down the transcriptional regulatory sequence of MDM2 using the KLF5 antibody. A total of 4 pieces of human MDM2 gene-binding candidate sequences were obtained after binding site prediction using the JASPAR database (Figure S1). In particular, we designed primers to cover the binding sequences, and the predicted first and third candidate binding sequences were 138 bp and 166 bp in length, respectively. Indeed, we were able to show that the KLF5 antibody pulled down two pieces of sequences which had the calibrated length close to those of the first and third KLF5-binding sequences (138 and 166 bp, respectively; Figure S1) in the transcription regulatory region of MDM2 (Figures 5(a) and 5(b)).

Finally, four pieces of mouse MDM2 gene candidate binding sequences for KLF5 were identified in the JASPAR database (Figure S2). We designed two sets of primers to amplify the binding sequences. Primer 1 amplified the first two binding sequences, and primer 2 amplified the third and fourth binding sequences. Using the KLF5 antibody, we were able to pull down the third and fourth KLF5 binding sequences from the MDM2 gene in chromatin immunoprecipitation assay, which was about the predicted size of 190 bp (Figure 5(c)).

4. Discussion

In this study, for the first time, we showed that AGEs *in vitro* could trigger the overexpression of MDM2 (Figure 2(a)) which directly bond to p53 and Rb, which led to Rb and p53 degradation (Figures 2(a) and 2(b)). Increase in MDM2 expression was also seen in a diabetic mouse model (Figure 4(b)). Furthermore, transcription factor KLF5 was found to directly transcribe MDM2 *in vitro* and *in vivo*, which was responsible for the increased MDM2 expression (Figures 4(e), 4(f), and 5(c)).

In diabetes, raised insulin and insulin-like growth factors stimulate cancer cell proliferation and metastasis. Increases in inflammatory cytokines in diabetes promote tumour development, which include interleukin-6 (IL-6), monocyte chemoattractant protein, plasminogen activator inhibitor-1 (PAI-1), adiponectin, leptin, and tumor necrosis factor-alpha [27]. Due to the increase in cytokines, several prooncogenes are hyperactivated in diabetes. Akt/mTOR is positively associated with diabetes cancer initiation and progression [28]. SIRT1 deacetylates and inactivates p53 and HIF1A,

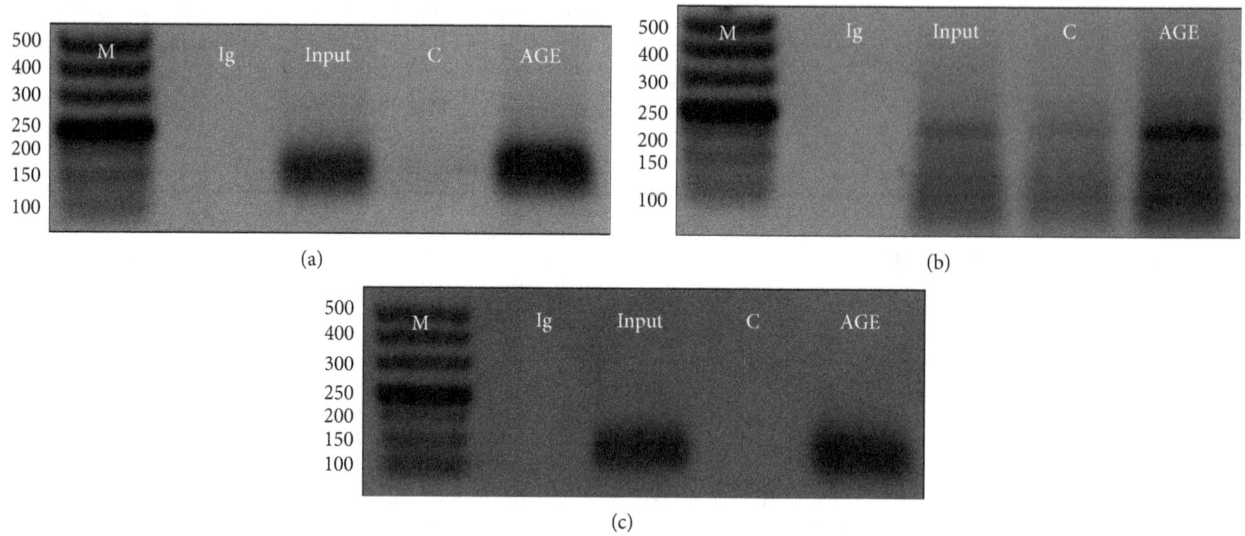

FIGURE 5: Evidence that KLF5 transcribed MDM2 *in vitro* and *in vivo* in a diabetic animal model. (a) Chromatin immunoprecipitation pulled down the first piece of KLF5-binding sequence (predicted 138 bp) in the human MDM2 gene. (b) Chromatin immunoprecipitation pulled down the third piece of the KLF5-binding sequence (predicted 166 bp) in the human MDM2 gene. (c) Chromatin immunoprecipitation pulled down the third and fourth KLF5-binding sequences in the mouse MDM2 gene, which was predicted to be 190 bp in size; H: healthy; D: diabetic. M: DNA size marker. Every experiment was repeated at least three times.

active liver X receptor proteins, peroxisome proliferator-activated receptor γ, and NFKB1 to promote cell proliferation [29]; RAS signaling, the excessive activation of which is associated with colon cancer initiation, is reported to promote cancer development in diabetes [30].

In normal cells, p53 are carefully controlled at a low concentration by MDM2 and MDMX, presented MDM2 are required for development and protect cells from cellular stress [31]. However, continued presence of MDM2 is required for cancer initiation [32] and results in sustained regression of tumors [33]. MDM2 is known as the main regulator of Rb and p53 in many human cancers [34]. MDM2 is able to mediate Rb degradation directly [35] or in an ubiquitin-independent manner [36]. MDM2 can directly interact with p53 through the N-terminal regions and promote p53 proteasomal degradation in the cytoplasm [37, 38]. Specifically in colon cancer, increases in MDM2 protein expression and gene amplification are observed [12, 39], which is associated with increased colorectal cancer risk and can be used as a prognostic marker [33]. Knockdown of MDM2 enhances the efficacy of cisplatin-based chemotherapy *in vitro* and *in vivo* [40] as well as radiotherapy [41]. In the present study, AGEs promote MDM2 expression which triggers Rb and p53 inactivation/degradation (Figures 2(a) and 2(b)). p53 function is impaired in 69.4% of colon cancer [42, 43]. Knockout or mutation of p53 *in vitro* or *in vivo* can cause tumorigenesis. Mutation of Rb is involved in cancer initiation in many types of human cancer [44]. Conditional depletion of Rb can disrupt the coordination between DNA replication and mitosis [45], induce missed regulation of pluripotency networks [46], and cause early-stage cancer [47]. In embryo cells with mutant p53, knockout of Rb is sufficient to initiate tumorigenesis [48]. Thus, dysregulation of oncogenes and tumor suppressors is implicated in cancer development, including cancer development in diabetes. Our results, more specifically, support a view that AGEs-caused MDM2 overexpression as well as inactivation of p53 and Rb contribute to the development of colon cancer in type 2 diabetes.

Cell stimulation with lysophosphatidic acid can increase the expression of MDM2; under experimental conditions, knockdown of SP1 but not KLF5 blocks the MDM2 overexpression [49]. This shows that, under experimental conditions, SP1 rather than KLF5 serves as the transcription factor for MDM2, which is different from our results that AGEs increased the MDM2 expression via KLF5 (Figure 4(d)). The difference is likely to be due to that different triggers activate different signaling pathways and/or transcription factors. AGEs is found to activate RAS and ERK1/2 in PC12 and colon cancer cells *in vitro* [50, 51]. In IEC6 cells, overexpression of KRAS upregulates KLF5 [52]. Sphingosine-1-phosphate enhances KLF5 expression through the G(i)-protein-Ras-ERK/p38 pathway in neointimal cells and vascular smooth muscle cells [53], indicating that the KLF5 transcriptional activity is closely related to MAPK signaling.

In HCT116 cells, AGEs did not increase the protein level of KLF5, but promoted the nuclear translocation (Figure 4(d)), whereas, in our diabetic mouse model, KLF5 protein level was increased (Figure 5(b)). This might be due to the different behaviors of KLF5 between nontransformed and cancerous cells. Indeed, in nontumorous cells (i.e., IEC8 and IMCE), overexpression of KLF5 enhances cyclin D expression, cell proliferation, and colony formation. In contrast, overexpression of KLF5 in colon cancer cell shows the opposite effects [54]. In cancer cells, microRNA mir-143 and mir-153 directly inhibit the expression of KLF5 [55, 56].

In conclusion, our results showed that KLF5 directly transcribed MDM2 *in vitro* in a cell model and *in vivo* in

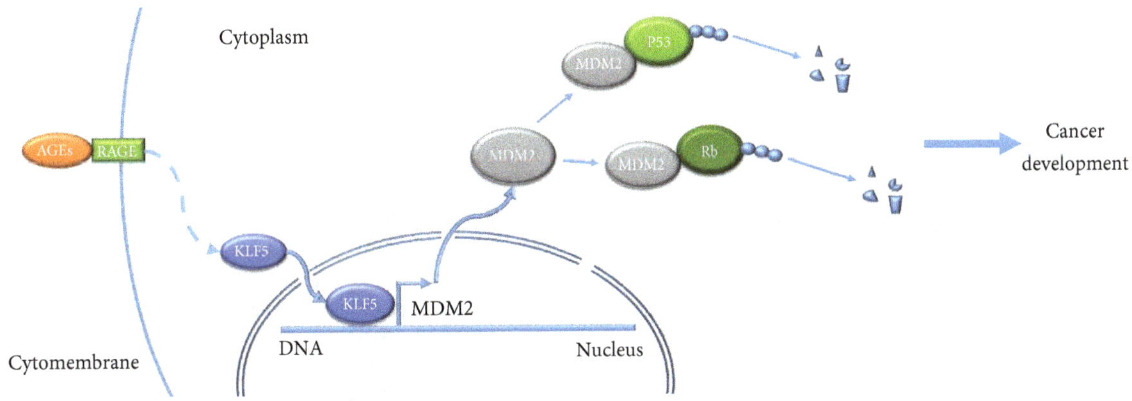

FIGURE 6: Conclusion figure of our research in this paper. Advanced glycation end products promote the nucleus translocation of transcription factor KLF5, which directly bind to the transcriptional regulatory region of MDM2 and promote its expression. Overexpressed MDM2 directly binds and promotes cancer suppressor Rb and p53 degradation via the ubiquitination pathway.

diabetes mouse colon, which was responsible for AGEs-increased expression of MDM2 (Figure 6). Overexpression of oncogene (i.e., MDM2) and inactivation of tumor suppressor (i.e., p53 and Rb) are a candidate biological link between type 2 diabetes and colon cancer development.

Conflicts of Interest

The authors declare no conflicts of interest.

Acknowledgments

The authors thank Dr. ZY Li for her help in establishing our cell culture facility. This work was supported by Shanxi University (nos. 113533901005 and 113545017; Talent Recruitment Fund) and the Department of Science and Technology of Shanxi Province (2015081034 and 201601D11066).

References

[1] NCD Risk Factor Collaboration (NCD-RisC), "Worldwide trends in diabetes since 1980: a pooled analysis of 751 population-based studies with 4.4 million participants," *The Lancet*, vol. 387, no. 10027, pp. 1513–1530, 2016.

[2] E. Giovannucci, D. M. Harlan, M. C. Archer et al., "Diabetes and cancer: a consensus report," *CA: A Cancer Journal for Clinicians*, vol. 60, no. 4, pp. 207–221, 2010.

[3] T. I. L. Nilsen and L. J. Vatten, "Prospective study of colorectal cancer risk and physical activity, diabetes, blood glucose and BMI: exploring the hyperinsulinaemia hypothesis," *British Journal of Cancer*, vol. 84, no. 3, pp. 417–422, 2001.

[4] F. B. Hu, J. E. Manson, S. Liu et al., "Prospective study of adult onset diabetes mellitus (type 2) and risk of colorectal cancer in women," *Journal of the National Cancer Institute*, vol. 91, no. 6, pp. 542–547, 1999.

[5] E. Weiderpass, G. Gridley, O. Nyrén, A. Ekbom, I. Persson, and H. O. Adami, "Diabetes mellitus and risk of large bowel cancer," *Journal of the National Cancer Institute*, vol. 89, no. 9, pp. 660-661, 1997.

[6] R. Singh, A. Barden, T. Mori, and L. Beilin, "Advanced glycation end-products: a review," *Diabetologia*, vol. 44, no. 2, pp. 129–146, 2001.

[7] V. P. Singh, A. Bali, N. Singh, and A. S. Jaggi, "Advanced glycation end products and diabetic complications," *The Korean Journal of Physiology & Pharmacology*, vol. 18, no. 1, pp. 1–14, 2014.

[8] S. Y. Kong, M. Takeuchi, H. Hyogo et al., "The association between glyceraldehyde-derived advanced glycation end-products and colorectal cancer risk," *Cancer Epidemiology, Biomarkers & Prevention*, vol. 24, no. 12, pp. 1855–1863, 2015.

[9] K. J. Lee, J. W. Yoo, Y. K. Kim, J. H. Choi, T. Y. Ha, and M. Gil, "Advanced glycation end products promote triple negative breast cancer cells via ERK and NF-κB pathway," *Biochemical and Biophysical Research Communications*, vol. 495, no. 3, pp. 2195–2201, 2018.

[10] H. Kuniyasu, Y. Chihara, and H. Kondo, "Differential effects between amphoterin and advanced glycation end products on colon cancer cells," *International Journal of Cancer*, vol. 104, no. 6, pp. 722–727, 2003.

[11] R. Deng, H. Wu, H. Ran et al., "Glucose-derived AGEs promote migration and invasion of colorectal cancer by up-regulating Sp1 expression," *Biochimica et Biophysica Acta*, vol. 1861, no. 5, pp. 1065–1074, 2017.

[12] J. Hernández-Monge, A. B. Rousset-Roman, I. Medina-Medina, and V. Olivares-Illana, "Dual function of MDM2 and MDMX toward the tumor suppressors p53 and RB," *Genes & Cancer*, vol. 7, no. 9-10, pp. 278–287, 2016.

[13] M. Hav, L. Libbrecht, L. Ferdinande et al., "MDM2 gene amplification and protein expressions in colon carcinoma: is targeting MDM2 a new therapeutic option?," *Virchows Archiv*, vol. 458, no. 2, pp. 197–203, 2011.

[14] M. Wade, Y. C. Li, and G. M. Wahl, "MDM2, MDMX and p53 in oncogenesis and cancer therapy," *Nature Reviews. Cancer*, vol. 13, no. 2, pp. 83–96, 2013.

[15] D. M. Gilkes, Y. Pan, D. Coppola, T. Yeatman, G. W. Reuther, and J. Chen, "Regulation of MDMX expression by mitogenic signaling," *Molecular and Cellular Biology*, vol. 28, no. 6, pp. 1999–2010, 2008.

[16] A. Gembarska, F. Luciani, C. Fedele et al., "MDM4 is a key therapeutic target in cutaneous melanoma," *Nature Medicine*, vol. 18, no. 8, pp. 1239–1247, 2012.

[17] N. A. Laurie, S. L. Donovan, C. S. Shih et al., "Inactivation of the p53 pathway in retinoblastoma," *Nature*, vol. 444, no. 7115, pp. 61–66, 2006.

[18] K. I. Pishas, F. Al-Ejeh, I. Zinonos et al., "Nutlin-3a is a potential therapeutic for Ewing sarcoma," *Clinical Cancer Research*, vol. 17, no. 3, pp. 494–504, 2011.

[19] J. McEvoy, A. Ulyanov, R. Brennan et al., "Analysis of MDM2 and MDM4 single nucleotide polymorphisms, mRNA splicing and protein expression in retinoblastoma," *PLoS One*, vol. 7, no. 8, article e42739, 2012.

[20] B. B. McConnell and V. W. Yang, "Mammalian Krüppel-like factors in health and diseases," *Physiological Reviews*, vol. 90, no. 4, pp. 1337–1381, 2010.

[21] J. T. Dong and C. Chen, "Essential role of KLF5 transcription factor in cell proliferation and differentiation and its implications for human diseases," *Cellular and Molecular Life Sciences*, vol. 66, no. 16, pp. 2691–2706, 2009.

[22] M. D. Conkright, M. A. Wani, K. P. Anderson, and J. B. Lingrel, "A gene encoding an intestinal-enriched member of the Krüppel-like factor family expressed in intestinal epithelial cells," *Nucleic Acids Research*, vol. 27, no. 5, pp. 1263–1270, 1999.

[23] S. M. Diakiw, R. J. D'Andrea, and A. L. Brown, "The double life of KLF5: Opposing roles in regulation of gene-expression, cellular function, and transformation," *IUBMB Life*, vol. 65, no. 12, pp. 999–1011, 2013.

[24] T. Nakaya, S. Ogawa, I. Manabe et al., "KLF5 regulates the integrity and oncogenicity of intestinal stem cells," *Cancer Research*, vol. 74, no. 10, pp. 2882–2891, 2014.

[25] J. Kaczynski, T. Cook, and R. Urrutia, "Sp1- and Krüppel-like transcription factors," *Genome Biology*, vol. 4, no. 2, p. 206, 2003.

[26] L. Duan, R. E. Perez, L. Chen, L. A. Blatter, and C. G. Maki, "p53 promotes AKT and SP1-dependent metabolism through the pentose phosphate pathway that inhibits apoptosis in response to Nutlin-3a," *Journal of Molecular Cell Biology*, 2017.

[27] R. C. M. van Kruijsdijk, E. van der Wall, and F. L. J. Visseren, "Obesity and cancer: the role of dysfunctional adipose tissue," *Cancer Epidemiology, Biomarkers & Prevention*, vol. 18, no. 10, pp. 2569–2578, 2009.

[28] S. L. Habib and S. Liang, "Hyperactivation of Akt/mTOR and deficiency in tuberin increased the oxidative DNA damage in kidney cancer patients with diabetes," *Oncotarget*, vol. 5, no. 9, pp. 2542–2550, 2014.

[29] J. Yang, R. Nishihara, X. Zhang, S. Ogino, and Z. R. Qian, "Energy sensing pathways: bridging type 2 diabetes and colorectal cancer?," *Journal of Diabetes and its Complications*, vol. 31, no. 7, pp. 1228–1236, 2017.

[30] J. K. Brewer, "Behavioral genetics of the depression/cancer correlation: a look at the Ras oncogene family and the 'cerebral diabetes paradigm'," *Journal of Molecular Neuroscience*, vol. 35, no. 3, pp. 307–322, 2008.

[31] J. K. Buolamwini, J. Addo, S. Kamath, S. Patil, D. Mason, and M. Ores, "Small molecule antagonists of the MDM2 oncoprotein as anticancer agents," *Current Cancer Drug Targets*, vol. 5, no. 1, pp. 57–68, 2005.

[32] A. Meye, P. Würl, M. Bache et al., "Colony formation of soft tissue sarcoma cells is inhibited by lipid-mediated antisense oligodeoxynucleotides targeting the human mdm2 oncogene," *Cancer Letters*, vol. 149, no. 1-2, pp. 181–188, 2000.

[33] I. Chaar, T. A. Arfaoui, E. H. O. el Amine et al., "Impact of MDM2 polymorphism: increased risk of developing colorectal cancer and a poor prognosis in the Tunisian population," *European Journal of Gastroenterology & Hepatology*, vol. 24, no. 3, pp. 320–327, 2012.

[34] D. B. S. Yap, J.-K. Hsieh, F. S. G. Chan, and X. Lu, "mdm2: a bridge over the two tumour suppressors, p53 and Rb," *Oncogene*, vol. 18, no. 53, pp. 7681–7689, 1999.

[35] C. Uchida, S. Miwa, K. Kitagawa et al., "Enhanced Mdm2 activity inhibits pRB function via ubiquitin-dependent degradation," *The EMBO Journal*, vol. 24, no. 1, pp. 160–169, 2005.

[36] P. Sdek, H. Ying, D. L. F. Chang et al., "MDM2 promotes proteasome-dependent ubiquitin-independent degradation of retinoblastoma protein," *Molecular Cell*, vol. 20, no. 5, pp. 699–708, 2005.

[37] S. M. Picksley, B. Vojtesek, A. Sparks, and D. P. Lane, "Immunochemical analysis of the interaction of p53 with MDM2;-fine mapping of the MDM2 binding site on p53 using synthetic peptides," *Oncogene*, vol. 9, no. 9, pp. 2523–2529, 1994.

[38] G. W. Yu, S. Rudiger, D. Veprintsev, S. Freund, M. R. Fernandez-Fernandez, and A. R. Fersht, "The central region of HDM2 provides a second binding site for p53," *Proceedings of the National Academy of Sciences of the United States of America*, vol. 103, no. 5, pp. 1227–1232, 2006.

[39] A. Forslund, Z. Zeng, L. X. Qin et al., "MDM2 gene amplification is correlated to tumor progression but not to the presence of SNP309 or TP53 mutational status in primary colorectal cancers," *Molecular Cancer Research*, vol. 6, no. 2, pp. 205–211, 2008.

[40] Y. Yu, P. Sun, L. C. Sun et al., "Downregulation of MDM2 expression by RNAi inhibits LoVo human colorectal adenocarcinoma cells growth and the treatment of LoVo cells with *mdm2*siRNA3 enhances the sensitivity to cisplatin," *Biochemical and Biophysical Research Communications*, vol. 339, no. 1, pp. 71–78, 2006.

[41] H. Wang, P. Oliver, Z. Zhang, S. Agrawal, and R. Zhang, "Chemosensitization and radiosensitization of human cancer by antisense anti-MDM2 oligonucleotides: *in vitro* and *in vivo* activities and mechanisms," *Annals of the New York Academy of Sciences*, vol. 1002, no. 1, pp. 217–235, 2003.

[42] J. Gao, B. A. Aksoy, U. Dogrusoz et al., "Integrative analysis of complex cancer genomics and clinical profiles using the cBioPortal," *Science Signaling*, vol. 6, no. 269, article pl1, 2013.

[43] E. Cerami, J. Gao, U. Dogrusoz et al., "The cBio cancer genomics portal: an open platform for exploring multidimensional cancer genomics data," *Cancer Discovery*, vol. 2, no. 5, pp. 401–404, 2012.

[44] Y. Song, D. Gilbert, T. N. O'Sullivan et al., "Carcinoma initiation via RB tumor suppressor inactivation: a versatile approach to epithelial subtype-dependent cancer initiation in diverse tissues," *PLoS One*, vol. 8, no. 12, article e80459, 2013.

[45] R. J. Bourgo, U. Ehmer, J. Sage, and E. S. Knudsen, "RB deletion disrupts coordination between DNA replication licensing

and mitotic entry in vivo," *Molecular Biology of the Cell*, vol. 22, no. 7, pp. 931–939, 2011.

[46] M. S. Kareta, L. L. Gorges, S. Hafeez et al., "Inhibition of pluripotency networks by the Rb tumor suppressor restricts reprogramming and tumorigenesis," *Cell Stem Cell*, vol. 16, no. 1, pp. 39–50, 2015.

[47] L. A. Maddison, B. W. Sutherland, R. J. Barrios, and N. M. Greenberg, "Conditional deletion of Rb causes early stage prostate cancer," *Cancer Research*, vol. 64, no. 17, pp. 6018–6025, 2004.

[48] S. Kitajima, S. Kohno, A. Kondoh et al., "Undifferentiated state induced by Rb-p53 double inactivation in mouse thyroid neuroendocrine cells and embryonic fibroblasts," *Stem Cells*, vol. 33, no. 5, pp. 1657–1669, 2015.

[49] S. J. Lee, Y. R. No, D. T. Dang et al., "Regulation of hypoxia-inducible factor 1α (HIF-1α) by lysophosphatidic acid is dependent on interplay between p53 and Krüppel-like factor 5," *Journal of Biological Chemistry*, vol. 288, no. 35, pp. 25244–25253, 2013.

[50] H. M. Lander, J. M. Tauras, J. S. Ogiste, O. Hori, R. A. Moss, and A. M. Schmidt, "Activation of the receptor for advanced glycation end products triggers a p21^{ras}-dependent mitogen-activated protein kinase pathway regulated by oxidant stress," *Journal of Biological Chemistry*, vol. 272, no. 28, pp. 17810–17814, 1997.

[51] K. Fukami, S. Yamagishi, M. T. Coughlan et al., "Ramipril inhibits AGE-RAGE-induced matrix metalloproteinase-2 activation in experimental diabetic nephropathy," *Diabetology and Metabolic Syndrome*, vol. 6, no. 1, p. 86, 2014.

[52] M. O. Nandan, B. B. McConnell, A. M. Ghaleb et al., "Krüppel-like factor 5 mediates cellular transformation during oncogenic KRAS-induced intestinal tumorigenesis," *Gastroenterology*, vol. 134, no. 1, pp. 120–130, 2008.

[53] S. Usui, N. Sugimoto, N. Takuwa et al., "Blood lipid mediator sphingosine 1-phosphate potently stimulates platelet-derived growth factor-A and -B chain expression through $S1P_1$-G_i-Ras-MAPK-dependent induction of Kruppel-like factor 5," *Journal of Biological Chemistry*, vol. 279, no. 13, pp. 12300–12311, 2004.

[54] N. W. Bateman, D. Tan, R. G. Pestell, J. D. Black, and A. R. Black, "Intestinal tumor progression is associated with altered function of KLF5," *Journal of Biological Chemistry*, vol. 279, no. 13, pp. 12093–12101, 2004.

[55] A. Pagliuca, C. Valvo, E. Fabrizi et al., "Analysis of the combined action of miR-143 and miR-145 on oncogenic pathways in colorectal cancer cells reveals a coordinate program of gene repression," *Oncogene*, vol. 32, no. 40, pp. 4806–4813, 2013.

[56] J. Y. Liu, J. B. Lu, and Y. Xu, "MicroRNA-153 inhibits the proliferation and invasion of human laryngeal squamous cell carcinoma by targeting KLF5," *Experimental and Therapeutic Medicine*, vol. 11, no. 6, pp. 2503–2508, 2016.

4

The Effect of Thyroid Dysfunction on the Cardiovascular Risk of Type 2 Diabetes Mellitus Patients in Ghana

Osei Sarfo-Kantanka[1] **Fred Stephen Sarfo,**[1,2] **Eunice Oparebea Ansah,**[1] **and Ishmael Kyei**[1]

[1]*Komfo Anokye Teaching Hospital, Kumasi, Ghana*
[2]*Kwame Nkrumah University of Science and Technology, Kumasi, Ghana*

Correspondence should be addressed to Osei Sarfo-Kantanka; osarfokantanka21@gmail.com

Academic Editor: Eusebio Chiefari

Background. Thyroid dysfunction is known to exaggerate the coronary heart disease (CHD) risk associated with type 2 diabetes mellitus (T2DM) among whites. The effect is yet to be studied among African populations. *Methods.* This is a cross-sectional study involving 780 T2DM patients enrolled in a diabetes clinic in Kumasi, Ghana. CHD risk was estimated using the Framingham and UKPDS risk scores. Risks were categorised as low (<10%), intermediate (10–19%), and high (≥20%). Associations between metabolic risk factors, thyroid dysfunction, and CHD risk were measured using Spearman's partial correlation analysis while controlling for age and gender. Differences were considered statistically significant at $p < 0.05$. *Results.* 780 T2DM patients (57.7% females), mean ± SD age of 57.4 ± 9.4 was analysed. The median (IQR) 10-year CHD score estimated using the Framingham and UKPDS risk engines for males and females was 12 (8–20), 9.4 (5.7–13.4), $p < 0.0001$ and 3 (1–6), 5.8 (3.4–9.6), $p < 0.0001$, respectively. Positive correlation was found between CHD risk and HbA1c, total cholesterol, low-density lipoprotein cholesterol, systolic blood pressure, and thyroid stimulating hormone. *Conclusion.* The presence of thyroid dysfunction significantly increased the CHD risk associated with T2DM patients in Ghana.

1. Introduction

There has been a remarkable surge in the worldwide prevalence of type 2 diabetes mellitus (T2DM) over the past two decades. Per estimates by the International Diabetes Federation (IDF), at least 415 million people worldwide had diabetes mellitus in 2015 [1]. Countries in sub-Saharan Africa (SSA) will suffer significantly, with a projection of over 30 million cases expected to be recorded over the next three decades [2]. Ghana, like in most SSA countries, has been affected by profound escalations in the rates of all traditional vascular risk factors including diabetes, hypertension, dyslipidemia, and obesity [3]. Currently, an estimated 6% of Ghanaian urban population has been affected by diabetes [4].

Patients with diabetes compared to nondiabetic individuals bear up to six-fold higher risk of future coronary heart disease (CHD), equivalent to nondiabetic patients with preexisting cardiovascular disease [5–8]. Part of this excess risk found in diabetes patients is attributed to a higher prevalence of other cardiovascular disease (CVD) risk factors such as obesity, dyslipidemia, and hypertension.

Thyroid conditions represent the second commonest endocrine disorder seen in adults [9]. The coexistence of both T2DM and thyroid diseases can further increase the CHD risk associated with T2DM [10]. Like T2DM, thyroid disorders can have deleterious effects on the cardiovascular system; thyrotoxicosis leads to a hyperdynamic state with increased heart rate, left ventricular contractility, and systolic hypertension and may also be complicated by atrial fibrillation [11, 12]. Hypothyroidism, on the other hand, can enhance CHD risk through multiple interactions with indices like dyslipidemia and hypertension [13–16]. Identifying the CHD risk in T2DM patients with thyroid dysfunction will be beneficial in the end since evidence points to patients benefiting from aggressive strategies in CVD risk reduction [17].

Despite a well-known association of thyroid dysfunction with T2DM, no known studies have been conducted in sub-Saharan Africa to investigate the effect of such relationship on CHD risk of T2DM patients. Our objective in this study was to identify the effect of thyroid dysfunction on the CHD risk of Ghanaian T2DM patients attending an outpatient diabetes clinic using the well-validated Framingham risk [18] and the United Kingdom Prospective Diabetes Study Scores (UKPDS) [19].

2. Methods

2.1. Study Design and Setting. This study is a hospital-based cross-sectional study conducted at the Diabetes Clinic of the Komfo Anokye Teaching Hospital, a tertiary referral medical center in Kumasi, Ghana. Kumasi is the second largest city in Ghana, with an estimated population of 4 million inhabitants. The Diabetes Clinic was established in 1992 and runs throughout the working week receiving referrals for adults > 16 years with diabetes disorders from 6 out of the 10 administrative regions of Ghana with an estimated population of 10 million.

2.2. Study Participants. Consecutive T2DM patients attending the Diabetes Clinic at KATH were approached for enrollment into the study after obtaining informed consent. Patients were diagnosed with T2DM when they fulfilled the World Health Organization (WHO) diagnostic criteria for diabetes: an elevated fasting plasma glucose level (≥7 mmol/L) on two occasions, or oral glucose tolerance test ≥ 11.1 mmol/L [20], and age 30 years or older at the time of diagnosis, had not undergone insulin therapy for a year after diagnosis, and had no history of diabetic ketoacidosis. Using a structured validated questionnaire and a review of medical records, we obtained the sociodemographic and clinical information of all participants. Because of their confounding effects on thyroid function, we excluded pregnant women, patients on amiodarone, lithium, and long-term corticosteroids, and those with an acute illness and history of hospitalisation less than six months from the day of recruitment.

2.3. Consent and Ethical Approval. We obtained ethical approval from the Committee on Human Research Publication and Ethics (CHRPE) of the School of Medical Sciences, Kwame Nkrumah University of Science and Technology, and the Komfo Anokye Teaching Hospital (KATH), Kumasi, Ghana. All participants gave an informed consent with those unable to understand or sign the consent forms excluded.

2.4. Study Measurements. Patients were interviewed using a well-validated questionnaire to obtain information such as age, gender, smoking, and alcohol consumption habits. Current smoking status and alcohol intake status were ascertained from either the patient or a responsible relative. Smokers were identified by self-report as those who had smoked at least 10 sticks of cigarettes per day for six months or more or those who smoked daily for one year or more regardless of the number of cigarettes smoked per day [21]. A high alcohol intake was defined as ≥14 U per week for women and ≥21 U per week for men [22].

2.5. Physical Measurements. The weight of study subjects was measured in kilograms using a scale, and the height in centimeters using a Stadiometer with the patient standing at the anatomical position. The weight and height measurements were used to calculate the BMI. Subjects with BMI ≥ 30 kg/m^2 were classified as obese [23].

Duplicate waist circumference (WC) measurements were taken, and the average was recorded using a plastic stretch-resistant anthropometric tape calibrated in centimeters and inches (made in Shanghai, China). The measurements were taken from the approximate midpoint between the lower margin of the last palpable rib and the superior border of the iliac crest at the level of the umbilicus in the midaxillary line with the participant erect and abdomen relaxed, arms by the side and heels together, and breathing normally. WC measurements > 80 cm and 94 cm were recorded as central obesity for females and males, respectively [23].

Blood pressure was measured thrice on the upper left arm using a validated automatic sphygmomanometer after at least 5 minutes of rest and the second and third readings averaged for analysis. Hypertension was diagnosed if the patient was on antihypertensive medications or if the patient had a systolic and diastolic blood pressure of 140/90 mmHg [24].

2.6. Laboratory Measurements of Biochemical Variables. Approximately ten milliliters (10 mL) of fasting venous samples was collected from each participant into Vacutainer tubes (Becton Dickinson, Rutherford, NJ) and Sequestrene bottles. Samples were manually processed and cryopreserved before transporting to the laboratory for analysis. Fasting plasma glucose (FPG), free thyroxine (FT4), free triiodothyronine (FT3), thyroid stimulating hormone (TSH), total cholesterol (TC), low-density lipoprotein cholesterol (LDL-C), high-density lipoprotein cholesterol (HDL-C), triglycerides (TG), urea, and creatinine levels were analysed on the serum obtained from each participant using a Cobras e 411 autoanalyzer® per manufacturer's instructions and previously described by Sarfo-Kantanka et al. [25].

Dyslipidemia was defined as a high TC, >5 mmol/L or LDL-cholesterol > 4 mmol/L, triglycerides > 1.7 mmol/L, or HDL-cholesterol < 1.30 mmol/L for women and <1.04 mmol/L for men or previous use of statin for dyslipidemia [26].

The reference ranges, intra-assay, and interassay coefficients of variation for thyroid hormones were as follows: TSH: 0.25–5.0 IU/mL, <2.1% and <2.4%; FT3: 3.7–10.4 pmol/L, 5.8% and 6.9% for FT3; and FT4: 7.5–21.1 pmol/L, 2.8% and 2.4%.

Thyroid function was classified as euthyroidism when free thyroxine (FT4), free triiodothyronine (FT3), and thyroid stimulating hormone (TSH) were within the normal range; clinical hypothyroidism when TSH level was greater than the upper limit of the reference range and FT4 or FT3 was lower than the lower limit of their reference ranges; subclinical hypothyroidism when TSH is greater than the upper limit of the reference range and FT4 and FT3 are within the normal range; clinical hyperthyroidism when TSH level was lower than the lower limit of the reference range and FT4 or FT3 was greater than the upper limit of their reference ranges; and subclinical hyperthyroidism when TSH level was lower than the lower limit of the reference range and FT3 and FT4 are within the normal range.

Glycated hemoglobin (HbA1c) measurements were performed using standardized high-performance liquid chromatography assay using Bio-Rad Variant. We followed the methodology described by Darko et al. [27].

2.7. Cardiovascular Risk Estimation. The Framingham risk engine and UKPDS questionnaire were administered to all eligible subjects and used to calculate the 10-year CHD risk of each participant. The Framingham risk questionnaire is a gender- and LDL-C-specific questionnaire and incorporates risk factors including age, sex, TC, HDL-C, SBP, DBP, smoking status, and presence of diabetes. UKPDS is an offline diabetes-specific risk engine used to estimate the 10-year CHD risk of an individual. The model is diabetes-specific and incorporates HbA1c, SBP, and lipid levels as risk factors, in addition to age, sex, ethnic group, smoking status, and time since diagnosis of diabetes. For the UKPDS risk estimation, participants were treated as African Caribbean. Estimated CHD risks were then categorised as low (<10%), intermediate (10–20%), and high (>20%).

2.8. Statistics. Data was entered into Microsoft Excel, and statistical analysis was performed using GraphPad Prism 5 software. Data normality was tested using D'Agostino and Pearson omnibus normality test. The statistical difference between means and medians was estimated by the Student t-tests and Mann-Whitney U test. Associations were measured by coefficients of Spearman's partial correlation whiles controlling for age and gender. Differences were considered statistically significant at $p < 0.05$.

3. Results

3.1. Demographic and Clinical Characteristics. 958 participants were approached, but 178 declined participation in the study. As shown in Table 1, 780 T2DM subjects, mean age 57.4 ± 9.4, were included in the analyses. Of these, 450 (57.7%) subjects were female. The median (IQR) age at diagnosis of participants was 50 (41–54), and the mean duration of T2DM was 9.8 ± 5.6 years. The predominant vascular risk factors identified included hypertension (77.9%), central obesity (74.6%), dyslipidemia (59.2%), and abnormal glycemic control, HbA1c > 7% (66.2%). Females had a significantly higher prevalence of central obesity, high BMI, and DBP. The median (IQR) 10-year CHD score estimated using the Framingham and UKPDS risk engines for males and females was 12 (8–20), 9.4 (5.7–13.4), $p < 0.0001$ and 3 (1–6), 5.8 (3.4–9.6), $p < 0.0001$, respectively. The median (IQR) CHD risk score estimated using the UKPDS engine was 4 (0.4–7): 9.4 (5.7–13.4) for males and 5.8 (3.4–9.6), $p < 0.0001$, for females.

3.2. CHD Score Based on Thyroid Status. Table 2 shows the median (IQR) Framingham risk score of T2DM patients with thyroid dysfunction significantly higher than for euthyroid T2DM patients: 11 (6–22) versus 4 (1–10), $p < 0.0001$. 8% of euthyroid T2DM subjects were identified as having high CHD risk using the Framingham risk score, 24% had intermediate risk, and 68% had low risk. Among those with thyroid dysfunction, 43% were identified as high risk, 28% as medium risk, and 25% as low risk. Of those identified with subclinical hyperthyroidism, 32% had high risk of CHD, 23% had an intermediate risk, and 44% had low risk. Of those with hyperthyroidism, 36% had high risk, 42% intermediate risk, and 22% low risk of CHD (Figure 1). In patients with subclinical hypothyroidism, 48% were classified as high risk, 29% as intermediate risk, and 23% as low risk; with hypothyroidism, 55% had high risk, 31% intermediate risk, and 14% low risk. The difference between the groups was highly significant ($p < 0.0001$). Using the UKPDS score, 4% of euthyroid T2DM subjects were identified as high risk, 44% as intermediate risk, and 52% as low risk. Among those with thyroid dysfunction, 26% were classified as high risk of CHD, 58% as intermediate risk, and 16% as low risk.

3.3. Correlates of Increased Cardiovascular Risk. As shown in Table 2, the demographic characteristics, vascular risk factor profile, and clinical features of T2DM subjects classified as having high CHD risk using the Framingham risk score were older, had female gender predisposition, older age at diagnosis, obese (general and central), had poorer glycemic control and lipid profiles, higher blood pressures, and higher rates of alcohol abuse compared to those with intermediate or low CHD risks.

3.3.1. Association between Biochemical and Physical Characteristics and Coronary Heart Disease Risk in T2DM Patients. A strong positive correlation was found between high Framingham CHD risk and HbA1c ($r = 0.51, p < 0.04$), TC ($r = 0.49, p < 0.0001$), LDL-C ($r = 0.37, p < 0.0001$), and TSH ($r = 0.27, p = 0.01$). Under the UKPDS scoring, a strong association was found between CHD risk and HbA1c ($r = 0.42, p < 0.0001$) and TSH ($r = 0.32, p < 0.02$) (Table 3).

4. Discussion

We have found in this study that T2DM subjects in Ghana possess high prevalence levels of modifiable vascular risk factors: 74.5% had central obesity, 77.9% had hypertension, and 59.2% had dyslipidemia. In addition, 30.0% abused alcohol and 7.4% smoked cigarette. In general terms, glycemic control was poorer among male T2DM subjects showing poorer controls compared to females. Females had higher prevalence of some important vascular risk factors. This is explained by the fact that female T2DM patients especially those who are menopausal have worse CVD risk factor profiles and mortalities compared to their male counterparts [28, 29]. This was illustrated by a meta-analysis of 37

TABLE 1: Demographic and clinical characteristics of 780 T2DM participants enrolled for the study.

Test parameters	Total	Male	Female	p value
Number (%)	780 (100)	330 (42.3)	450 (57.7)	
Age, mean ± SD	57.4 ± 9.4	57.8 ± 9.5	57.3 ± 9.3	0.65
Age at diagnosis, median (IQR)	50 (43–56)	51 (43–60)	50 (43–78)	0.08
Duration of diabetes, mean ± SD	9.8 ± 5.6	9.9 ± 3.2	9.6 ± 8.9	0.09
Body mass index (kg/m), median (IQR)	27.5 (24.8–30.9)	27.0 (24–30.3)	27.9 (25.1–31.5)	0.04*
General obesity (%)	262 (33.6)	92 (27.9)	170 (37.8)	0.04*
Waist circumference, cm, median (IQR)	97 (87–105)	94 (84–101)	98 (90–106)	<0.001*
Central obesity, n (%)	582 (74.6)	156 (47.3)	426 (94.7)	<0.001*
Fasting blood glucose, median (IQR)	8.8 (6.7–12.6)	8.6 (6 .7–12.2)	9.1 (6.8–13.5)	0.4
Hba1c (%), median (IQR)	8.1 (6.8–9.6)	8.1 (6.6–9.8)	8.1 (6.9–9.6)	0.92
Abnormal glycemic control (>7%)	716 (66.2)	220 (66.7)	286 (63.6)	0.85
Total cholesterol mmol/L, median (IQR)	5.0 (4.1–6.0)	5 (4.2–5.9)	5 (4–6.1)	0.63
Hypercholesterolemia, n (%)	400 (51.3)	164 (49.7)	236 (52.4)	0.15
Triglycerides (mmol/L), median (IQR)	1.2 (0.9–1.6)	1.16 (0.85–1.6)	1.24 (0.94–1.57)	0.22
Hypertriglyceridemia, n (%)	170 (21.8)	66 (20.0)	104 (23.1)	0.44
LDL-C, median (IQR)	3.2 (2.1–3.9)	3.1 (2.2–3.8)	3.2 (2 .1–4.0)	0.92
High LDL, n (%)	470 (60.3)	186 (56.4)	284 (63.1)	0.18
HDL-C, median (IQR)	1.2 (1–1.5)	1.1 (1–1.4)	1.2 (1.0–1.5)	0.2
Low HDL-C, n (%)	54 (6.9)	32 (9.6)	22 (4.9)	0.007*
Dyslipidemia, n (%)	462 (59.2)	196 (59.4)	266 (59.1)	0.12
Systolic blood pressure, median (IQR)	140 (130–150)	140 (129–150)	140 (130–150)	0.43
Diastolic blood pressure, median (IQR)	80 (70–90)	80 (70–90)	80 (80–90)	0.01*
Hypertension, n (%)	602 (77.9)	272 (82.4)	330 (73.3)	0.03*
Alcohol, n (%)	234 (30.0)	200 (60.6)	34 (7.6)	<0.001*
Current smokers, n (%)	58 (7.4)	56 (17.0)	2 (0.4)	<0.001*
Framingham CHD risk, %, median (IQR)	6 (2–12)	12 (8–20)	3 (1–6)	<0.001*
UKPDS CHD risk score, median (IQR)	4 (0.4–7)	9.4(5.7–13.4)	5.8 (3.4–9.6)	<0.001*
Subclinical hypothyroidism	64 (8.2)	14 (4.2)	50 (11.1)	0.02*
Subclinical hyperthyroidism	22 (2.8)	14 (4.2)	8 (1.8)	<0.001
Hypothyroidism	12 (1.6)	2 (0.6)	10 (2.2)	0.08
Hyperthyroidism	4 (0.5)	2 (0.6)	2 (0.4)	0.21
Euthyroidism	678 (86.9)	298 (90.3)	380 (84.4)	0.02

CHD: coronary heart disease; HbA1c: glycated hemoglobin; HDL-C: high-density lipoprotein cholesterol; IQR: interquartile range; LDL-C: low-density lipoprotein cholesterol; UKPDS: United Kingdom Prospective Diabetes Study; SD: standard deviation. *$p < 0.05$ statistically significant.

prospective cohort studies where the risk of fatal CHD was 50% higher in female T2DM patients compared to males [30]. The reason for this postmenopausal T2DM female predilection towards increased CHD risk is multifactorial. Principally, it has been demonstrated that chronic hyperglycemia alters the estrogen-related protective mechanisms that leave premenopausal woman at a lower CVD risk compared to males. This leads to notable adverse changes in CVD risk factors leading to enhanced atherogenesis in females even premenopausal [31, 32]. Additionally, postmenopausal T2DM females have been shown to possess a relatively heavier risk factor burden [32] as well as a significant array and involvement of inflammatory factors [33], smaller size of coronary vessels, and disordered angiogenesis [34, 35]. The removal of the protective effect of female sex on the risk of CHD in people with diabetes warrants aggressive screening and treatment of females with this risk [36].

The proportion of patients with high CHD risk (18.7%) recorded in this present study is comparable to that found in similar studies involving African American [37] and non-Hispanic white T2DM subjects [38] who were assessed using the Framingham risk scoring. However, among Brazilian T2DM subjects where UKPDS was used in risk assessment, a significantly higher CHD risk was recorded [39]. It is unknown whether these differences observed in CHD risk prevalence are due to the different methods used

TABLE 2: Demographic and clinical characteristics of T2DM participants based on CHD risk.

Test parameters	Total	CHD risk Low	 Moderate	 High	p
Number (%)	780 (100)	424 (54.4)	210 (26.9)	146 (18.7)	
Age, mean ± SD	59.2 ± 8.6	56.6 ± 7.9	61.6 ± 8.5	62.9 ± 8.4	<0.0001*
Female gender, n (%)	450 (57.7)	326 (76.9)	124 (59.0)	52 (35.6)	<0.0001*
Age at diagnosis, mean ± SD	51.3 ± 9.0	47.4 ± 7.2	52.8 ± 7.9	54.2 ± 10.2	<0.0004*
BMI, median (IQR)	27 (24.1–30.8)	27 (24–29.5)	26.7 (23–30.9)	27 (24–30.9)	0.37
Waist circumference, median (IQR)	98 (88–108)	87.3 (95.5–105)	107 (99–114)	95 (85–109)	<0.0001*
Central obesity, n (%)	582 (74.6)	256 (60.4)	190 (90.5)	136 (93.2)	<0.0001*
Fasting glucose, median (IQR)	8.6 (6.7–13.0)	8.2 (6.7–12.9)	8.6 (6–12.5)	9.4 (7.1–14)	0.37
Hba1c (%), median (IQR)	8.2 (7–9.8)	7.9 (6.9–9.5)	8.7 (6.9–9.9)	8.4 (7.3–10)	<0.0001*
Abnormal glycemic control (>7%)	516 (66.2)	232 (54.7)	160 (76.2)	124 (84.9)	<0.001*
Total cholesterol, median (IQR)	5.3 (4.3–6.65)	5.0 (4.1–5.9)	5.7 (4.7–6.9)	6.1 (6–7.9)	<0.0001*
Hypercholesterolemia, n (%)	400 (51.3)	196 (46.2)	112 (53.3)	92 (63.0)	<0.0001*
Triglycerides, median (IQR)	0.95 (1.22–1.6)	1.2 (0.9–1.5)	1.2 (1.0–1.7)	1.4 (1.0–1.7)	0.06
LDL-C, median (IQR)	3.3 (2.3–4.2)	3.2 (2.2–3.8)	3.6 (2.6–4.4)	4.19 (3.2–5)	<0.0001*
High LDL, n (%)	470 (60.3)	216 (50.9)	136 (64.8)	118 (80.8)	<0.0001*
HDL-C, median (IQR)	1.2 (1–1.43)	1.2 (1–1.5)	1.2 (1–1.4)	1.1 (1–1.32)	0.14
Low HDL-C, n (%)	108 (13.8)	26 (6.1)	38 (18.1)	44 (30.1)	<0.0001*
Dyslipidemia, n (%)	462 (59.2)	212 (50.0)	124 (59.1)	126 (86.3)	<0.00001*
Systolic blood pressure, median (IQR)	140 (130–152)	140 (130–150)	140 (130–154)	148 (130–160)	0.14
Diastolic blood pressure, median (IQR)	80 (80–90)	80 (80–90)	80 (70–90)	80 (80–90)	0.78
Hypertension, n (%)	602 (77.9)	304 (71.7)	158 (75.2)	140 (95.9)	<0.001*
Alcohol, n (%)	234 (30.0)	108 (25.5)	62 (29.5)	64 (43.8)	<0.0001*
Current smokers, n (%)	58 (7.4)	26 (6.1)	16 (7.6)	18 (12.3)	<0.0001*

CHD: coronary heart disease; HbA1c: glycated hemoglobin; HDL-C: high-density lipoprotein cholesterol; IQR: interquartile range, LDL-C: low-density lipoprotein cholesterol; SD: standard deviation. $^*p < 0.05$ statistically significant.

for assessment and study sample sizes. A high risk of CHD was seen among Caucasians and South Americans [38, 39]. This applies particularly to men, where both morbidity and mortality from heart disease are about half that of the general population [40]. Data on African Americans from the United States conflict this finding, showing higher CHD rates than US whites [41]. This appears to be in part explained by the degree of acculturation and miscegenation, as birthplace within or outside the USA was a strong determinant of mortality risk [35]. Furthermore, African men have been shown to be less centrally obese than their Caucasian counterparts [37].

Thus, with this present study, which to the best of our knowledge is the first among West Africans, we have shown a higher CHD risk in T2DM subjects with thyroid dysfunction compared with those who were euthyroid. This we attribute to the significantly higher risk factor burden of CHD seen in T2DM subjects with thyroid dysfunction compared to their euthyroid counterparts recorded in the study. Moreover, this effect is better explained by the higher CHD risk seen among patients with hypothyroidism compared to those with other forms of thyroid dysfunction and euthyroidism. It is well known that patients with hypothyroidism possess significant incidence of inflammatory factors, hypercholesterolemia, and diastolic blood pressures compared to those with other forms of thyroid dysfunction [38].

A significantly positive linear association found in T2DM subjects between TSH and CHD risk could be attributed to the increasing association of thyroid dysfunction with high inflammatory markers, dyslipidemia, and poor glycemic control [39]. It has been postulated that high inflammatory state induced by thyroid dysfunction produces oxidative stress, insulin resistance, cell apoptosis, vascular endothelial injury, platelet activation, and neuroendocrine disorders which all promote the development of atherosclerosis [40, 41]. For this reason, it is now recognised that subclinical hypothyroidism together with hypothyroidism are risk factors for increased CHD risk and mortality in the general population as well as diabetics even after accounting for traditional vascular risk factors [42].

Some inherent limitations were associated with this study including our sample size composition. We had fewer males with T2DM relative to females which may have influenced

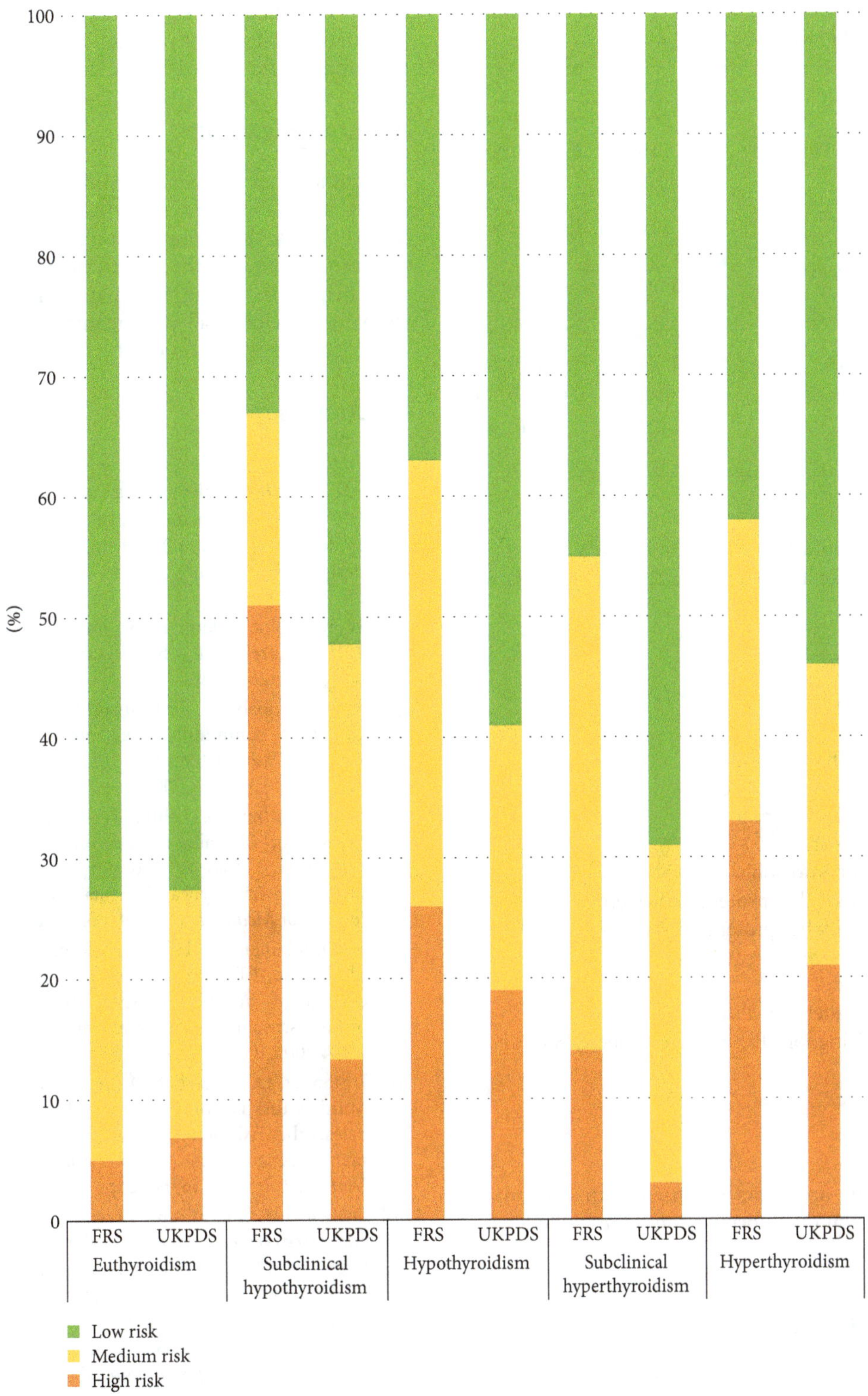

Figure 1: Variation of coronary heart disease risk per Framingham and UKPDS Scores.

the results. Moreover, confounders such as physical activity and dietary patterns were not explored in this study even though they could have influenced the CHD risk. Secondly, the cross-sectional study design means that the associations observed between thyroid dysfunction and CHD risk could not be interpreted as causal relationships.

5. Conclusion

We conclude that our T2DM patients with thyroid dysfunction compared to their euthyroid counterparts have a significantly higher CHD risk. A significant association of CHD risk has been shown with HbA1c and dyslipidemia.

Table 3: Pearson bivariate correlation between ten-year coronary heart disease risk and independent variables.

Test parameters	Framingham	UKPDS
Waist circumference	0.12 (0.061)	−0.08 (0.42)
Glycated hemoglobin, HbA1c	0.51 (0.041)	0.42 (<0.0001)
Total cholesterol	0.49 (0.0001)	0.14 (<0.51)
Low-density lipoprotein cholesterol	0.37 (<0.0001)	0.10 (0.04)
High-density lipoprotein cholesterol	0.02 (0.21)	−0.06 (0.12)
Triglycerides	0.12 (0.02)	0.11 (0.06)
Systolic blood pressure	0.12 (0.12)	0.10 (0.04)
Thyroid stimulating hormone	0.27 (0.0006)	0.32 (0.02)
Free triiodothyronine	0.07 (0.23)	0.10 (0.34)
Free thyroxine	0.11 (0.09)	0.13 (0.15)

Physicians taking care of these patients should have a high index of suspicion for thyroid dysfunction in patients with high CVD risk.

Abbreviations

CHD: Coronary heart disease
CVD: Cardiovascular disease
FT3: Free triiodothyronine
FT4: Free thyroxine
HbA1c: Glycated hemoglobin
HDL: High-density lipoprotein cholesterol
LDL-C: Low-density lipoprotein cholesterol
TC: Total cholesterol
TG: Triglycerides
T2DM: Type 2 diabetes mellitus
UKPDS: United Kingdom Prospective Diabetes Study.

Consent

All participants gave an informed consent with those unable to understand or sign the informed consent excluded.

Conflicts of Interest

There is no competing interest involving any of the authors of this study.

Authors' Contributions

Osei Sarfo-Kantanka conceived the study, participated in its design, and drafted the manuscript. Fred Stephen Sarfo contributed in the study design and helped in the manuscript preparation and statistical analysis. Eunice Oparebea Ansah contributed in conducting the field and manuscript preparation. Ishmael Kyei participated in the manuscript preparation and helped in the analysis of data.

Acknowledgments

The authors acknowledge the immense role played by the nurses and laboratory scientists at the Diabetes Clinic, KATH. The authors also appreciate the contribution of the staff at the office of the Department of Medicine, KATH, who helped in typing the manuscript. The authors are eternally grateful to all participants for participating in the study. This study was funded by Osei Sarfo-Kantanka.

References

[1] "International Diabetes Federation IDF diabetes atlas," March 2017, http://www.diabetesatlas.org/resources/2015-atlas.htlm.

[2] L. Chen, D. J. Magliano, and P. Z. Zimmet, "The worldwide epidemiology of type 2 diabetes mellitus–present and future perspectives," *Nature Reviews Endocrinology*, vol. 8, no. 4, pp. 228–236, 2012.

[3] WHO, "Global status report on non-communicable diseases 2010," March 2017, http://www.who.int/nmh/publications/ncd_report2010/en/.

[4] A. G. Amoah, S. K. Owusu, and S. Adjei, "Diabetes in Ghana: a community-based prevalence study in Greater Accra," *Diabetes Research and Clinical Practice*, vol. 56, no. 3, pp. 197–205, 2002.

[5] S. M. Haffner, S. Lehto, T. Ronnemaa, K. Pyörälä, and M. Laakso, "Mortality from coronary heart disease in subjects with type 2 diabetes and non-diabetic subjects with and without prior myocardial infarction," *The New England Journal of Medicine*, vol. 339, no. 4, pp. 229–234, 1998.

[6] A. Juutilainen, S. Lehto, T. Rönnemaa, K. Pyörälä, and M. Laakso, "Type 2 diabetes as a "coronary heart disease equivalent": an 18-year prospective population-based study in Finnish subjects," *Diabetes Care*, vol. 28, no. 12, pp. 2901–2907, 2005.

[7] J. Stamler, O. Vaccaro, J. D. Neaton, D. Wentworth, and The Multiple Risk Factor Intervention Trial Research Group, "Diabetes, other risk factors, and 12-yr cardiovascular mortality for men screened in the multiple risk factor intervention trial," *Diabetes Care*, vol. 16, no. 2, pp. 434–444, 1993.

[8] Diabetes drafting group, "Prevalence of small vessel disease and large vessel disease in diabetic patients from 14 centers. The World Health Organization Multinational Study of Vascular Disease in diabetics," *Diabetologia*, vol. 28, Supplement 1, pp. 615–640, 1985.

[9] R. Sathish and V. Mohan, "Diabetes and thyroid diseases-a review," *International Journal of Diabetes in Developing Countries*, vol. 23, no. 4, pp. 120–123, 2003.

[10] S. Danzi and I. Klein, "Thyroid hormone and blood pressure regulation," *Current Hypertension Reports*, vol. 5, no. 6, pp. 513–520, 2003.

[11] E. A. Palmieri, S. Fazio, G. Lombardi, and B. Biondi, "Subclinical hypothyroidism and cardiovascular risk: a reason to treat?," *Treatments in Endocrinology*, vol. 3, no. 4, pp. 233–244, 2004.

[12] S. A. Chubb, W. A. Davis, and Z. Inman, "Prevalence and progression of subclinical hypothyroidism in women with

type 2 diabetes: the Fremantle diabetes study," *Clinical Endocrinology*, vol. 62, no. 4, pp. 480–486, 2005.

[13] P. Haentjens, A. Van Meerhaeghe, K. Poppe, and B. Velkeniers, "Subclinical thyroid dysfunction and mortality: an estimate of relative and absolute excess all-cause mortality based on time-to-event data from cohort studies," *European Journal of Endocrinology*, vol. 159, no. 3, pp. 329–341, 2008.

[14] T. Sathyapalan, A. M. Manuchehri, A. S. Rigby, and S. L. Atkin, "Subclinical hypothyroidism is associated with reduced all-cause mortality in patients with type 2 diabetes," *Diabetes Care*, vol. 33, no. 3, article e37, 2010.

[15] N. Ochs, R. Auer, D. C. Bauer et al., "Meta-analysis: subclinical thyroid dysfunction and the risk of coronary heart disease and mortality," *Annals of Internal Medicine*, vol. 148, no. 11, pp. 832–845, 2008.

[16] S. Razvi, A. Shakoor, M. Vanderpump, J. U. Weaver, and S. H. S. Pearce, "The influence of age on the relationship between subclinical hypothyroidism and ischemic heart disease: a metaanalysis," *The Journal of Clinical Endocrinology & Metabolism*, vol. 93, no. 8, pp. 2998–3007, 2008.

[17] F. J. del Canizo-Gomez and M. N. Moreira-Andres, "Stick control of modifiable risk factors for type 2 diabetes," *The New England Journal of Medicine*, vol. 348, no. 5, pp. 383–393, 2003.

[18] R. B. D'Agostino Sr., R. S. Vasan, M. J. Pencina et al., "General cardiovascular risk profile for use in primary care: the Framingham heart study," *Circulation*, vol. 117, no. 6, pp. 743–753, 2008.

[19] The University of Oxford, Diabetes trial unit, "The Oxford Centre for Diabetes, Endocrinology and Metabolism, UKPDS risk engine," February 2017, http://www.dtu.ox.ac.uk/riskengine/download.php.

[20] WHO/NCD/NCS/99.2, *WHO Consultation. Definition, Diagnosis and Classification of Diabetes Mellitus and Its Complications: Report of a WHO Consultation Part 1: Diagnosis and Classification of Diabetes Mellitus*, World Health Organization, Geneva, 1999, Publication no. WHO/NCD/NCS/99.2.

[21] S. G. Wannamethee, A. G. Shaper, and I. J. Perry, "British regional heart study: smoking as a modifiable risk factor for type 2 diabetes in middle-aged men," *Diabetes Care*, vol. 204, no. 9, pp. 1590–1595, 2001.

[22] A. G. Shaper, G. Wanathee, and M. Walker, "Alcohol and mortality in British: explaining the U shaped curve," *The Lancet*, vol. 332, no. 8623, pp. 1267–1273, 1988.

[23] World Health Organisation, *Obesity: Prevention and Managing the Global Epidemic. Report of a WHO Consultation*, WHO Technical Report Series 894, Geneva, 2000, http://www.who.int/nutrition/publications/obesity/WHO_TRS_894/en/.

[24] J. Chalmers, S. McMahon, G. Mancia et al., "1999 World Health Organisation-International Society of Hypertension Guidelines for treatment of hypertension," *Clinical and Experimental Hypertension*, vol. 21, no. 5-6, pp. 1009–1060, 1999.

[25] O. Sarfo-Kantanka, F. S. Sarfo, E. O. Ansah et al., "Frequency and determinants of thyroid autoimmunity in Ghanaian type 2 diabetes patients: a case-control study," *BMC Endocrine Disorders*, vol. 17, no. 1, p. 2, 2017.

[26] P. W. Wilson, R. B. D'Agostino, D. Levy, A. M. Belanger, H. Silbershatz, and W. B. Kannel, "Prediction of coronary heart disease using risk factor categories," *Circulation*, vol. 97, no. 18, pp. 1837–1847, 1998.

[27] S. N. Darko, D. D. Yar, E. Owusu-Dabo et al., "Variations in levels of IL-6 and TNF-α in type 2 diabetes mellitus between rural and urban Ashanti Region of Ghana," *BMC Endocrine Disorders*, vol. 15, no. 1, p. 50, 2015.

[28] G. Hu, P. Jousilahti, Q. Qiao, S. Katoh, and J. Tuomilehto, "Sex differences in cardiovascular and total mortality among diabetic and non-diabetic individuals with or without a history of myocardial infarction," *Diabetologia*, vol. 48, no. 5, pp. 856–861, 2005.

[29] W. L. Lee, A. M. Cheung, D. Cape, and B. Zinman, "Impact of diabetes on coronary artery disease in women and men: a meta-analysis of prospective studies," *Diabetes Care*, vol. 23, no. 7, pp. 962–968, 2000.

[30] R. Huxley, F. Barzi, and M. Woodward, "Excess risk of coronary heart diseases associated with diabetes in men and women: meta-analysis of 37 prospective cohort studies," *BMJ*, vol. 332, no. 7533, pp. 73–78, 2006.

[31] I. Martin-Timon, C. Sevillano- Collantes, A. Sejura-Galindo, and F. J. Del Cañizo-Gómez, "Type 2 diabetes and cardiovascular disease: have all the risk factors the same strength?," *World Journal of Diabetes*, vol. 5, no. 4, pp. 444–470, 2014.

[32] H. O. Steinberg, G. Paradisi, J. Cronin et al., "Type II diabetes abrogates sex differences in endothelial function in premenopausal women," *Circulation*, vol. 101, no. 17, pp. 2040–2046, 2000.

[33] A. M. Kanaya, D. Grady, and E. Barrett-Connor, "Explaining the sex difference in coronary heart disease mortality among patients with type 2 diabetes mellitus: a meta-analysis," *Archives of Internal Medicine*, vol. 162, no. 15, pp. 1737–1745, 2002.

[34] A. A. Rivellese, G. Riccardi, and O. Vaccaro, "Cardiovascular risk in women with diabetes," *Nutrition, Metabolism & Cardiovascular Diseases*, vol. 20, no. 6, pp. 474–480, 2010.

[35] C. S. Fox, "Cardiovascular disease risk factors, type 2 diabetes mellitus and the Framingham free heart study," *Trends in Cardiovascular Medicine*, vol. 20, no. 3, pp. 90–95, 2010.

[36] A. R. Cappola, L. P. Fried, A. M. Arnold et al., "Thyroid status, cardiovascular risk, and mortality in older adults," *JAMA*, vol. 295, no. 9, pp. 1033–1041, 2006.

[37] A. Adeniye, A. R. Folson, F. Z. Brancati, M. Desvorieux, J. S. Pankow, and H. Taylor, "Incidence and risk factors of African American with diabetes: atherosclerosis risk in communities (ARIC) study," *Journal of the National Medical Association*, vol. 94, no. 12, pp. 1025–1035, 2002.

[38] G. Iervasi, S. Molinaro, P. Landi et al., "Association between increased mortality and mild thyroid dysfunction in cardiac patients," *Archives of Internal Medicine*, vol. 167, no. 14, pp. 1526–1532, 2007.

[39] M. B. Gomes, D. Giannella-Neto, M. Faria et al., "Estimating cardiovascular risk in patients with type 2 diabetes: a national multicenter study in Brazil," *Diabetology & Metabolic Syndrome*, vol. 1, no. 1, p. 22, 2009.

[40] M. Laakso, "Cardiovascular disease in type 2 diabetes from population to man to mechanisms," *Diabetes Care*, vol. 33, no. 2, pp. 442–449, 2010.

[41] S. Y. Gebreab and A. V. Diez Roux, "Exploring racial disparities in CHD mortality between blacks and whites across the United States: a geographically weighted regression approach," *Health & Place*, vol. 18, no. 5, pp. 1006–1014, 2012.

[42] I. L. G. Todorova, K. L. Tucker, M. P. Jimenez, A. K. Lincoln, S. Arevalo, and L. M. Falcón, "Determinants of self-rated health and the role of acculturation: implications for health inequalities," *Ethnicity & Health*, vol. 18, no. 6, pp. 563–585, 2013.

5

Association of Wrist Circumference and Waist-to-Height Ratio with Cardiometabolic Risk Factors among Type II Diabetics in a Ghanaian Population

Christian Obirikorang,[1] Yaa Obirikorang,[2] Emmanuel Acheampong,[1] Enoch Odame Anto,[1,3] Emmanuel Toboh,[4] Evans Adu Asamoah,[5] Bright Amakwaa,[1] Emmanuella Nsenbah Batu,[1] and Peter Brenya[1]

[1]*Department of Molecular Medicine, School of Medical Sciences, Kwame Nkrumah University of Science and Technology (KNUST), Kumasi, Ghana*
[2]*Department of Nursing, Faculty of Health and Allied Sciences, Garden City University College (GCUC), Kenyasi, Kumasi, Ghana*
[3]*School of Medical and Health Sciences, Edith Cowan University, Joondalup, WA, Australia*
[4]*Diagnostic Unit, Dansoman Polyclinic, Ghana Health Service, Accra, Ghana*
[5]*Department of Medical Laboratory Technology, Faculty of Allied Health Sciences, KNUST, Kumasi, Ghana*

Correspondence should be addressed to Emmanuel Acheampong; emmanuelachea1990@yahoo.com

Academic Editor: Rajesh Vedanthan

The study determined the association of wrist circumference (WrC) and waist-to-height ratio (WHtR) with cardiometabolic risk factors among diabetics in a Ghanaian population. This cross-sectional study involved 384 diabetic patients at Begoro District Hospital, Ghana. Blood pressure, anthropometrics, and biochemical indices were measured. The overall prevalence of dyslipidaemia, metabolic syndrome (MetS), and hypertension was 42.4%, 76.3%, and 39.8%, respectively. The optimum cut-off range of WrC to identify individuals at increased cardiometabolic risk was 17.5 to –17.8 cm for men and 16.0 to 16.7 cm for women while that of WHtR was 0.52 to 0.61 for men and 0.53 to 0.59 for women. WrC for women was a significant independent predictor for MetS [aOR = 3.0 (1.39–6.72), $p = 0.005$] and systolic blood pressure [aOR = 2.08 (1.17–3.68), $p = 0.012$]. WHtR was a significant positive predictor for triglycerides [aOR = 3.23 (0.10–3.82), $p = 0.001$] for women. Using Framingham risk scores, 61% of the subjects had elevated 10-year risk of developing cardiovascular diseases (CVDs), with no significant difference in gender prevalence. WrC [aOR = 6.13 (0.34–111.4), $p = 0.107$] and WHtR [aOR = 2.52 (0.42–15.02), $p = 0.309$] were associated with statistically insignificant increased odds of moderate-to-high risk of developing CVDs in 10 years. The use of gender-specific cut-offs for WrC and WHtR may offer putative markers for early identification of CRFs.

1. Introduction

Diabetes mellitus (DM) is one of the major public health problems worldwide, not only due to the increasing number of affected people, but also according to its relation with disability and premature mortality and not neglecting the costs involved in its treatment and prevention [1, 2]. Africa alone accounted for 14 million diagnosed cases of diabetes; as at 2015, Ghana recorded 266,200 cases with a prevalence rate of 1.9% in adults (20–79 years). About 4790 deaths recorded in the same year aside the many undiagnosed cases in Africa, type II diabetes mellitus (T2DM) accounted for 90–95% of all diagnosed cases [3, 4]. The relationship between obesity and diabetes has been well documented in the Ghanaian population [5, 6]. A study among urban and rural settlers in a Ghanaian population found an increased cardiometabolic risk factors among urban settlers due to their increased sedentary and unhealthy dietary habits [7]. In sub-Saharan Africa, hypertension followed by obesity was the commonly known cardiometabolic risk factors associated with the general adult population [8]. Obesity and overweight are associated with an increased cardiometabolic risk; however, this may vary significantly by age, dietary habits, gender, and even among participants with morbid obesity [9]. However, the argument about the most effective anthropometric index associated with cardiometabolic risk factors among diabetics remains unresolved. Cardiovascular disease (CVD) risk factors such as obesity, hypertension, and dyslipidaemia are common in patients with DM, placing them at increased risk for cardiac events [10, 11]. In addition, many studies have found biological mechanisms associated with DM that independently increase the risk of CVD in diabetic patients [10–12]. Body mass index (BMI) being the most studied anthropometric index has been reported to be significantly related to CVD risk factors as demonstrated by several prospective and cross-sectional studies [13–15]. However, there are cumulative doubts about its role in predicting CVD risk factors. This has led to an increasing evidence for abdominal obesity indices such as waist circumference (WC), waist-to-hip ratio (WHR), and waist-to-height ratio (WHtR) as predictors of CVD [16, 17]. In a study among South African blacks, WHtR was found as a significant predictor for all cardiometabolic risk components after 5 years in an adult population [18]. The application of WHtR provides an alternative anthropometric index of central obesity that avoids the limitations of WC because the inclusion of height into the index enhances the avoidance of any potential confounding of cardiometabolic risk by height [19]. Previous studies have found similar WHtR cut-offs for increased cardiometabolic risk among Caucasian and Asian populations as well as men and women [20]. WrC is a simple anthropometric tool for the measurement of skeletal frame size. It has recently been suggested in several studies to be associated with insulin resistance in obese children and adults [21, 22], its consideration as a measurement of peripheral fat distribution has attracted much attention [23]. Moreover, it is an easy tool to detect measures of skeletal frame size without being severely confounded by body fat variation [22].

Various other anthropometric indexes such as WC, hip circumference (HC), and WHR have been used to determine the index more closely related to cardiometabolic risk factors among diabetics. To our knowledge, no study has been done to determine the association of WrC and WHtR with cardiometabolic risk factors among diabetics in a Ghanaian population. In contrast to the routine management requirement, individual risk stratification is highly recommended, and there is the need to elucidate proper anthropometric measurement that defines individuals who are at risk of cardiometabolic complications. To fill this gap, the present study sought to determine the association between WrC and WHtR with cardiometabolic risk factors and ascertain WrC and WHtR predictive values for cardiovascular risk burden using FS10 lipid risk score system.

2. Methodology

2.1. Study Design and Setting. This was a cross-sectional study conducted among diabetic patients attending Begoro District Hospital diabetic clinic on a weekly basis. The diabetic clinic at Begoro District Hospital is the only hospital in Fanteakwa North District in the Eastern Region of Ghana that runs a diabetic clinic. Moreover, it is located in Begoro and records attendance of 110,134 people per annum from over 157 communities within the district. It also serves as the main referral facility for Community Health-based Planning Service (CHPS, i.e., a community health officer-led program widely implemented across Ghana, notable for its impact on under-5 and maternal mortality [24]) centers, Clinics and Health centers in the Fanteakwa District, and the adjoining districts. Therefore, sampling was without bias but with fair distribution covering the ethnic groups, the majority being Akans and Ga-dangmes within the district.

2.2. Study Population and Subject Selection. Using a nonprobability convenience sampling, a total of 384 diabetics were recruited for the study. Selection of subject was done using a structured questionnaire. Trained nurses were placed at the Out-Patient Department (OPD) to administer the questionnaires regarding lifestyle (including smoking and drinking), medical history (including past illness history and medication history), physiological conditions (including pregnancy and fasting time), and sociodemographics, to all subjects during their health check-up. The researcher verified the completion of each questionnaire prior to collection. Subjects with incomplete data as well as those who were pregnant or had a chronic disease that may affect the metabolic status or body composition (e.g., thyroid or hypothalamic disease, chronic hepatitis, and cirrhosis) were excluded from the study. The sample used for the current analysis consisted of 147 men and 237 women. The protocol for the selection of subject is shown in Figure 1.

2.3. Inclusion and Exclusion Criteria. All diabetic individuals with complete data on sociodemographic and lifestyle characteristics without any chronic disease reviewed from their medical history were included in the study.

2.4. Sample Size Determination. A total of 384 diabetics were recruited from an estimated diabetic population of 1870, using a proportionate rate of 20.5%, confidence level of 95% (*z*-score 1.96), and margin of error of 5%. Using Cochran's formula [25], the minimum size required was 300; however, to accommodate a nonresponse rate of 10.0% and stronger statistical power and effect size, the samples were projected to 384 students.

2.5. Blood Pressure Measurement. Blood pressure (BP) was recorded after 5 minutes of rest with the subject being in the seated position using manual and an automated

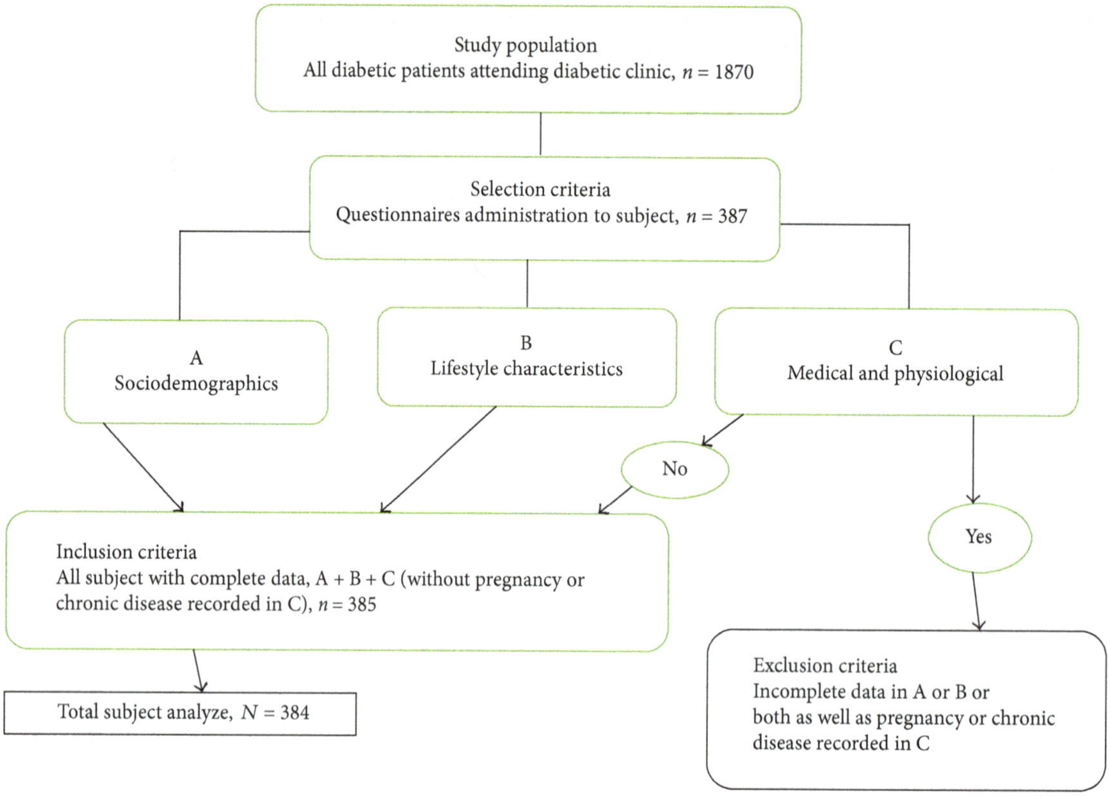

Figure 1: Flowchart of the protocol for the selection of subject.

sphygmomanometer placed on the subject's right arm. This was measured three times, and the average reading was recorded. Individuals were deemed hypertensive if they were taking antihypertensive medications, if they self-reported a diagnosis of hypertension, if their systolic pressure was above 140 mmHg, if their diastolic pressure was above 90 mmHg, or a combination of these features.

2.6. Anthropometric Measurements. Body weight, expressed in 0.1 kg intervals, was measured at fasting state in the morning using automated scale. Portable height rod stadiometers were used for body height to the nearest centimeters. The subject stood straight, with feet placed together and flat on the ground, heels, buttocks, and scapulae against the vertical backboard, and arms loose and relaxed with the palms facing medially. Their heads were carefully positioned in the Frankfurt plane, with the lower margins of the orbit in the same horizontal plane as the upper margin of the external auditory meatus. BMI was calculated as body weight divided by height squared (kg/m^2).

WrC was measured with subjects in a seated position using a tape measure positioned over the Lister tubercle of the distal radius and over the distal ulna. HC was measured at the level of maximal gluteal protrusion and waist circumference at the midpoint between the anterior superior iliac crest and the lowest rib using a tape measure while the subject stood with feet 25–30 cm apart. The tape measure was placed directly on the skin. Patients were allowed to breathe out normally, and measurements were taken. The tape was held lightly so as not to compress the skin. WHtR and WHR were calculated WC (cm) divided by Ht (cm) and HC, respectively. Body adiposity index (BAI) was calculated as the size of the hips compared to the patient's height [26].

$$\text{BAI} = \text{HC}\,(\text{cm}) \div [\text{height}\,(\text{m})]^{1.5} - 18. \quad (1)$$

The conicity index (CI) was determined from the measurements of weight, height, and waist circumference [27].

$$\text{Conicity index} = \frac{\text{WC}\,(\text{m})}{0.109 \times \sqrt{\text{weight}\,(\text{kg})/\text{height}\,(\text{m})}}. \quad (2)$$

Abdominal volume index (AVI) was derived from the measurements of waist circumference (WC) and hip circumferences (HC) [28].

$$\text{AVI} = \frac{2[\text{WC}\,(\text{cm})]^2 + 0.7[\text{WC}\,(\text{cm}) - \text{HC}\,(\text{cm})]^2}{1000}. \quad (3)$$

Visceral adiposity index (VAI) uses the study participant's waist circumference (WC), BMI, triglyceride (TG), and HDL-C levels [29].

$$\text{VAI for females} = \frac{\text{WC}}{36.58} + (1.89 \times \text{BMI}) \times \left(\frac{\text{TG}}{0.81}\right) \times \left(\frac{1.52}{\text{HDL}}\right),$$
$$\text{VAI for males} = \frac{\text{WC}}{39.68} + (1.88 \times \text{BMI}) \times \left(\frac{\text{TG}}{1.03}\right) \times \left(\frac{1.31}{\text{HDL}}\right). \quad (4)$$

All measurement was done by two (2) health technicians, one being the examiner and the other being the recorder.

2.7. Biochemical Analysis. Subjects fasted for a minimum of 12 hours and avoided a high-fat diet and alcohol consumption for at least 24 h prior to phlebotomy. Fasting blood glucose was measured using the One Touch glucometer and recorded. A fasting venous blood sample was obtained between 6:00 am and 11:00 am into a gel separator tube; sample allowed to clot and centrifuged at 5000 rpm room temperature for 5 minutes. Serum was then separated into a plain tube and stored in a 4°C refrigerator prior to analysis in the hospital laboratory. Clinical chemistry workup included total cholesterol (TC), high-density lipoprotein cholesterol (HDL-C), very-low-density lipoprotein (VLDL-C), low-density lipoprotein (LDL-C), and triglycerides (TG) using the COBAS INTEGRA® 400 plus automated chemistry analyzer. Other parameters like the coronary risk were calculated by dividing TC by HDL-C. A diagnosis of MetS was defined as central obesity plus either dyslipidaemia and hypertension or raised plasma glucose as illustrated in Table 1. Cardiometabolic risk was defined as a cluster of hypertension, metabolic syndrome, and an enhanced waist circumference (above 102 cm in males and 88 cm in females) accompanied by the alterations in lipid profile quoted above (HDL cholesterol below <1.03 mmol/L in males and <1.29 mmol/L in females, and serum triglycerides above ≥1.7 mmol/L).

2.8. Statistical Analysis. All statistical analyses were performed separately according to sex by using the Statistical Package for Social Science (SPSS version 12.0). The basic characteristics were presented by descriptive analysis as means and standard deviations (SD) for continuous data and as frequencies for categorical data. Comparisons between men and women were made using independent samples *t*-tests for continuous data and chi-square tests for categorical data. Pearson's correlation coefficients were used to determine the correlation between anthropometric indices and cardiometabolic risk factors. Receiver operating characteristic (ROC) curves were used to demonstrate the discriminatory ability of an anthropometric index over the entire range of possible values in the detection of a cardiometabolic outcome as quantified by the area under the curve (AUC). The optimal cut-off point for each anthropometric variable in the prediction of a given cardiometabolic outcome was established based on the highest combination of sensitivity and specificity. p values of less than 0.05 were considered to indicate statistical significance.

3. Ethical Consideration

The investigations were approved by the Committee on Human Research Publications and Ethics (CHRPE) at School of Medical Sciences, Kwame Nkrumah University of Science and Technology (KNUST), Kumasi, Ghana, in collaboration with the management of Begoro District Hospital. Participation was voluntary, and written informed consent was obtained from each participant according to Helsinki Declaration. Respondents were assured that the information gathered was to be used strictly for research and academic purpose only. In addition, respondents were given the freedom to opt out at any time they thought they could not continue with the study.

4. Results

The basic characteristics and prevalence of cardiometabolic risk factors of the study sample are presented in Table 2. The results found that mean age of men was significantly higher compared to the age of the women (60.8 ± 11.5 versus 55.0 ± 13.3, $p = 0.029$). Male participant had significantly larger wrist size than females (17.4 ± 0.8 versus 16.4 ± 1.0, p value < 0.0001). The variation was also seen among men and women where mean value for central adiposity (WHR) was significantly higher among men (0.96 ± 0.07 versus 0.91 ± 0.06, p value $= 0.002$). However, significantly higher TC and LDL-C levels were recorded in women compared with men (7.2 ± 1.4 versus 5.9 ± 1.6 and 5.15 ± 1.35 versus 3.89 ± 1.42, respectively, p value < 0.0001). BAI was also significantly higher in women compared to men (32.8 ± 6.2 versus 27.6 ± 3.6, p value < 0.0001). The study population was comparable in terms of cardiometabolic risk prevalence and anthropometric parameters other than the variations noted above (all p values > 0.05).

Table 3 illustrates the regression analysis of wrist circumference for dyslipidaemia and haemodynamic parameters. Regarding women, WrC was observed to be the significant positive predictors for MetS [aOR = 3.0 (1.39–6.72), $p = 0.005$] and SBP [aOR = 2.08 (1.17–3.68), $p = 0.012$]. The coefficients of determination were 0.221 and 0.481, which means WrC was significantly responsible for 22.1% and 48.1% for MetS and SBP. However, WrC was observed not to be statistically significant predictors for dyslipidaemia and haemodynamic indices in relation to men. WHtR was observed to be the significant positive predictors for TG [aOR = 3.23 (0.10–3.82), $p = 0.001$] for women not men.

Table 4 depicts the AUC of each anthropometric index in the prediction of multiple cardiometabolic risk among men and women. Each index apart from visceral adiposity index (VAI) was at its best in the prediction of MetS in both sexes ranging from 0.68 to 1.00 at 95% confidence interval, p values < 0.05. Among men and women, VAI was the best predictor of dyslipidaemia (TG and low HDL-C). The AUC of BAI in the prediction of TC was only significant in male subjects. However, the AUC of WrC, WHtR, AVI, VAI, CI, BAI, and BMI were best predictors of multiple cardiometabolic risk factors (hypertension, MetS, and dyslipidaemia) among male and female subjects, p values < 0.05.

Table 1: IDF definition of metabolic syndrome (IDF, 2006).

According to IDF, for a person to be defined as having cardiometabolic risk, the person must have a WC of >90 cm for men and >80 cm for women or BMI > 30 kg/m^2 and any two of the following.		
Dyslipidaemia	Raised triglyceride, TG	≥1.7 mmol/L or specific treatment for this lipid abnormality
	Reduced HDL-C	<1.03 mmol/L in males <1.29 mmol/L in females or specific treatment for this lipid abnormality
Hypertension	Systolic blood pressure	≥130 mmHg
	Diastolic blood pressure	≥85 mmHg or treatment of previously diagnosed hypertension
Raised fasting plasma glucose		(FPG) ≥ 5.6 mmol/L or previously diagnosed diabetes

Table 2: Descriptive of anthropometric indices, haemodynamic indices, and lipid parameters of study participants.

Variables	Total (n = 384)	Men (n = 147)	Women (n = 237)	p value
Age (years)	56.4 ± 13.1	60.8 ± 11.5	55.0 ± 13.3	**0.029**
Duration of diabetes (years)	9.3 ± 7.5	10.9 ± 8.0	8.8 ± 7.3	0.228
WrC (cm)[a]	16.5 ± 1.1	17.4 ± 0.8	16.4 ± 1.0	**<0.0001**
WC (cm)[a]	91.9 ± 10.7	92.4 ± 10.2	91.8 ± 10.9	0.794
WHR[a]	0.9 ± 0.1	1.0 ± 0.1	0.9 ± 0.1	**0.002**
WHtR[a]	0.6 ± 0.1	0.6 ± 0.1	0.6 ± 0.1	0.152
BMI[a]	26.2 ± 4.9	24.9 ± 3.4	26.6 ± 5.3	**0.047**
VAI[a]	3.4 ± 4.0	2.9 ± 2.9	3.6 ± 4.2	0.320
AVI[a]	17.2 ± 3.9	17.3 ± 3.7	17.2 ± 3.9	0.877
BAI (%)[a]	31.5 ± 6.1	27.6 ± 3.6	32.8 ± 6.2	**<0001**
CI[a]	1.3 ± 0.1	1.32 ± 0.1	1.30 ± 0.1	0.309
SBP (mmHg)[a]	133.3 ± 19.7	135.7 ± 16.2	132.6 ± 20.7	0.404
DBP (mmHg)[a]	82.0 ± 16.2	85.7 ± 10.0	80.8 ± 9.9	0.065
FBS (mmol/L)[a]	10.5 ± 4.2	10.8 ± 4.2	10.4 ± 4.2	0.700
TC (mmol/L)[a]	6.9 ± 1.6	5.9 ± 1.6	7.2 ± 1.4	**<0.0001**
TG (mmol/L)[a]	1.9 ± 0.9	1.9 ± 0.9	1.8 ± 0.9	0.972
HDL-C (mmol/L)[a]	1.2 ± 0.4	1.1 ± 0.4	1.3 ± 0.4	0.071
LDL-C (mmol/L)[a]	4.9 ± 1.5	3.9 ± 1.4	5.1 ± 1.4	**<0.0001**
VLDL (mmol/L)[a]	0.9 ± 0.4	0.8 ± 0.4	0.8 ± 0.4	0.972
Coronary risk[a]	6.1 ± 2.7	5.8 ± 3.1	6.1 ± 2.5	0.591
High SBP, n (%)[b]	260 (67.8)	110 (75.0)	155 (65.6)	0.350
High DBP, n (%)[b]	153 (39.8)	68 (46.4)	89 (37.8)	0.414
High TG, n (%)[b]	178 (46.4)	68 (46.4)	110 (46.7)	0.982
Low HDL, n (%)[b]	205 (53.4)	58 (39.3)	137 (57.8)	0.087
MetS IDF, n (%)[b]	293 (76.3)	99 (64.3)	189 (80.0)	0.088
MetS WHO, n (%)[b]	289 (75.4)	101 (75.0)	179 (75.6)	0.952
MetS AACE, n (%)[b]	303 (78.8)	116 (78.6)	187 (78.9)	0.917
MetS NHLBI, n (%)[b]	296 (77.1)	105 (71.4)	187 (78.9)	0.412
MetS NCEP ATP III, n (%)[b]	296 (77.1)	105 (71.4)	187 (78.9)	0.412

All numbers are means ± standard deviation unless specified. [a]t-tests. [b]Chi-square tests. BMI: body mass index; WC: waist circumference; WHtR: waist-to-height ratio; WHR: waist-to-hip ratio; BAI: body adiposity index; VAI: visceral adiposity index; CI: conicity index; AVI: abdominal volume index; MetS: metabolic syndrome; FBG: fasting blood sugar; SBP: systolic blood pressure; DBP: diastolic blood pressure; TC: total cholesterol; TG: triglycerides; HDL-C: high-density lipoprotein cholesterol. $p < 0.05$ = statistically significant.

The cut-off value of WrC predictive of cardiometabolic risk factors was higher in male compared to that of female (17.5 to 17.8 versus 16.0 to 16.7). However, that of BAI was higher in women (30.5 to 32.8) than in men (24.2 to 29.5) in predicting cardiometabolic risk factors. Table 5 presents the cut-off values, sensitivities, and specificities of anthropometric indices predictive of cardiometabolic risk factors.

Multiple logistic analyses of lipid profile, haemodynamic indices, and anthropometric indices for predicting incidence

TABLE 3: Cross-sectional association and predictability of baseline wrist circumference (WrC) for dyslipidaemia and haemodynamic indices.

Variable	Men				Women			
	β (SE)	R^2	aOR (95% CI)	p value	β (SE)	R^2	aOR (95% CI)	p value
					WrC			
MetS*	0.80 (0.67)	0.45	2.23 (0.60–8.28)	0.230	1.118 (0.402)	0.221	3.06 (1.39–6.72)	**0.005**
TC$^{\theta}$	0.02 (0.54)	0.18	1.02 (0.35–2.95)	0.969	0.355 (0.424)	0.143	1.43 (0.63–3.28)	0.403
TG$^{\theta}$	0.24 (0.54)	0.06	0.98 (0.36–2.68)	0.963	0.021 (0.210)	0.01	1.02 (0.67–1.54)	0.919
HDL-C$^{\theta}$	1.42 (0.81)	0.29	4.14 (0.85–20.24)	0.079	0.201 (0.239)	0.027	1.22 (0.77–1.95)	0.401
CR*	0.78 (0.72)	0.22	2.19 (0.54–8.90)	0.273	0.148 (0.217)	0.051	1.16 (0.76–1.77)	0.495
SBP*	0.42 (0.54)	0.09	1.52 (0.52–4.38)	0.436	0.730 (0.292)	0.481	2.08 (1.17–3.68)	**0.012**
DBP*	1.31 (0.71)	0.24	0.27 (0.07–1.08)	0.064	0.360 (0.244)	0.061	1.42 (0.89–2.31)	0.140
					WHtR			
MetS*	**0.53 (0.81)**	**0.08**	**1.70 (0.40–2.01)**	**0.283**	**0.014 (0.102)**	**0.091**	**1.01 (0.43–1.07)**	**0.381**
TC$^{\theta}$	**0.17 (0.90)**	**0.13**	**1.19 (0.30–2.91)**	**0.558**	**0.243 (0.183)**	**0.074**	**1.28 (0.39–2.18)**	**0.459**
TG$^{\theta}$	**0.43 (0.81)**	**0.08**	**1.14 (0.31–2.22)**	**0.601**	**1.173 (0.228)**	**0.375**	**3.23 (0.10–3.82)**	**0.001**
HDL-C$^{\theta}$	**−0.30 (0.81)**	**0.21**	**0.74 (0.20–8.34)**	**0.815**	**0.293 (0.197)**	**0.058**	**1.34 (0.05–1.99)**	**0.431**
CR*	**0.37 (0.75)**	**0.30**	**1.45 (0.17–2.83)**	**0.339**	**0.153 (0.216)**	**0.092**	**1.17 (0.53–1.95)**	**0.503**
SBP*	**0.31 (0.54)**	**0.05**	**1.36 (0.12–2.19)**	**0.407**	**0.527 (0.191)**	**0.329**	**1.69 (0.51–2.25)**	**0.425**
DBP*	**0.03 (0.21)**	**0.02**	**1.03 (0.18–1.25)**	**0.591**	**0.278 (0.37)**	**0.101**	**1.32 (0.51–1.72)**	**0.595**

*Adjusted for fasting blood glucose, duration of diabetes, history of hypertension, and age. $^{\theta}$Adjusted for fasting blood glucose, duration of diabetes, and age. CR: coronary risk.

of 10-year CVD risk level among diabetic patients after controlling for age duration of diabetes and history of hypertension are shown in Tables 5 and 6. Subjects with poor controlled of FBS are significantly more likely to develop CVD [aOR = 5.0 (1.09–22.82), $p = 0.038$]. Similarly, increased likelihood was observed among patients with high TC [aOR = 2.65 (0.51–13.83)], TG [aOR = 2.26 (0.41–12.28)], LDL-C [aOR = 2.0 (0.46–8.72)], and MetS [aOR = 3.69 (0.98–13.86)] but was statistically not significant ($p > 0.05$). The presence of MetS [aOR = 4.53 (1.14–17.99), $p = 0.031$] and diagnosed as hypertensive using SBP [aOR = 68.2 (3.41–136.50), $p = 0.0002$] were associated with significant increased risk of CVD.

As shown in Table 7, larger wrist circumference was associated with increased odds [aOR = 6.13 (0.34–111.4)] of developing CVD in 10 years but was statistically not significant ($p > 0.05$). Similarly, increased odds were observed in other anthropometric indices for both moderated-to-high risk of 10-year incidence of CVD but did not show any significant results ($p > 0.05$).

5. Discussion

Cardiometabolic risk has commonly been used to describe the aggregate risk of developing cardiovascular disease. Although there is a general agreement upon such a risk, differences in the diagnosis of central obesity still exist [30]. In this study, in addition to conventional indices of central obesity, the recently introduced WrC and WHtR were included.

In this present study, WrC was significantly associated with MetS and hypertension (using SBP > 140) in diabetic female subjects, but no significant association was found in male subject. Moreover, WrC was a significant predictor of MetS and hypertension among female subjects even after controlling for subject's age, duration of diabetes, history of hypertension, and FBS (glycaemic control) (Table 3). This is inconsistent with the findings from a cross-sectional study by Jahangiri et al. [21] among Iranian population. The study found a significant positive association between WrC and MetS in both genders. In women population, WrC is independent from general and central obesity measures in the prediction of cardiometabolic abnormalities [16]. This could be expounded by the presence of "bone-fat-pancreas" axis that regulates energy hemostasis and coordinates energy partitioning between bone and adipose tissue and impacts insulin sensitivity [23]. In another cross-sectional study by Capizzi et al. [22] conducted among overweight and obese children and adolescents to identify WrC as a marker for insulin resistance, they found a significant positive association between WrC, its bone component, and insulin resistance, which is similar to our findings. Several other studies have also presented results corroborating our findings in this present study [23, 31]. WHtR was observed to be the significant positive predictors for TG for women not men in this study, which is in concordance with the findings from previous studies [18, 32, 33].

Differences between the two genders regarding the association between wrist circumference and cardiometabolic risk factors occurrence could be due to the effects of sex steroid hormones and their interaction with bone metabolism and glucose homeostasis [21]. In a meta-analysis conducted by Ma et al. [34] to evaluate association between bone mineral density (BMD) and type 2 diabetes mellitus, they concluded that overall individuals with T2DM have about 25–50% SD higher BMD compared to nondiabetic control subjects. Physiologically, insulin has an anabolic effect on

Table 4: AUC for various anthropometric indices and cardiometabolic risk factors in men and women.

(a)

Risk factor	WrC	VAI	WHR	WHtR
Men (n = 147)				
Hypertension	**0.59 (0.41–0.77)***	0.59 (0.37–0.81)	0.55 (0.34–0.76)	**0.67 (0.47–0.86)***
Mets IDF	**0.69 (0.55–0.84)***	0.59 (0.39–0.79)	**0.85 (0.72–0.98)***	**0.99 (0.99–0.99)***
High TC	0.57 (0.24–0.89)	0.50 (0.24–0.76)	0.54 (0.28–0.80)	0.57 (0.29–0.85)
High TG	0.59 (0.39–0.78)	**0.94 (0.90–0.98)***	**0.70 (0.49–0.90)***	0.53 (0.32–0.74)
Low HDL-C	**0.70 (0.56–0.84)***	**0.95 (0.95–0.95)***	0.50 (0.30–0.71)	0.57 (0.35–0.78)
Women (n = 237)				
Hypertension	**0.67 (0.67–0.67)***	0.53 (0.41, 0.65)	0.59 (0.47–0.71)	**0.66 (0.57–0.79)***
Mets IDF	**0.73 (0.66–0.81)***	**0.71 (0.58–0.84)***	**0.68 (0.52–0.83)***	**0.87 (0.77–0.97)***
High TC	0.54 (0.48–0.61)	0.56 (0.43–0.69)	0.54 (0.38–0.55)	0.57 (0.44–0.71)
High TG	0.52 (0.52–0.52)	**0.95 (0.92–0.99)***	0.51 (0.38–0.63)	0.53 (0.41–0.65)
Low HDL-C	**0.60 (0.60–0.60)***	**0.85 (0.78–0.93)***	0.60 (0.48–0.71)	0.52 (0.40–0.64)

(b)

Risk factor	AVI	CI	BAI	BMI
Men (n = 147)				
Hypertension	**0.66 (0.47–0.85)***	**0.61 (0.41–0.82)***	**0.72 (0.54–0.91)***	**0.69 (0.50–0.88)***
Mets IDF	**1.00 (1.0-1.0)***	**1.0 (1.0-1.0)***	**0.78 (0.62–0.94)***	**0.81 (0.66–0.96)***
High TC	0.53 (0.28–0.77)	0.51 (0.26–0.74)	**0.76 (0.54–0.98)***	0.58 (0.32–0.84)
High TG	0.56 (0.35–0.77)	0.57 (0.37–0.78)	0.55 (0.34–0.77)	0.50 (0.29–0.72)
Low HDL-C	0.54 (0.33–0.75)	0.56 (0.35–0.76)	0.66 (0.45–0.86)	0.54 (0.33–0.75)
Women (n = 237)				
Hypertension	**0.66 (0.54–0.77)***	**0.61 (0.49–0.73)***	**0.63 (0.51–0.74)***	**0.68 (0.57–0.79)***
Mets IDF	**0.83 (0.71–0.96)***	**0.68 (0.53–0.84)***	**0.81 (0.69–0.94)***	**0.88 (0.78–0.98)***
High TC	0.58 (0.45–0.71)	0.59 (0.45–0.72)	0.57 (0.45–0.70)	0.58 (0.46–0.71)
High TG	0.54 (0.42–0.65)	0.52 (0.40–0.64)	0.58 (0.47–0.70)	0.56 (0.45–0.68)
Low HDL-C	0.50 (0.38–0.62)	0.51 (0.39–0.63)	0.51 (0.39–0.63)	0.50 (0.38–0.62)

Data are AUC (95% confidence interval). ∗ represents positive test if test variable < threshold. All values in bold are significant, p value <0.05.

Table 5: WrC and WHtR as a selected discriminator of cardiometabolic risk factors.

Discriminator	AUC	Cut-off	Sensitivity, %	Specificity, %	Kappa
Women					
WrC ∗ SBP	0.67	16.7 cm	43	84	0.05
WrC ∗ MetS	0.73	16.3 cm	61	72	0.23
WrC ∗ HDL-C	0.60	16.0 cm	39	82	0.04
WHtR ∗ SBP	0.67	0.55	80	53	0.24
WHtR ∗ MetS	0.99	0.53	90	78	0.58
Men				72	
WrC ∗ MetS	0.69	17.8 cm	50	90	0.315
WrC ∗ HDL-C	0.70	17.5 cm	55	77	0.18
WrC ∗ MetS	0.73	16.3 cm	61	74	—
WHtR ∗ SBP	0.66	0.61	39	100	0.402
WHtR ∗ MetS	0.87	0.52	100	90	0.837

TABLE 6: Multiple logistic analyses of lipid profile and haemodynamic indices for predicting incidence of 10-year CVD risk level among diabetic patients.

Variable	Moderate to high aOR (95% CI)	p value
TC		
Low	1	
High	3.0 (0.65–13.74)	0.157
TG		
Low	1	
High	4.73 (0.93–23.82)	0.060
HDL-C		
High	1	
Low	2.0 (0.39–10.16)	0.067
LDL-C		
Low	1	
High	4.13 (0.99–17.28)	0.052
CR	1	
Normal	1	
Risk	3.78 (0.75–19.06)	0.107
FBS		
Poor control	2.79 (0.73–10.72)	**0.038**
Good control	1	
SBP		
Normal	1	
Prehypertension	2.71 (0.59–12.31)	0.196
Hypertension	68.2 (3.41–136.5)	**0.0002**
MetS		
No	1	
Yes	4.53 (1.14–17.99)	**0.031**
Dyslipidaemia		
No	1	
Yes	2.92 (0.69–12.19)	0.142
Duration of disease		
<5	1	
05–10	0.52 (0.12–2.35)	0.398
>10	3.68 (0.36–37.92)	0.273

aOR: adjusted odds ratio; CI: confidence interval; FBG: fasting blood sugar; SBP: systolic blood pressure; DBP: diastolic blood pressure; TC: total cholesterol; TG: triglycerides; HDL-C: high-density cholesterol; MetS: metabolic syndrome.

TABLE 7: Multiple logistic analyses of anthropometric indices for predicting the incidence of 10-year CVD risk level among diabetic patients.

Variables	Moderate to high aOR (95% CI)	p value
WrC		
Normal	1	
Larger	6.13 (0.34–111.4)	0.107
WC		
Normal	1	
Risk	0.95 (0.18–4.94)	0.951
BMI		
Underweight	—	
Normal	1	
Overweight	0.97 (0.25–3.70)	0.959
Obese	5.41 (0.27–104.7)	0.302
CI		
Normal	1	
Risk	1.01 (0.26–3.90)	0.987
VAI		
Q1	1	
Q2	2.43 (0.39–15.27)	0.344
Q3	2.29 (0.36–14.43)	0.379
Q4	3.57 (0.58–22.02)	0.170
WHR		
Normal	1	
Overweight	1.33 (0.10–17.99)	0.827
Obese	1.19 (0.12–11.41)	0.880
WHtR		
Underweight	—	
Normal	1	
Overweight	3.67 (0.27–49.29)	0.327
Obese	2.52 (0.42–15.02)	0.309

aOR: adjusted odds ratio; CI: confidence interval; BMI: body mass index; WC: waist circumference; WHtR: waist-to-height ratio; WHR: waist-to-hip ratio; BAI: body adiposity index; VAI: visceral adiposity index; CI: conicity index; AVI: abdominal volume index.

bone due to its structural homology to IGF-1 by interacting with the IGF-1 receptor, which is present on osteoblasts [34].

The current study identified the gender-stratified cut-off points of potent anthropometric indices that proved to be better predictors of cardiometabolic risk factors. The optimal cut-off value of WrC to identify individuals at increased cardiometabolic risk is between 17.5 and 17.8 cm for men and 16.0 and 16.7 cm for women while that of WHtR was between 0.52 and 0.61 for men and 0.53 and 0.59 for women. Consistency in risk estimation using established cut-off was poor to fair for WrC estimation; high systolic pressure, kappa (0.05) for women; and metabolic syndrome, kappa (0.23) for women and (0.32) for men. Consistency with WHtR was good for SBP, kappa (0.24 and 0.40) for men and women, respectively, to very good for metabolic syndrome, kappa (0.58) for men and (0.84) for women, respectively. The current study reported a 10-year risk of developing CVD among diabetes patients and the plausible risk factors. Using the Framingham risk scores, 61% of the subjects had an elevated 10-year risk of developing cardiovascular diseases (CVDs). Both male and female subjects showed descry prevalence of prejudicial cardiovascular risk and moderate to higher risk of developing CVD in the future. Cohering the results of this present study in part is a multicenter study in Brazil among patients with type II diabetes by Gomes et al. [35]. In another study among diabetic patients in Manipur, Northeast India, Tungdim et al. [36] found similar results that corroborate our present finding. Several other studies have reported a higher risk of CVD among women. Accumulating evidence from recent findings has demonstrated alterations in estrogen-related protective mechanism by diabetes [21, 37]. This poses adverse changes in cardiovascular risk leading to enhanced atherogenesis in females [36]. In a meta-analysis by Agatisa et al. [38] and Kanaya et al. [39] among T2DM patients, they also reported that although the odds of CVD mortality were higher among women than men, the number of excess deaths attributable to diabetes was higher among men after controlling for CVD risk. The high incidence of moderate-to-high incidence of 10-year cardiovascular among subjects could be explained in terms of their lifestyle without exercise, poor glycaemic control (74.6%), prevalence of hypertension (42.4%), high LDL (80.5%), and MetS (76.3%).

Literature has provided several contradicting findings concerned with detrimental effect of hyperglycaemia on cardiovascular risk profile. High blood glucose level leads to oxidative stress and mitochondrial overproduction of superoxide, which have been acknowledged in the pathogenesis of diabetic micro- and macrovascular complications [40]. Regular physical exercise has been reported to be associated with lower risk of cardiovascular morbidity and mortality, both in the primary and secondary prevention [41], while elevation of small dense LDL particles and ApoB in type II diabetes mellitus (T2DM) patients is a predictor of cardiovascular risk [42]. The results of this present study found that larger WrC was associated with increased odds of moderate and high risk of developing CVD in 10 years (Table 5). In a cohort study by Mohebi et al. [23], they reported that WrC was independently associated with hypertension and CVD outcome. WHtR was also a plausible risk marker for CVD events with increasing odds of moderate and high 10-year CVD incidence (Table 6). The WrC was assumed to be a possible surrogate of body bone status and did not measure any bone status measures; thus, we could not evaluate the true predictive power of bone status in relation to CVD outcomes. Notwithstanding that findings in this study are comparable to reports from previous studies, the sample size was small, and the use of nonprobability sampling approach may have affected the statistical power and introduced sampling bias.

6. Conclusion

Using gender-specific cut-offs for WrC may offer putative marker for early detection of cardiometabolic risk factors among diabetic patients; therefore, being a simple and easy-to-detect measure, WrC and WHtR could be regarded as a new anthropometric assessment for prediction of cardiovascular and metabolic complications. Moreover, considering central and general obesity measurements, increasing wrist circumference highlighted an independent risk for incident cardiometabolic risk factors only among diabetic women. Further study needs to be done to include measurements of bone status and body fat stores to evaluate the true predictive power of bone status in relation to cardiometabolic risk outcome in a larger population.

Conflicts of Interest

The authors declare that there is no conflict of interest regarding the publication of this paper.

Acknowledgments

The authors would like to acknowledge the management and staff of Begoro District Hospital, Department of Molecular Medicine, for allowing them to carry out this work in their departments.

References

[1] World Health Organization, *Global Status Report on Noncommunicable Diseases. Geneva: 2010*, World Health Organization, 2015, February 2012, http://www.who.int/nmh/publications/ncd_report2010/en.

[2] World Health Organization, *Global Health Risks: Mortality and Burden of Disease Attributable to Selected Major Risks*, World Health Organization, 2009.

[3] IDF, *Global Diabetes Scorecard: Tracking Progress for Action*, International Diabetes Federation Brussels, 2015.

[4] IDF, *Global Diabetes Scoreboard: Ghana at a Glance*, International Diabetes Federation Diabetes Atlas, 2013.

[5] K. Opare-Asamoah, S. Majeed, L. Quaye et al., "Assessing the prevalence of hypertension and obesity among diabetics in the Tamale Metropolis, Ghana," *British Journal of Medicine and Medical Research*, vol. 20, no. 9, pp. 1–9, 2017.

[6] Y. Obirikorang, C. Obirikorang, E. Odame Anto et al., "Knowledge and lifestyle-associated prevalence of obesity among newly diagnosed type II diabetes mellitus patients attending diabetic clinic at Komfo Anokye Teaching Hospital, Kumasi, Ghana: a hospital-based cross-sectional study," *Journal of Diabetes Research*, vol. 2016, Article ID 9759241, 10 pages, 2016.

[7] C. Obirikorang, D. N. M. Osakunor, E. O. Anto, S. O. Amponsah, and O. K. Adarkwa, "Obesity and cardio-metabolic risk factors in an urban and rural population in the Ashanti Region-Ghana: a comparative cross-sectional study," *PLoS One*, vol. 10, no. 6, article e0129494, 2015.

[8] S. Kingue, S. Rakotoarimanana, N. Rabearivony, and F. L. Bompera, "Prevalence of selected cardiometabolic risk factors among adults in urban and semi-urban hospitals in four sub-Saharan African countries," *Cardiovascular Journal of Africa*, vol. 28, no. 3, pp. 147–153, 2017.

[9] G. A. Nichols, M. Horberg, C. Koebnick et al., "Cardiometabolic risk factors among 1.3 million adults with overweight or obesity, but not diabetes, in 10 geographically diverse regions of the United States, 2012–2013," *Preventing Chronic Disease*, vol. 14, article 160438, 2017.

[10] A. S. de Mattos Matheus, L. R. M. Tannus, R. A. Cobas, C. C. Sousa Palma, C. A. Negrato, and M. B. Gomes, "Impact of diabetes on cardiovascular disease: an update," *International Journal of Hypertension*, vol. 2013, Article ID 653789, 15 pages, 2013.

[11] A. Rivellese, G. Riccardi, and O. Vaccaro, "Cardiovascular risk in women with diabetes," *Nutrition, Metabolism and Cardiovascular Diseases*, vol. 20, no. 6, pp. 474–480, 2010.

[12] D. A. Chyun and L. H. Young, "Diabetes mellitus and cardiovascular disease," *Nursing Clinics of North America*, vol. 41, no. 4, pp. 681–695, 2006.

[13] C. A. Monteiro, M. D. A. Benicio, W. Conde, and B. Popkin, "Shifting obesity trends in Brazil," *European Journal of Clinical Nutrition*, vol. 54, no. 4, pp. 342–346, 2000.

[14] S. Yusuf, S. Hawken, S. Ôunpuu et al., "Effect of potentially modifiable risk factors associated with myocardial infarction in 52 countries (the INTERHEART study): case-control study," *The Lancet*, vol. 364, no. 9438, pp. 937–952, 2004.

[15] A. Pietrobelli and K. Steinbeck, "Paediatric obesity: what do we know and are we doing the right thing?," *International Journal of Obesity*, vol. 28, no. 1, pp. 2-3, 2004.

[16] D. Freedman, L. Khan, M. Serdula, W. Dietz, S. Srinivasan, and G. Berenson, "Inter-relationships among childhood BMI, childhood height, and adult obesity: the Bogalusa Heart Study," *International Journal of Obesity*, vol. 28, no. 1, pp. 10–16, 2004.

[17] S.-Y. Ho, T.-H. Lam, and E. D. Janus, "Waist to stature ratio is more strongly associated with cardiovascular risk factors than other simple anthropometric indices," *Annals of Epidemiology*, vol. 13, no. 10, pp. 683–691, 2003.

[18] L. Ware, K. Rennie, H. S. Kruger et al., "Evaluation of waist-to-height ratio to predict 5 year cardiometabolic risk in sub-Saharan African adults," *Nutrition, Metabolism & Cardiovascular Diseases*, vol. 24, no. 8, pp. 900–907, 2014.

[19] R. Y. Sung, H.-K. So, K.-C. Choi et al., "Waist circumference and waist-to-height ratio of Hong Kong Chinese children," *BMC Public Health*, vol. 8, no. 1, p. 324, 2008.

[20] M. Ashwell and S. D. Hsieh, "Six reasons why the waist-to-height ratio is a rapid and effective global indicator for health risks of obesity and how its use could simplify the international public health message on obesity," *International Journal of Food Sciences and Nutrition*, vol. 56, no. 5, pp. 303–307, 2005.

[21] Y. Jahangiri Noudeh, F. Hadaegh, N. Vatankhah et al., "Wrist circumference as a novel predictor of diabetes and prediabetes: results of cross-sectional and 8.8-year follow-up studies," *The Journal of Clinical Endocrinology & Metabolism*, vol. 98, no. 2, pp. 777–784, 2013.

[22] M. Capizzi, G. Leto, A. Petrone et al., "Wrist circumference is a clinical marker of insulin resistance in overweight and obese children and adolescents," *Circulation*, vol. 123, no. 16, pp. 1757–1762, 2011.

[23] R. Mohebi, A. Mohebi, F. Sheikholeslami, F. Azizi, and F. Hadaegh, "Wrist circumference as a novel predictor of hypertension and cardiovascular disease: results of a decade follow up in a West Asian cohort," *Journal of the American Society of Hypertension*, vol. 8, no. 11, pp. 800–807, 2014.

[24] F. K. Nyonator, J. K. Awoonor-Williams, J. F. Phillips, T. C. Jones, and R. A. Miller, "The Ghana community-based health planning and services initiative for scaling up service delivery innovation," *Health Policy and Planning*, vol. 20, no. 1, pp. 25–34, 2005.

[25] W. G. Cochran, *Sampling Techniques-3*, 1977.

[26] D. S. Freedman, J. C. Thornton, F. X. Pi-Sunyer et al., "The body adiposity index (hip circumference ÷ height$^{1.5}$) is not a more accurate measure of adiposity than is BMI, waist circumference, or hip circumference," *Obesity*, vol. 20, no. 12, pp. 2438–2444, 2012.

[27] F. Shidfar, F. Alborzi, M. Salehi, and M. Nojomi, "Association of waist circumference, body mass index and conicity index with cardiovascular risk factors in postmenopausal women: cardiovascular topic," *Cardiovascular Journal of Africa*, vol. 23, no. 8, pp. 442–445, 2012.

[28] V. C. Patil, G. Parale, P. Kulkarni, and H. V. Patil, "Relation of anthropometric variables to coronary artery disease risk factors," *Indian Journal of Endocrinology and Metabolism*, vol. 15, no. 1, pp. 31–37, 2011.

[29] M. C. Amato, C. Giordano, M. Pitrone, and A. Galluzzo, "Cut-off points of the visceral adiposity index (VAI) identifying a visceral adipose dysfunction associated with cardiometabolic risk in a Caucasian Sicilian population," *Lipids in Health and Disease*, vol. 10, no. 1, p. 183, 2011.

[30] M. Numan Ahmad and F. Halim Haddad, "Suitability of visceral adiposity index as a marker for cardiometabolic risks in Jordanian adults," *Nutricion Hospitalaria*, vol. 32, no. 6, pp. 2701–2709, 2015.

[31] A. Amini, B. I. Noureddin Soltanian, G. Askari et al., "Association of wrist circumference with cardio metabolic risk factors," *Journal of the Pakistan Medical Association*, vol. 62, no. 3, Supplement 1, pp. S34–S36, 2012.

[32] C. S. W. Miralles, L. M. Wollinger, D. Marin, J. P. Genro, V. Contini, and S. M. Dal Bosco, "Waist-to-height ratio (WHtR) and triglyceride to HDL-c ratio (TG/HDL-c) as predictors of cardiometabolic risk," *Nutricion Hospitalaria*, vol. 31, no. 5, pp. 2115–2121, 2015.

[33] X. Ren, Z. A. Chen, S. Zheng et al., "Association between triglyceride to HDL-C ratio (TG/HDL-C) and insulin resistance in Chinese patients with newly diagnosed type 2 diabetes mellitus," *PLoS One*, vol. 11, no. 4, article e0154345, 2016.

[34] L. Ma, L. Oei, L. Jiang et al., "Association between bone mineral density and type 2 diabetes mellitus: a meta-analysis of observational studies," *European Journal of Epidemiology*, vol. 27, no. 5, pp. 319–332, 2012.

[35] M. B. Gomes, D. Giannella-Neto, M. Faria et al., "Estimating cardiovascular risk in patients with type 2 diabetes: a national multicenter study in Brazil," *Diabetology & Metabolic Syndrome*, vol. 1, no. 1, p. 22, 2009.

[36] M. G. Tungdim, T. Ginzaniang, G. P. Kabui, D. Verma, and S. Kapoor, "Risk of cardiovascular disease among diabetic patients in Manipur, Northeast India," *Journal of Anthropology*, vol. 2014, Article ID 421439, 9 pages, 2014.

[37] W. L. Lee, A. M. Cheung, D. Cape, and B. Zinman, "Impact of diabetes on coronary artery disease in women and men: a meta-analysis of prospective studies," *Diabetes Care*, vol. 23, no. 7, pp. 962–968, 2000.

[38] P. K. Agatisa, R. B. Ness, J. M. Roberts, J. P. Costantino, L. H. Kuller, and M. K. McLaughlin, "Impairment of endothelial function in women with a history of preeclampsia: an indicator of cardiovascular risk," *American Journal of Physiology-Heart and Circulatory Physiology*, vol. 286, no. 4, pp. H1389–H1393, 2004.

[39] A. M. Kanaya, D. Grady, and E. Barrett-Connor, "Explaining the sex difference in coronary heart disease mortality among patients with type 2 diabetes mellitus: a meta-analysis," *Archives of Internal Medicine*, vol. 162, no. 15, pp. 1737–1745, 2002.

[40] M. Laakso, "Cardiovascular disease in type 2 diabetes from population to man to mechanisms," *Diabetes Care*, vol. 33, no. 2, pp. 442–449, 2010.

[41] M. Tanasescu, M. F. Leitzmann, E. B. Rimm, and H. FB, "Physical activity in relation to cardiovascular disease and total mortality among men with type 2 diabetes," *Circulation*, vol. 107, no. 19, pp. 2435–2439, 2003.

[42] I. Martín-Timón, C. Sevillano-Collantes, A. Segura-Galindo, and F. J. del Cañizo-Gómez, "Type 2 diabetes and cardiovascular disease: have all risk factors the same strength?," *World Journal of Diabetes*, vol. 5, no. 4, pp. 444–470, 2014.

6

Predicting Type 2 Diabetes Mellitus Occurrence using Three-Dimensional Anthropometric Body Surface Scanning Measurements

Ming-Kuo Ting,[1] Pei-Ju Liao,[2] I-Wen Wu,[3] Shuo-Wei Chen,[4] Ning-I Yang,[5] Tzu-Yu Lin,[6] and Kuang-Hung Hsu[6,7,8,9]

[1]*Division of Endocrinology and Metabolism, Chang Gung Memorial Hospital, Keelung, Taiwan*
[2]*Department of Health Care Administration, Oriental Institute of Technology, New Taipei City, Taiwan*
[3]*Division of Nephrology, Chang Gung Memorial Hospital, Keelung, Taiwan*
[4]*Division of Gastroenterology and Hepatology, Chang Gung Memorial Hospital, Keelung, Taiwan*
[5]*Division of Cardiology, Chang Gung Memorial Hospital, Keelung, Taiwan*
[6]*Healthy Aging Research Center, Chang Gung University, Taoyuan, Taiwan*
[7]*Laboratory for Epidemiology, Department of Health Care Management, Chang Gung University, Taoyuan, Taiwan*
[8]*Department of Emergency Medicine, Chang Gung Memorial Hospital, Taoyuan, Taiwan*
[9]*Department of Urology, Chang Gung Memorial Hospital, Taoyuan, Taiwan*

Correspondence should be addressed to Kuang-Hung Hsu; khsu@mail.cgu.edu.tw

Academic Editor: Brunella Capaldo

Background. An accurate and comprehensive anthropometric measure for predicting type 2 diabetes mellitus (T2DM) has not yet been depicted. *Methods.* A total of 8450 nondiabetic participants were recruited during 2000–2010 in Taiwan. The cohort was followed up to the end of 2013, over an average of 8.87 years. At recruitment, participants completed a questionnaire related to basic demographics, lifestyle variables, personal disease history, and family disease history. 3D body surface scanning was used to obtain 35 anatomical measurements. A Cox proportional hazard model was used to conduct multivariable analyses. *Results.* A total of 2068 T2DM cases at an incidence rate of 27.59×10^{-3} (year^{-1}) were identified during the follow-up period. Multivariable-adjusted hazard ratios (HRs) demonstrated that neck circumference (NC) (HR = 1.048; 95% CI = 1.033–1.064), waist width (WW) (HR = 1.061; 95% CI = 1.040–1.081), and left thigh circumference (TC) (HR = 0.984; 95% CI = 0.972–0.995) were significant predictors of the occurrence of T2DM. While dividing body measurement into median high/low groups, an increased risk of T2DM was observed among participants with a larger NC and smaller TC (HR = 1.375; 95% CI = 1.180–1.601) and a larger WW and smaller TC (HR = 1.278; 95% CI = 1.085–1.505) relative to other participants. *Conclusions.* This study suggests that as well as using traditional waist and TC measurements, NC can be used as an indicator to provide an early prediction of developing T2DM, while providing clues for future mechanistic investigations of T2DM.

1. Introduction

Type 2 diabetes mellitus (T2DM) is currently the fastest growing chronic disease in the world. According to WHO calculations, the number of people affected by diabetes will have increased 114% by 2030 relative to the year 2000 [1], and Asia is the region where diabetes is growing the fastest [1, 2]. Chronic complications from the disease result in major health care burdens and affect patient longevity and quality of life. Therefore, knowledge of early markers to predict the disease and the implementation of associated preventive strategies is vital for ameliorating this global problem.

Literature indicates that groups at a high risk for T2DM have a family history of the disease, are overweight or obese, do less exercise, have metabolic syndrome, or have had gestational diabetes mellitus [3]. People with T2DM are at risk of hypertension, hyperlipidemia, and cardiovascular disease. Central obesity, or abdominal visceral fat accumulation, is a major body shape phenotype used to predict the risk of T2DM and is related to an inflammatory response mechanism and insulin resistance [4]. One meta-analysis indicated that body mass index, waist circumference (WC), and waist/hip ratio are three major obesity markers associated with the incidence of T2DM [5]. Another meta-analysis indicated that the use of the waist-to-height ratio (WHtR) may also predict several cardiometabolic risk factors, particularly in diabetes, and is superior to the use of the BMI [6]. Furthermore, other studies have shown that four anthropometric indices (BMI, WC, W/HR, and WHtR) are markers of obesity and may predict the future onset of diabetes, and a number of studies have documented the wide use of WC measurements to approximate abdominal visceral fat accumulation, which is documented as being associated with insulin resistance and cardiometabolic risk [7–10]. However, the neck circumference (NC) has also been used as an alternative measure of upper-body subcutaneous fat, which correlates with whole-body adiposity and abdominal adiposity [7–9, 11]. Taking NC measurements has been demonstrated as practical in a relatively large population [12–14] and is a better predictor of metabolic syndrome than WC [15]. Moreover, the thigh circumference (TC) or waist-to-thigh ratio is reported to be associated with T2DM [16–18], and low subcutaneous thigh fat has been documented as a risk factor for hyperlipidemia and hyperglycemia [19].

Previous literature has demonstrated the use of noninvasive three-dimensional (3D) scanning technology to cross-sectionally associate body measurements, such as waist-to-thigh, with T2DM [18, 20] but no longitudinal studies with long-term follow-up have been performed to date. Therefore, this study investigated selected 3D body measurements in the evaluation of HRs for developing T2DM during an average 8.87-year follow-up in an established cohort.

2. Methods

2.1. Study Samples. A total of 8450 participants (4431 men and 4019 women) without diabetes were recruited from the Department of Health Promotion and Examination of Chang Gung Memorial Hospital in Taiwan. The study follow-up period spanned from February 2000 to December 2013 (a total of 13 years and 11 months), and the average follow-up period was 8.87 years. This study was approved by the Institutional Review Board of Chang Gung Medical Foundation (97-2538 B).

2.2. Anthropometrical Parameters. 3D body surface measurements were collected by using whole-body 3D laser scanning according to previously published methods [20, 21]. In addition to body height, body weight, and BMI, 35 measurements from four anatomical regions were found. The trunk region included the chest profile area, chest circumference, chest width, waist profile area, WC, waist width (WW), trunk volume, and trunk surface area. The head and neck region included the head volume, head surface area, head circumference, and NC. The hip to the lower limbs included the hip profile area, hip circumference, hip width, left leg volume, left leg surface area, left calf circumference, right leg volume, right leg surface area, right calf circumference, left TC, right TC, left leg length, and right leg length. The upper limb region included the left arm volume, left arm surface area, left arm length, right arm volume, right arm surface area, right arm length, left upper arm circumference, right upper arm circumference, left forearm circumference, and right forearm circumference. In addition to whole measures of the trunk, the trunk dimension was further classified into chest and waist measures due to the distinguishably anatomic and physiological characteristics. The 3D laser scanning machine (LT3DCam) was built by Logistic Technology Company (LTC, Hsinchu, Taiwan) and was proven with high standard of accuracy due to the objective and comprehensive ways of measuring human body surface. The standard procedure of measuring is to require a subject to remove all outer clothes except for underwear in preparation for scanning (women with bras in addition to pants) and to stand still on the stage for scanning (a total scanning time is about 10 seconds) [19]. The software system will collect, realign, construct, and measure a subject's whole-body digital stature and selected information. The measurement error of the 3D scanner in measuring human surface body has been checked, and the error in the x- and y-axis is approximately 1 mm (1.2%), and in the z-axis it is less than 0.1 mm (0.2%) [22].

2.3. Data Collection. Upon recruitment, a questionnaire was administered that requested the following information: date of birth; sex; education; marital status; occupation; history of cigarette smoking, alcohol drinking, and betel nut chewing; personal history of disease (including diabetes, hypertension, heart disease, chronic kidney disease, liver cirrhosis, and chronic hepatitis); and family history of T2DM. A medical chart review confirmed the answers provided. For those with no history of diabetes, a fasting blood glucose level was obtained. Diabetes was defined according to ADA guidelines. For those without a history of hypertension, blood pressure was measured with a mercury sphygmomanometer on the left arm after the patient had been resting for 20 minutes in a seated position. Hypertension was defined according to the guidelines of the Joint National Committee on Detection, Evaluation, and Treatment of High Blood Pressure (systolic blood pressure $\geq$ 140 mmHg, diastolic blood pressure $\geq$ 90 mmHg, or the use of antihypertensive medication) [23]. Heart disease was based on medical chart findings and defined using the ICD-9 Clinical Modification (ICD-9-CM) codes 390–398, 410–141, and 420–429. Renal disease, liver cirrhosis, and chronic hepatitis were coded as ICD-9-CM 580–583, ICD-9-CM 571.2 and 571.5, and ICD-9-CM 571.4, respectively. The occurrence of T2DM was determined using the national registration database and then further confirmed with insurance claim data. Patients diagnosed as ICD-9-CM code 250.00 and administered with DM-related drug prescriptions at least three times during the first diagnosis year were identified.

2.4. Statistical Analyses. Two independent sample t-tests were used to compare differences between the continuous variables of the groups, and results were presented as the mean ± SD. The χ^2 test was used to differentiate between the distribution of categorical variables, and results were expressed using frequencies and percentages between the groups. 3D body surface measurements were screened using a two-sample t-test by comparing differences between patients and controls. To avoid collinearity in the regression analysis, one body measurement with the lowest p value was selected from each anatomic dimension for subsequent multivariable analysis. A Cox proportional hazard model was used to determine the strength of the association between the selected body measurements and the incidence of T2DM. In addition to the forced-in sociodemographic variables, a backward model selection with $p < 0.1$ was used to determine variables, including lifestyles, body measures, and underlying diseases, to be retained in the regression model. Results were expressed as hazard ratios (HRs) adjusted for confounding variables, including age, sex, education, marital status, occupation, betel nut chewing, and hypertension history. For stratified analysis, selected body measurements were further categorized into high and low levels, according to the median result. A combination of two body measurements was generated to examine high-risk body shape characteristics. The statistical software used for the analyses in this study was SPSS 22.0 (IBM Corporation, Armonk, NY).

3. Results

Out of the 8450 participants (a total of 74964.5 person-years with an average of 8.87 years ranging from 0 to 13.80 years) in this study, a total of 2068 cases of T2DM were identified during the follow-up period, with an incidence rate of 0.02759 per year (Table 1). An increased incidence of disease occurrence was found for participants older than 50.7 years (median) (HR 1.52; 95% CI = 1.36–1.70) compared with younger participants. The study sample consisted of 4431 (52.4%) men and 4019 (47.6%) women who were at risk for developing T2DM. Results showed that participants who had a lower level of education were at a higher risk of developing T2DM. T2DM occurrence was associated with occupational categories: farmers and housekeeping and others were at the highest risk. Among lifestyle variables, betel nut chewers had a higher risk of developing T2DM (HR = 1.26; 95% CI = 1.08–1.47). In addition, participants with a personal disease history of hypertension (HR = 1.98; 95% CI = 1.79–2.18) and heart disease (HR = 1.39; 95% CI = 1.202–1.611) were more likely to develop T2DM (Table 1).

The results of almost all selected body measurements were statistically significant between cases and controls. In general, T2DM cases had larger body measurements than controls (Table 2). Multivariable analyses indicated that NC (HR = 1.05; 95% CI = 1.03–1.06), WW (HR = 1.06; 95% CI = 1.04–1.08), and left TC (HR = 0.984; 95% CI = 0.972–0.995) were significantly associated with the occurrence of T2DM when adjusted for age, sex, education, marital status, occupation, betel nut chewing, and personal hypertension disease history (Table 3). The three body measurements were then further categorized into median high and median low groups, and combinations of NC/left TC and WW/left TC were made to further explore an association with high-risk groups. The results demonstrated a monotonic trend in multivariable-adjusted HRs for lower NC/lower TC (HR = 1.09; 95% CI = 0.96–1.24), higher NC/higher TC (HR = 1.29; 95% CI = 1.13–1.49), and higher NC/lower TC (HR = 1.38; 95% CI = 1.18–1.60), compared with lower NC/higher TC. The combination of WW and left TC followed a dose-dependent relationship according to lower WW/higher TC (HR = 1.00), lower WW/lower TC (HR = 1.09; 95% CI = 0.94–1.26), higher WW/higher TC (HR = 1.28; 95% CI = 1.11–1.47), and higher WW/lower TC (HR = 1.28; 95% CI = 1.09–1.51) (Figure 1).

4. Discussion

The results of this prospective cohort analysis indicate that NC, WW, and TC measurements can be used as alternative biomarkers for predicting the incidence of T2DM in the Taiwanese population. In addition to waist measurements, this study demonstrates that NC, TC, and NC/TC ratio are good independent predictors of the occurrence of T2DM (Appendix A (available here)). We did analyses on models with both prevalent and incident T2DM cases and only incident T2DM cases to ascertain the reliability of selected body measures and found NC, WW, and TC to be consistency predictors to T2DM. During the analyses, our study finds that NC has a positive correlation with WC ($r = 0.61$; $p < 0.0001$) and BMI ($r = 0.59$; $p < 0.0001$) and exhibits a strong association with the occurrence of T2DM. It is considered that NC measurements could be used as an alternative biomarker to WC in predicting T2DM. However, WW could be used as a supplementary measurement to NC, as it reflects the visceral fat capacity. Although the literature indicates that TC is negatively associated with the prevalence of T2DM, it was confirmed as a long-term predictor of the occurrence of T2DM in this study [20]. The present study proposes using a combination of neck, waist, and thigh measurements as reliable biomarkers for predicting the occurrence of T2DM.

NC has been positively and significantly associated with higher age, weight, BMI, WC, and hip circumference in both men and women [12–14]. In addition, NC may present as an alternative predictive factor for being overweight and obese and is correlated with central obesity. A larger NC has also been associated with a higher WC and values and levels of metabolic syndrome components, including SBP, DBP, dyslipidemia, and hyperglycemia [14–16]. Studies have demonstrated that NC is positively associated with the incidence of T2DM [24, 25] and that a larger NC has been associated with increased insulin resistance and various cardiometabolic risk factors, such as decreasing HDL levels and increasing plasma triglyceride levels among healthy Chinese adults [26]. Notably, insulin resistance is the core etiology of metabolic syndromes and is one of the principal pathogeneses of T2DM. Another study reported that NC may well predict the occurrence of gestational diabetes in Chinese women [27].

Table 1: Basic demographics, lifestyle variables, and personal and family disease history between study groups.

	Total (%)	Person-years	Number of T2DM	Incidence density ($year^{-1}$)	Hazard ratio (HR)	95% CI
Demographics						
Age group	51.1 ± 11.9* (18.0, 90.7)	74964.5	2068	0.027586		
≤50.7275	4229 (50.1%)	39576.2	747	0.018875	1.000	—
>50.7275	4221 (50.0%)	35388.3	1321	0.037329	1.976	(1.806, 2.161)
Sex						
Female	4019 (47.6%)	36696.7	1030	0.028068	1.000	—
Male	4431 (52.4%)	38267.8	1038	0.027125	0.971	(0.891, 1.058)
Education						
Junior high school & below	3244 (38.4%)	27775.2	1011	0.036399	1.000	—
Senior high school	1719 (20.3%)	15,413	357	0.023162	0.639	(0.567, 0.721)
College/university & above	2813 (33.3%)	25843.9	528	0.020430	0.562	(0.506, 0.625)
Unknown	674 (8.0%)	5932.49	172	0.028993	0.798	(0.679, 0.938)
Marital status						
Married	6448 (76.3%)	57,660	1573	0.027281	1.000	—
Unmarried	1354 (16.0%)	11633.3	315	0.027077	0.994	(0.880, 1.122)
Unknown	648 (7.7%)	5671.25	180	0.031739	1.164	(0.997, 1.358)
Occupation						
Government	1169 (13.8%)	11724.5	291	0.024820	1.000	—
Farmers	587 (7.0%)	4745.08	160	0.033719	1.373	(1.132, 1.665)
Labourers	1065 (12.6%)	9581.96	199	0.020768	0.852	(0.711, 1.020)
Business	2559 (30.3%)	22030.3	555	0.025193	1.034	(0.897, 1.193)
Housekeeping & others	1933 (22.9%)	16640.2	575	0.034555	1.411	(1.225, 1.625)
Unknown	1137 (13.5%)	10242.4	288	0.028118	1.146	(0.974, 1.349)
Lifestyle variables						
Cigarette smoking						
No	6301 (74.6%)	56419.3	1553	0.027526	1.000	—
Yes	2149 (25.4%)	18545.2	515	0.027770	1.011	(0.915, 1.117)
Alcohol drinking						
No	6147 (72.8%)	54,897	1518	0.027652	1.000	—
Yes	2303 (27.3%)	20067.5	550	0.027407	0.994	(0.902, 1.096)
Betel nut chewing						
No	7826 (92.6%)	69575.5	1884	0.027078	1.000	—
Yes	624 (7.4%)	5388.99	184	0.034144	1.261	(1.084, 1.467)
Underlying diseases						
Hypertension						
No	6895 (81.6%)	62848.7	1515	0.024105	1.000	—
Yes	1423 (16.8%)	11150.4	531	0.047622	1.976	(1.790, 2.182)
Unknown	132 (1.6%)	965.437	22	0.022788	0.974	(0.639, 1.484)
Heart disease						
No	7700 (91.1%)	68690.6	1847	0.026889	1.000	—
Yes	618 (7.3%)	5308.45	199	0.037487	1.391	(1.202, 1.611)
Unknown	132 (1.6%)	965.437	22	0.022788	0.87	(0.571, 1.325)
Family disease history						
Hypertension						
No	5515 (65.3%)	49469.2	1333	0.026946	1.000	—
Yes	2845 (33.7%)	24865.1	721	0.028996	1.078	(0.984, 1.180)
Unknown	90 (1.1%)	630.259	14	0.022213	0.847	(0.500, 1.435)

Table 1: Continued.

	Total (%)	Person-years	Number of T2DM	Incidence density ($year^{-1}$)	Hazard ratio (HR)	95% CI
Diabetes						
No	6613 (78.3%)	59774.9	1515	0.025345	1.000	—
Yes	1747 (20.7%)	14555.9	539	0.037030	1.466	(1.329, 1.617)
Unknown	90 (1.1%)	633.752	14	0.022091	0.897	(0.530, 1.520)
Stroke						
No	7197 (85.2%)	63978.1	1745	0.027275	1.000	—
Yes	1164 (13.8%)	10362.1	309	0.029820	1.093	(0.968, 1.233)
Unknown	89 (1.1%)	624.331	14	0.022424	0.844	(0.499, 1.429)
Heart disease						
No	7304 (86.4%)	64926.4	1783	0.027462	1.000	—
Yes	1056 (12.5%)	9403.82	271	0.028818	1.049	(0.923, 1.192)
Unknown	90 (1.1%)	634.366	14	0.022069	0.825	(0.488, 1.397)

*Mean ± SD (min, max).

In this study, further evidence was found in the literature to support the association between NC and T2DM. A previous study proposed that using NC as a proxy indicator of upper-body fat may be superior to using it as a proxy indicator of whole-body fat in reflecting ectopic fat deposition and indicating cardiometabolic risk [9]. The measurement has also been shown to have a higher association with HOMA, low HDL-C, and triglycerides, compared with the use of WC [28]. Overall, NC is documented as a marker of upper-body subcutaneous adipose tissue distribution and a risk indicator of insulin resistance that may result in hyperglycemia and subsequent diabetes mellitus. Because it is easy to obtain, NC is becoming an alternative measurement; it not only exhibits a strong correlation with other body markers (such as WHR and BMI) but also is associated with physiological and biochemical measurements [29]. It is thus feasible for use as an innovative measurement in clinical practice and epidemiological surveys in large population communities.

Studies have indicated that larger hip and thigh circumferences are associated with a lower risk of T2DM, independent of age, BMI, and WC [28, 30]. The soft tissue in the thigh is mostly composed of muscle mass and subcutaneous fat. The skeletal muscles are the key target organ for insulin action and the site of insulin resistance [31]. Insulin resistance, the pathogenesis of T2DM, may interfere with glucose regulation and homeostasis, eventually resulting in hyperglycemia and leading to diabetes. Because a larger TC is related to a greater area of muscle mass, it is associated with a lower risk of diabetes [32]. A larger TC indicates not only a larger muscle mass but also an increased femoral subcutaneous fat mass. This is highly beneficial for the muscles and the liver and is free from high exposure to free fatty acid uptake and storage, thereby providing better insulin sensitivity and a superior lipid profile [33]. A lower muscle mass and less subcutaneous fat in the thighs may be associated with insulin resistance and eventually result in hyperglycemia and diabetes [19].

Our study also differs from those using traditional measurements because we used a combination of the NC/TC and WW/TC ratios to compare the HRs of T2DM incidence. These ratios may be useful as future screening measurements for identifying individuals at a high risk for diabetes. In our cohort study, a small NC and larger TC had a negative relationship with the incidence of diabetes. In addition, a small TC, in addition to being associated with diabetes, was associated with the development of heart disease or premature death [34].

WC and WHR are frequently used in current practice to estimate body fat accumulation on the trunk, and they represent an acknowledged risk factor for many metabolic disorders. The WHR offers a measurement of the relative accumulation of abdominal fat compared with the size of the body and is more widely adopted than using WC alone. Traditionally, WC has been a popular and useful body index for evaluating whether an individual was overweight and obese. One study showed that WC explains obesity-related health risk better than BMI and that for a given WC value, overweight, obese, and normal-weight persons have comparable health risks [35]. In this study, however, NC might be an alternative measure of a certain part of visceral fat and could provide a supplement to more comprehensive amount of body fat on the upper body. In addition, WC was replaced by WW as an indicator of the trunk's capacity to accumulate abdominal fat. Therefore, using a combination of WW and NC may offer a better indicator of upper-body fat accumulation in relation to subsequent long-term adverse effects.

Studies have demonstrated that other parameters, such as body weight, BMI, WC, and WHR, are associated with T2DM [5]. However, in this cohort study, NC, TC, and WW were the most significant predictors of T2DM in an Asian population. Many studies have shown that BMI is associated with obesity and metabolic syndrome, but the association is varied across ethnic groups [36–38]. The use of BMI to indicate body fat distribution is less reliable when used as an anthropometric index to predict adverse effects

Table 2: Three-dimensional body surface measurements of T2DM cases and controls.

	Control Mean ± SD	T2DM Mean ± SD	p value
Whole body			
Height (cm)	161.4 ± 8.6	159.9 ± 8.5	<0.0001
Weight (kg)	63.9 ± 11.5	66.8 ± 12.1	<0.0001
Body mass index	24.4 ± 3.4	26.0 ± 3.6	<0.0001
Head & neck			
Head circumference (cm)	58.9 ± 2.0	58.9 ± 1.9	0.3969
Head surface area (cm^2)	1337.3 ± 203.5	1313.0 ± 223.3	<0.0001
Head volume (cm^3)	4720.5 ± 531.4	4765.7 ± 536.5	0.0016
Neck circumference (cm)	36.9 ± 4.0	37.9 ± 4.1	<0.0001
Trunk			
Chest			
Chest circumference (cm)	95.5 ± 9.2	99.2 ± 9.2	<0.0001
Waist circumference (cm)	86.3 ± 10.3	91.0 ± 11.0	<0.0001
Chest width (cm)	31.9 ± 2.8	32.4 ± 2.9	<0.0001
Waist			
Waist width (cm)	30.2 ± 3.1	31.2 ± 3.2	<0.0001
Chest sectional area (cm^2)	636.0 ± 121.1	689.7 ± 126.3	<0.0001
Waist sectional area (cm^2)	568.7 ± 137.6	632.5 ± 150.5	<0.0001
Trunk surface area (cm^2)	6646.4 ± 1642.4	6712.4 ± 1928.5	0.1875
Trunk volume (cm^3)	37859.3 ± 7921.9	40685.6 ± 8550.9	<0.0001
Upper limbs			
Arm length (cm)			
Right	56.4 ± 3.5	56.1 ± 3.4	0.0112
Left	55.8 ± 3.5	55.5 ± 3.4	0.0028
Upper arm circumference (cm)			
Right	29.8 ± 3.8	31.0 ± 4.0	<0.0001
Left	30.2 ± 4.0	31.3 ± 4.2	<0.0001
Forearm circumference (cm)			
Right	24.2 ± 2.5	24.9 ± 2.7	<0.0001
Left	24.4 ± 2.8	24.9 ± 2.8	<0.0001
Arm surface area (cm^2)			
Right	1512.8 ± 275.5	1487.9 ± 259.0	0.0002
Left	1526.5 ± 316.8	1487.8 ± 297.8	<0.0001
Arm volume (cm^3)			
Right	2338.2 ± 479.0	2421.9 ± 478.3	<0.0001
Left	2392.4 ± 544.4	2437.3 ± 541.8	0.0011
Hip			
Hip circumference (cm)	96.6 ± 6.2	98.5 ± 6.6	<0.0001
Hip width (cm)	34.3 ± 2.5	34.8 ± 2.4	<0.0001
Hip sectional area (cm^2)	675.4 ± 105.1	711.9 ± 110.7	<0.0001
Lower limbs			
Leg length (cm)			
Right	68.8 ± 5.0	67.7 ± 5.0	<0.0001
Left	68.8 ± 5.0	67.7 ± 5.0.	<0.0001
Thigh circumference (cm)			
Right	50.9 ± 4.9	52.0 ± 5.0	<0.0001
Left	50.8 ± 5.0	52.0 ± 5.1	<0.0001

Table 2: Continued.

	Control Mean ± SD	T2DM Mean ± SD	p value
Calf circumference (cm)			
Right	33.6 ± 3.5	34.0 ± 3.4	<0.0001
Left	33.5 ± 3.5	34.0 ± 3.5	<0.0001
Leg surface area (cm^2)			
Right	2282.3 ± 415.4	2246.4 ± 420.3	0.0007
Left	2244.8 ± 378.4	2214.5 ± 364.4	0.0011
Leg volume (cm^3)			
Right	6035.9 ± 1373.0	6166.2 ± 1370.1	0.0002
Left	5990.5 ± 1373.6	6141.9 ± 1368.3	<0.0001

Table 3: Factors associated with the occurrence of T2DM by multiple Cox regression analysis.

	HR	95% CI	p value
Age			
≤50.7275	1.000	—	—
>50.7275	1.521	(1.364, 1.695)	<0.0001
Sex			
Female	1.000	—	—
Male	0.727	(0.639, 0.827)	<0.0001
Education			
Junior high school & below	1.000	—	—
Senior high School	0.835	(0.727, 0.958)	0.0101
College/university & above	0.711	(0.617, 0.819)	<.0001
Unknown	0.872	(0.712, 1.069)	0.1874
Marital status			
Married	1.000	—	—
Unmarried	1.038	(0.911, 1.183)	0.5734
Unknown	1.163	(0.952, 1.420)	0.1395
Occupation			
Government	1.000	—	—
Farmers	0.821	(0.654, 1.030)	0.0877
Labourers	0.730	(0.595, 0.896)	0.0026
Business persons	0.847	(0.718, 1.000)	0.0496
Housewives/husbands & other categories	0.854	(0.713, 1.022)	0.0853
Unknown	0.766	(0.624, 0.939)	0.0102
Betel nut chewing			
No	1.000	—	—
Yes	1.291	(1.093, 1.525)	0.0027
Neck circumference	1.048	(1.033, 1.064)	<.0001
Waist width	1.061	(1.040, 1.081)	<.0001
Left thigh circumference	0.984	(0.972, 0.995)	0.0055
Right upper arm circumference	1.030	(1.016, 1.045)	<0.0001
Hypertension			
No	1.000	—	—
Yes	1.466	(1.315, 1.633)	<0.0001
Unknown	0.770	(0.494, 1.200)	0.2482

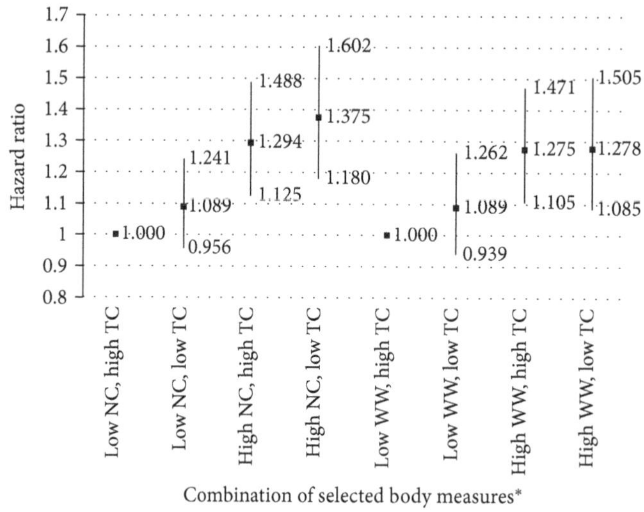

FIGURE 1: Association between body measurement combinations and HRs of T2DM occurrence. *NC: neck circumference; WW: waist width; TC: thigh circumference. Multivariable-adjusted HRs performed by Cox proportional hazard model adjusted for age, sex, education, marital status, occupation, betel nut chewing, and hypertension history.

due to its inability to sufficiently relate to visceral fat. The WHR is useful to determine body size or muscular mass (using the hip circumference). However, it has been criticized because it can be biased by pelvic skeletal structure and width.

This study proposes a combination of NC and WW corrected using TC, as superior, comprehensive, and feasible measurements that can be used to predict future disease, such as insulin resistance and T2DM. Anthropometry is a feasible method that has a well-documented association with body fat distribution and metabolic complications. It is also cheap and easy to practice [39–41] in large population surveys and provides a reliable predictor of an individual's risk of adverse outcomes. Therefore, the measurements proposed in this study could be extended into both clinical practice and preventive medicine in the future.

To increase the accuracy of disease diagnosis, this study used accurate measuring techniques such as comprehensive whole-body scanning, computer-based technology (which reduced measurement errors), a longitudinal cohort analysis (which avoided temporal ambiguity), and national health insurance data tracking. Nevertheless, this study contains certain limitations. First, accurate radiographic measurements were not used to identify and quantify fat deposits; therefore, this study was unable to differentiate between fat tissue and muscular tissue using surface scanning. Secondly, the findings were derived from an Asian population, which serves inferences to the billions of people in Asia (such as in China), but generalizing to Western populations should be done with caution. Thirdly, there are confounders related to the information obtained in relation to the questionnaire and medical records. Some factors such as health-seeking behaviour, psychological measurements, and health knowledge were not determined, but nondifferential misclassification was assumed in this study. Finally, only one-shot measurements of 3D whole-body scanning were obtained, and therefore a study could be designed in the future that employs repeated measurements or records body changes.

5. Conclusions

NC, WW, and TC were found to be comprehensive and innovative measurements for use in independently predicting the occurrence of T2DM over the long term. A combination of NC and WW corrected by TC could be useful measurements for predicting an individual's future risk of developing T2DM. The body measurements shown in this study provide mechanistic conjectures for the early screening and diagnosis of T2DM in clinical practice.

Conflicts of Interest

The authors declare no competing interests.

Authors' Contributions

Ming-Kuo Ting and Pei-Ju Liao contributed equally to this research.

Acknowledgments

This work was supported by the Chang Gung Medical Foundation (CMRPD3F0021, CMRPD3F0022, CMRPD3F0023, CMRPG2F0071, CMRPG2F0072, CMRPG2F0073, CMRPG2F0081, CMRPG2F0082, CMRPG2F0083, and CMRPD3G0101) and the Healthy Aging Research Center of Chang Gung University (EMRPD1H0371, EMRPD1H0551). The authors were indebted to the support, in part, provided by the Wang Jhan-Yang Public Trust Fund (WJY 2017-HR-01, WJY 2018-HR-01). The authors also acknowledged the supports of data linkage by Health and Welfare Data Center, Ministry of Health and Welfare, Taiwan.

References

[1] S. H. Wild, G. Roglic, A. Green, R. Sicree, and H. King, "Global prevalence of diabetes: estimates for the year 2000 and projections for 2030: response to Rathman and Giani," *Diabetes Care*, vol. 27, no. 10, pp. 2569-2570, 2004.

[2] J. C. N. Chan, V. Malik, W. Jia et al., "Diabetes in Asia: epidemiology, risk factors, and pathophysiology," *JAMA*, vol. 301, no. 20, pp. 2129–2140, 2009.

[3] D. E. Laaksonen, H. M. Lakka, L. K. Niskanen, G. A. Kaplan, J. T. Salonen, and T. A. Lakka, "Metabolic syndrome and development of diabetes mellitus: application and validation of recently suggested definitions of the metabolic syndrome in a prospective cohort study," *American Journal of Epidemiology*, vol. 156, no. 11, pp. 1070–1077, 2002.

[4] A. Tchernof and J. P. Després, "Pathophysiology of human visceral obesity: an update," *Physiological Reviews*, vol. 93, no. 1, pp. 359–404, 2013.

[5] G. Vazquez, S. Duval, D. R. Jacobs, and K. Silventoinen, "Comparison of body mass index, waist circumference, and waist/hip ratio in predicting incident diabetes: a meta-analysis," *Epidemiologic Reviews*, vol. 29, no. 1, pp. 115–128, 2007.

[6] S. C. Savva, D. Lamnisos, and A. Kafatos, "Predicting cardiometabolic risk: waist-to-height ratio or BMI. A meta-analysis," *Diabetes, Metabolic Syndrome and Obesity*, vol. 6, pp. 403–419, 2013.

[7] S. R. Preis, J. M. Massaro, S. J. Robins et al., "Abdominal subcutaneous and visceral adipose tissue and insulin resistance in the Framingham Heart Study," *Obesity*, vol. 18, no. 11, pp. 2191–2198, 2010.

[8] M. de Onis and J. P. Habicht, "Anthropometric reference data for international use: recommendations from a World Health Organization Expert Committee," *The American Journal of Clinical Nutrition*, vol. 64, no. 4, pp. 650–658, 1996.

[9] M. C. Pouliot, J. P. Després, S. Lemieux et al., "Waist circumference and abdominal sagittal diameter: best simple anthropometric indexes of abdominal visceral adipose tissue accumulation and related cardiovascular risk in men and women," *The American Journal of Cardiology*, vol. 73, no. 7, pp. 460–468, 1994.

[10] S. R. Preis, J. M. Massaro, U. Hoffmann et al., "Neck circumference as a novel measure of cardiometabolic risk: the Framingham Heart Study," *The Journal of Clinical Endocrinology & Metabolism*, vol. 95, no. 8, pp. 3701–3710, 2010.

[11] M.-A. Cornier, J.-P. Després, N. Davis et al., "Assessing adiposity: a scientific statement from the American Heart Association," *Circulation*, vol. 124, no. 18, pp. 1996–2019, 2011.

[12] L. L. Ben-Noun, E. Sohar, and A. Laor, "Neck circumference as a simple screening measure for identifying overweight and obese patients," *Obesity*, vol. 9, no. 8, pp. 470–477, 2001.

[13] L. L. Ben-Noun and A. Laor, "Relationship of neck circumference to cardiovascular risk factors," *Obesity*, vol. 11, no. 2, pp. 226–231, 2003.

[14] L. L. Ben-Noun and A. Laor, "Relationship between changes in neck circumference and cardiovascular risk factors," *Experimental & Clinical Cardiology*, vol. 11, no. 1, pp. 14–20, 2006.

[15] A. Onat, G. Hergenç, H. Yüksel et al., "Neck circumference as a measure of central obesity: associations with metabolic syndrome and obstructive sleep apnea syndrome beyond waist circumference," *Clinical Nutrition*, vol. 28, no. 1, pp. 46–51, 2009.

[16] C. Li, E. S. Ford, G. Zhao, H. S. Kahn, and A. H. Mokdad, "Waist-to-thigh ratio and diabetes among US adults: the Third National Health and Nutrition Examination Survey," *Diabetes Research and Clinical Practice*, vol. 89, no. 1, pp. 79–87, 2010.

[17] M. B. Snijder, J. M. Dekker, M. Visser et al., "Associations of hip and thigh circumferences independent of waist circumference with the incidence of type 2 diabetes: the Hoorn Study," *The American Journal of Clinical Nutrition*, vol. 77, no. 5, pp. 1192–1197, 2003.

[18] K. H. Hsu, C. P. Shih, and P. J. Liao, "Waist-to-thigh ratio is a predictor of internal organ cancers in humans: findings from a cohort study," *Annals of Epidemiology*, vol. 23, no. 6, pp. 342–348, 2013.

[19] M. B. Snijder, M. Visser, J. M. Dekker et al., "Low subcutaneous thigh fat is a risk factor for unfavourable glucose and lipid levels, independently of high abdominal fat. The Health ABC Study," *Diabetologia*, vol. 48, no. 2, pp. 301–308, 2005.

[20] Y.-C. Chuang, K.-H. Hsu, C.-J. Hwang, P.-M. Hu, T.-M. Lin, and W.-K. Chiou, "Waist-to-thigh ratio can also be a better indicator associated with type 2 diabetes than traditional anthropometrical measurements in Taiwan population," *Annals of Epidemiology*, vol. 16, no. 5, pp. 321–331, 2006.

[21] J. D. Lin, W. K. Chiou, H. F. Weng, Y. H. Tsai, and T. H. Liu, "Comparison of three-dimensional anthropometric body surface scanning to waist–hip ratio and body mass index in correlation with metabolic risk factors," *Journal of Clinical Epidemiology*, vol. 55, no. 8, pp. 757–766, 2002.

[22] C. Y. Yu, Y. H. Lo, and W. K. Chiou, "The 3D scanner for measuring body surface area: a simplified calculation in the Chinese adult," *Applied Ergonomics*, vol. 34, no. 3, pp. 273–278, 2003.

[23] National High Blood Pressure Education Program, "The fifth report of the Joint National Committee on Detection, and Treatment of High Blood Pressure (JNC V)," *Archives of Internal Medicine*, vol. 153, pp. 154–183, 1992.

[24] N. H. Cho, T. J. Oh, K. M. Kim et al., "Neck circumference and incidence of diabetes mellitus over 10 years in the Korean Genome and Epidemiology Study (KoGES)," *Scientific Reports*, vol. 5, no. 1, article 18565, 2015.

[25] M. Khalangot, V. Gurianov, N. Okhrimenko, I. Luzanchuk, and V. Kravchenko, "Neck circumference as a risk factor of screen-detected diabetes mellitus: community-based study," *Diabetology & Metabolic Syndrome*, vol. 8, no. 1, p. 12, 2016.

[26] J. Liang, F. Teng, Y. Li et al., "Neck circumference and insulin resistance in Chinese adults: the Cardiometabolic Risk in Chinese (CRC) study," *Diabetes Care*, vol. 36, no. 9, pp. e145–e146, 2013.

[27] F. He, H. He, W. Liu et al., "Neck circumference might predict gestational diabetes mellitus in Han Chinese women: a nested case–control study," *Journal of Diabetes Investigation*, vol. 8, no. 2, pp. 168–173, 2017.

[28] K. Joshipura, F. Muñoz-Torres, J. Vergara, C. Palacios, and C. M. Pérez, "Neck circumference may be a better alternative to standard anthropometric measures," *Journal of Diabetes Research*, vol. 2016, Article ID 6058916, 8 pages, 2016.

[29] A. Ramachandran, R. C. Wan Ma, and C. Snehalatha, "Diabetes in Asia," *The Lancet*, vol. 375, no. 9712, pp. 408–418, 2010.

[30] K. J. Jung, H. Kimm, J. E. Yun, and S. H. Jee, "Thigh circumference and diabetes: obesity as a potential effect modifier," *Journal of Epidemiology*, vol. 23, no. 5, pp. 329–336, 2013.

[31] J. C. Seidell, T. S. Han, E. J. M. Feskens, and M. E. J. Lean, "Narrow hips and broad waist circumferences independently contribute to increased risk of non-insulin-dependent diabetes mellitus," *Journal of Internal Medicine*, vol. 242, no. 5, pp. 401–406, 1997.

[32] B. A. Larsen, C. L. Wassel, S. B. Kritchevsky et al., "Association of muscle mass, area, and strength with incident diabetes in older adults: the Health ABC Study," *The Journal of Clinical Endocrinology & Metabolism*, vol. 101, no. 4, pp. 1847–1855, 2016.

[33] R. E. van Pelt, E. M. Evans, K. B. Schechtman, A. A. Ehsani, and W. M. Kohrt, "Contributions of total and regional fat mass to risk for cardiovascular disease in older women," *American Journal of Physiology-Endocrinology and Metabolism*, vol. 282, no. 5, pp. E1023–E1028, 2002.

[34] B. L. Heitmann and P. Frederiksen, "Thigh circumference and risk of heart disease and premature death: prospective cohort study," *BMJ*, vol. 339, article b3292, 2009.

[35] I. Janssen, P. T. Katzmarzyk, and R. Ross, "Waist circumference and not body mass index explains obesity-related health risk," *The American Journal of Clinical Nutrition*, vol. 79, no. 3, pp. 379–384, 2004.

[36] B. Falkner and N. D. F. H. Cossrow, "Prevalence of metabolic syndrome and obesity-associated hypertension in the racial ethnic minorities of the United States," *Current Hypertension Reports*, vol. 16, no. 7, p. 449, 2014.

[37] S. Rampal, S. Mahadeva, E. Guallar et al., "Ethnic differences in the prevalence of metabolic syndrome: results from a multi-ethnic population-based survey in Malaysia," *PLoS One*, vol. 7, no. 9, article e46365, 2012.

[38] M. D. DeBoer, "Ethnicity, obesity and the metabolic syndrome: implications on assessing risk and targeting intervention," *Expert Review of Endocrinology & Metabolism*, vol. 6, no. 2, pp. 279–289, 2011.

[39] T. Yoshizumi, T. Nakamura, M. Yamane et al., "Abdominal fat: standardized technique for measurement at CT," *Radiology*, vol. 211, no. 1, pp. 283–286, 1999.

[40] K. Van der Kooy and J. C. Seidell, "Techniques for the measurement of visceral fat: a practical guide," *International Journal of Obesity*, vol. 17, no. 4, pp. 187–196, 1993.

[41] T. Rankinen, S. Y. Kim, L. Pérusse, J. P. Després, and C. Bouchard, "The prediction of abdominal visceral fat level from body composition and anthropometry: ROC analysis," *International Journal of Obesity*, vol. 23, no. 8, pp. 801–809, 1999.

7

Effect of Diacerein on Metabolic Control and Inflammatory Markers in Patients with Type 2 Diabetes using Antidiabetic Agents

Glaucia S. Tres,[1,2] Sandra C. Fuchs,[1] Fabiana Piovesan,[1,2] Patricia Koehler-Santos,[3] Fernanda dos S. Pereira,[3] Suzi Camey,[1,4,5] Hugo K. Lisboa,[2] and Leila B. Moreira[1]

[1]*Postgraduate Program in Cardiology, School of Medicine, Universidade Federal do Rio Grande do Sul (UFRGS), R. Ramiro Barcelos 2600, 90035-003 Porto Alegre, RS, Brazil*
[2]*Hospital São Vicente de Paulo, School of Medicine, Universidade de Passo Fundo (UPF), R. Teixeira Soares 808, 99010-080 Passo Fundo, RS, Brazil*
[3]*Unidade de Análises Moleculares e de Proteínas (UAMP), Hospital de Clinicas de Porto Alegre, Universidade Federal do Rio Grande do Sul (UFRGS), R. Ramiro Barcelos 2350, 90035-903 Porto Alegre, RS, Brazil*
[4]*Department of Statistics, Mathematics Institute, Universidade Federal do Rio Grande do Sul, R. Ramiro Barcelos 2350, 90035-903 Porto Alegre, RS, Brazil*
[5]*Biostatistics Unit, GPPG, Hospital de Clinicas de Porto Alegre, Universidade Federal do Rio Grande do Sul (UFRGS), R. Ramiro Barcelos 2350, 90035-903 Porto Alegre, RS, Brazil*

Correspondence should be addressed to Leila B. Moreira; lbmoreira@hcpa.edu.br

Academic Editor: Craig S. Nunemaker

Introduction. Studies have shown that T2DM is an inflammatory disease. Thus, the present study was aimed at evaluating whether diacerein could improve the metabolic and inflammatory profile among patients with T2DM under long-term treatment with glucose-lowering agents. *Methods.* This is a double-blind, parallel, placebo-controlled trial with 72 participants randomly assigned to diacerein 50 mg or placebo for 12 weeks. The primary endpoint was the between-group difference in change in HbA1c. Secondary endpoints included the proportion of patients achieving metabolic control [HbA1c ≤ 7.0% (53 mmol/mol)] and change in inflammatory mediators. *Results.* Participants in the diacerein group had greater reductions in mean HbA1c level in comparison to placebo (−0.98; 95% CI: −2.02 to 0.05, $P = 0.06$), independently of confounding factors. The difference in HbA1c level was −1.3 (95% CI: −2.3 to −0.4) in favor of diacerein ($P = 0.007$) in those with <14 years of diabetes duration versus 0.05 (−0.7 to 0.8; $P = 0.9$) in those with longer duration. The diacerein group had a 50% increase in the number of participants at the lowest TNF-α level (≤1.46 pg/mL). *Conclusions.* In patients with long-established T2DM under long-term treatment with glucose-lowering agents, diacerein improves metabolic control as measured by HbA1c level and has a favorable impact on inflammatory profile. *Clinical Trial Registry.* This trial is registered with Brazilian Clinical Trials Registry (ReBEC) number RBR-29j956.

1. Introduction

Type 2 diabetes mellitus (T2DM) and obesity-related insulin resistance (IR) have been involved in a state of low-grade chronic inflammation and activation of the immune system [1]. The size of adipocytes might play a role in IR and lipolytic activity, since larger ones release less adiponectin and more inflammatory cytokines [2]. The immune changes that occur in diabetes—changes in the number and activation state of leukocyte populations, increased apoptosis and tissue fibrosis, abnormal cytokine production, elevated levels of acute-phase proteins, and other mediators—have been shown to activate inflammatory pathways [3–5]. Inflammation is related to insulin resistance, which increases pancreatic islet cell mass and insulin secretory activity until insulin deficiency develops [4, 6].

Several mechanisms contribute to beta-cell dysfunction and insulin resistance in T2DM. These mechanisms are strongly interlinked and contribute to tissue inflammation. The main dysfunctions affecting beta cells are glucotoxicity, lipotoxicity, oxidative stress, and amyloid deposition. All lead to activation of the immune system in adipose tissues, liver, pancreatic islets, the vasculature, and leukocytes. Immune adaptations alter levels of cytokines and chemokines, activate leukocyte populations, and increase apoptosis and tissue fibrosis [4].

The inflammatory pathway of T2DM has led to the investigation of drugs that act at different points of the inflammatory orbit. Anti-inflammatory treatment appears to improve insulin sensitivity and glycemic control in insulin-resistant patients with T2DM or inflammatory conditions [7]. In addition, glucose-lowering agents have been associated with anti-inflammatory effects, although it is not known whether this results from better glucose control or their intrinsic pharmacological effect [8]. Recent trials [9–11] of the anti-inflammatory agent diacerein conducted in patients with T2DM have shown improvement on metabolic control in both drug-naïve patients [9] and those under glucose-lowering therapy [10, 11]. Furthermore, diacerein seems to slow deterioration of metabolic control in patients with T2DM and chronic kidney disease [12].

However, most of these studies enrolled T2DM patients within a limited range of age and diabetes duration. In addition, there are few studies assessing the impact of diacerein on the metabolic and anti-inflammatory profile among patients with established disease undergoing long-term treatment, including with insulin. Within this context, the present study was aimed at evaluating whether diacerein could improve the metabolic and inflammatory profile of patients with T2DM under long-term treatment with glucose-lowering agents.

2. Materials and Methods

Patients with T2DM were recruited from the outpatient diabetes clinic of a university hospital in Passo Fundo, Southern Brazil. This randomized, double-blind, parallel, placebo-controlled trial enrolled participants aged 34 to 79 years, who had glycated hemoglobin (HbA1c) $\geq$ 7.4% (57.4 mmol/mol) and <11.0% (97 mmol/mol) and did not have kidney disease. Exclusion criteria included pregnancy, chronic inflammatory diseases such as rheumatoid arthritis and osteoarthritis, use of anti-inflammatory agents for more than five days in the last three months, previous diagnosis of pancreatitis, hypersensitivity to rhein and anthraquinone derivatives, liver disease (transaminases > 2.5 times the upper limit of normal), severe gastrointestinal disease/persistent diarrhea, signs of intercurrent infection, participation in another randomized controlled trial in the last 30 days, or inability to follow the protocol.

The protocol was registered into the Plataforma Brasil clinical trial registry as a precondition for Ethics Committee submission. It was approved by the Ethics Committee of Hospital de Clínicas de Porto Alegre (GPPG number 120482, on December 17, 2012), which is accredited by the US Office of Human Research Protections as an Institutional Review Board. The trial was subsequently registered in the Brazilian Clinical Trials Registry platform (available at http://www.ensaiosclinicos.gov.br/rg/RBR-29j956). Written informed consent was obtained from all participants, according to the principles expressed in the Declaration of Helsinki. This trial was designed, implemented, and described following the provisions of the CONSORT statement.

Participants were randomly assigned in a 1 : 1 ratio to receive either diacerein 50 mg or placebo, twice daily for 12 weeks. The randomization sequence was generated by a web-based randomization software (Random Allocation Software) with permuted-block allocation, with block sizes of four and six. This was done before the start of the trial by an epidemiologist not involved with clinical procedures. Diacerein and placebo capsules, identical in appearance, were stored in bottles labeled using an alphanumeric code. The bottles were stored out of the clinical site, with access controlled by a research assistant. After confirmation of eligibility, each participant received a bottle, ensuring allocation concealment and blinding of intervention to participants, care providers, and those assessing outcomes. Diacerein and placebo were manufactured by a pharmaceutical company (TRB Pharma, Campinas, SP, Brazil). Participants were asked to return for follow-up visits on days 7, 30, 60, and 90 after randomization to verify adherence to treatment and monitor adverse events. Patients in both groups were instructed to maintain their prescribed glucose-lowering agents and dietary recommendations. Adherence to treatment was self-reported and measured by counting the number of pills that were returned at each visit. The trial ended on day 90, when baseline measures were repeated.

The primary endpoint was the difference in change in HbA1c (end of trial minus baseline level), between the placebo and diacerein groups. Secondary endpoints included the proportion of patients achieving metabolic control [HbA1c $\leq$ 7.0% (53 mmol/mol)] and the difference between the two treatment arms in plasma levels of fasting glucose (mg/dL), inflammatory mediators [IL-1β, tumor necrosis factor- (TNF-) α, IL-6, and IL-10], and lipids [high-density lipoprotein cholesterol (HDLc), low-density lipoprotein cholesterol (LDLc), total cholesterol (TC), and triglycerides (TGs)], homeostasis model assessment of insulin resistance (HOMA1-IR), and rate of adverse events. Blood samples were collected after a 12-hour fast by venipuncture from all participants at baseline and at the end of the study. The samples were centrifuged and aliquoted for later analysis. Interleukin levels were measured using a customized Luminex® Human Ultrasensitive magnetic bead panel. Fasting glucose was measured by an enzymatic and colorimetric method and HbA1c by immunoturbidimetric assay.

The assessment included anthropometric measures, 24-hour ambulatory blood pressure monitoring (ABPM), use of statins, and blood pressure-lowering agents. Changes in the dose of glucose-lowering agents were collected in order to identify cointerventions that could affect the efficacy of the study intervention. Hypertension was defined as office

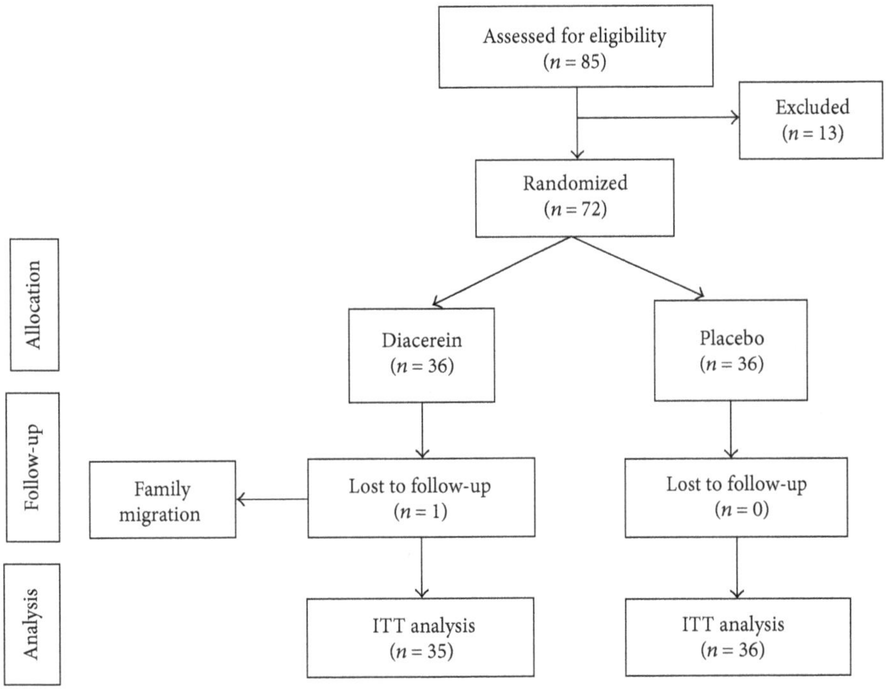

FIGURE 1: Flow diagram of participant selection, randomization, and follow-up.

systolic blood pressure (SBP) ≥ 140 mmHg or diastolic blood pressure (DBP) ≥ 90 mmHg or current treatment with blood pressure-lowering agents.

2.1. Sample Size Calculation and Statistical Analysis. A sample size of 31 participants in each group was estimated to detect a difference of 1.0% (SD ± 1.5) in HbA1c between diacerein and placebo arms, assuming a two-tailed test with significance of 0.05 and power of 80%. To account for possible losses to follow-up during the trial, 36 participants were included in each group. Outcomes were analyzed following the intention-to-treat approach.

Characteristics of the sample were compared between the two groups using Student's *t*-test for continuous variables or Pearson's chi-square test for categorical variables. A general linear model for baseline and end-of-trial measures was applied to analyze the effect of diacerein, and the change from baseline was estimated using analysis of covariance (ANCOVA) with control of baseline values for age, gender, diabetes duration, and change in dosage of glucose-lowering agents during the trial. P values < 0.05 were considered statistically significant. Because of the wide range of diabetes duration, analysis of HbA1c was stratified by diabetes duration (1–13 and 14–30 years) to explore the effect of diacerein in long-established diabetes mellitus. The levels of HbA1c were adjusted for gender and age. Considering the nonnormal distribution of inflammatory markers, they were categorized at the 25th or 75th percentile for baseline and end-of-trial values. The baseline 25th percentile was defined as the cutoff point for IL-6, IL-8, IL-10, leptin, selectin, and adiponectin, as well as the 75th percentile for IL-1β. For TNF-α, the 50th percentile (or median) baseline value was defined as the cutoff point. Poisson regression with a robust estimator was performed to verify the effect of diacerein on inflammatory markers, using the values at the end of the trial as outcomes and adjusting for baseline values. Relative risk and 95% CIs were used to express the association. All analyses were performed using SPSS for Windows (version 17.0; SPSS Inc., Chicago, IL, USA).

3. Results

Among 85 patients with T2DM assessed for eligibility, 72 were enrolled in the trial (36 in each group) and 71 completed the study. Participants attended all scheduled visits, but one participant in the diacerein group moved to another city and did not complete the baseline assessment (Figure 1). The trial was conducted from September 2013 to March 2014.

The baseline characteristics of the participants are shown in Table 1. The mean (SD) age was 62 (8) years in the diacerein group versus 59 (11) years in the placebo group. In both groups, participants, on average, completed six years of formal education, were obese, and had long-established diabetes, hypertension, and well-controlled blood pressure on 24-hour ABPM. Participants in the diacerein group were, on average, older, women, and with higher HbA1c levels, but used metformin less often than those who were taking placebo. About half of all participants were using insulin. Self-reported adherence to the study drug was high in both groups (diacerein, 93.7% ± 14.3; placebo, 92.7% ± 14.8), as well as pill counting, with 88.6% of diacerein-treated patients versus 86% of placebo-treated patients reporting 90% or more intake of the capsules. Although patients were advised to continue their glucose-lowering treatment as at baseline, one patient in the diacerein group and four in the placebo group had treatment modifications.

Table 1: Baseline characteristics of participants randomized to diacerein and placebo.

Characteristics	Diacerein ($n = 35$)	Placebo ($n = 36$)	P value
Age (years)	62 ± 8.0	59 ± 11.3	0.12
Male	20 (57.1)	27 (75.0)	0.11
Years at school	6.4 ± 4.1	5.6 ± 3.0	0.4
Chronic complications of diabetes	18 (51.4)	13 (36.1)	0.19
Cardiovascular disease	14 (40.0)	13 (36.1)	0.7
Hypertension	29 (82.9)	31 (86.1)	0.7
24 h systolic blood pressure (mmHg)	120.3 ± 11.5	123.1 ± 11.4	0.7
24 h diastolic blood pressure (mmHg)	75.0 ± 8.4	72.3 ± 8.1	0.3
Duration of diabetes (years)	14.0 ± 6.7	14.8 ± 6.6	0.7
Duration of diabetes 14–30 years	19 (54.3)	23 (63.9)	0.4
Use of oral hypoglycemic agents‡			
Sulfonylureas	13 (37.1)	12 (33.3)	0.7
Metformin	25 (71.4)	31 (86.1)	0.13
Use of insulin	17 (48.6)	22 (61.1)	0.3
Use of other antidiabetics#	1 (2.9)	4 (11.1)	0.17
Metabolic profile			
HbA1c (%)	9.1 ± 1.4	8.6 ± 1.0	0.11
HbA1c (mmol/mol)	76.7 ± 2.4	71.2 ± 2.4	0.11
Fasting glucose (mg/dL)	142.0 ± 69.5	138.7 ± 58.2	0.8
HOMA-IR	5.4 ± 1.0	6.5 ± 1.0	0.4
Lipids			
Total cholesterol (mg/dL)	149 ± 32.7	152.7 ± 34.8	0.6
HDLc (mg/dL)	42.1 ± 7.4	42.8 ± 8.0	0.7
LDLc (mg/dL)	73.0 ± 35.6	78.5 ± 35.5	0.3
Triglycerides (mg/dL)	200.5 ± 124.4	202.4 ± 210.5	1.0
Renal			
Creatinine (mg/dL)	0.93 ± 0.15	0.87 ± 0.17	0.11
eGFR (mL/min/1.73 m^2)	77.0 ± 13.1	83.5 ± 23.5	0.13
Urinary albumin/creatinine ratio (mg/24 h)	9.9 ± 6.6	10.8 ± 6.8	0.6
Hepatic			
ALT (units/L)	23.5 ± 11.1	23.1 ± 11.3	0.9
AST (units/L)	24.7 ± 11.8	21.9 ± 8.1	0.2
Gamma-glutamyltransferase (units/L)	43.4 ± 26.4	36.1 ± 20.6	0.2
Hematologic/inflammatory			
Hematocrit (%)	42.0 ± 4.9	41.7 ± 4.3	0.8
Platelet count ($\times 10^9$ cells/L)	215.0 ± 55.7	221.8 ± 60.0	0.6
C-reactive protein (mg/L)	7.0 ± 6.2	9.0 ± 16.4	0.5
Anthropometric assessment			
Weight (kg)	80.3 ± 19.8	78.7 ± 13.1	0.7
Height (m)	1.62 ± 0.10	1.59 ± 0.07	0.16
Body mass index (kg/m^2)	30.8 ± 6.9	31.3 ± 5.2	0.7

Data expressed as mean ± SD and n (%). ‡Numbers exceed 100% due to use of more than one agent. #Alpha-glucosidase inhibitors, meglitinides, DPP4 inhibitors, and amylin mimetics.

Table 2 shows that participants in the diacerein group had greater reduction in mean HbA1c level compared to the placebo arm, independently of age, gender, duration of diabetes, and addition of a new antidiabetic drug. The adjusted difference in mean change (−0.98; 95% CI: −2.02 to 0.05) had a P value of 0.06. As shown on exploratory analysis (Figure 2), the most striking reduction in glycated hemoglobin was observed among participants in the diacerein group who had shorter duration of diabetes mellitus. The difference in HbA1c level was −1.3 (95% CI: −2.3 to −0.4) in favor of diacerein ($P = 0.007$) in the <14 years of diabetes duration versus 0.05 (−0.7 to 0.8), with $P = 0.9$, in

TABLE 2: Mean values during the 12-week treatment and adjusted differences in mean changes between diacerein and placebo for the trial outcomes (mean ± SE).

	Diacerein ($n = 35$)		Placebo ($n = 36$)		Adjusted difference in mean change (diacerein-placebo)*	P value
	End of trial	Change from baseline	End of trial	Change from baseline		
Metabolic profile						
HbA1c (%)	8.1 ± 0.2	−0.98 ± 0.2	8.1 ± 0.2	−0.52 ± 0.2	−0.98 (−2.02 to 0.05)	0.06
HbA1c (mmol/mol)	65.9 ± 2.6	−10.8 ± 2.4	65.5 ± 2.6	−5.7 ± 2.3	−10.8 (−22.0 to 0.5)	0.06
Fasting glucose (mg/dL)	146.3 ± 13.1	4.3 ± 11.9	150.4 ± 12.9	11.8 ± 11.8	−19.8 (−78.3 to 38.5)	0.5
HOMA-IR	5.3 ± 0.8	−0.18 ± 0.7	6.2 ± 0.8	−0.27 ± 0.7	1.0 (−2.6 to 4.6)	0.6
Lipids						
Total cholesterol (mg/dL)	148.7 ± 5.5	−0.3 ± 4.6	151.1 ± 5.2	−1.6 ± 4.5	−0.12 (−22.9 to 22.6)	1.0
HDLc (mg/dL)	41.3 ± 1.3	−0.8 ± 0.9	42.8 ± 6.9	−0.03 ± 0.8	−2.2 (−6.4 to 2.1)	0.3
LDLc (mg/dL)	79.9 ± 5.1	6.8 ± 6.1	78.2 ± 5.0	−3.2 ± 6.0	20.1 (−10.4 to 50.5)	0.19
Triglycerides (mg/dL)	153.1 ± 17.7	−47.4 ± 23.2	164.7 ± 17.4	−37.7 ± 22.9	−78.7 (−193.4 to 36.1)	0.18
Renal						
Creatinine (mg/dL)	1.0 ± 0.04	0.06 ± 0.03	1.0 ± 0.04	0.03 ± 0.03	0.12 (−0.03 to 0.26)	0.11
eGFR (mL/min/1.73 m^2)	73.9 ± 3.2	−3.1 ± 1.9	81.7 ± 3.2	−1.8 ± 1.9	−7.7 (−17.3 to 1.9)	0.12
Urinary albumin/creatinine ratio (mg/24 h)	24.0 ± 5.6	14.1 ± 5.2	27.3 ± 5.5	16.5 ± 5.2	6.0 (−19.4 to 31.4)	0.6
Hepatic						
ALT (units/L)	24.4 ± 2.4	0.9 ± 1.6	25.1 ± 2.4	2.0 ± 1.5	0.5 (−6.5 to 7.5)	0.8
AST (units/L)	27.1 ± 2.3	2.4 ± 1.5	26.2 ± 2.3	4.3 ± 1.5	−0.6 (−8.0 to 6.8)	0.9
Gamma-glutamyltransferase (units/L)	44.9 ± 4.9	1.5 ± 2.4	39.3 ± 4.8	3.2 ± 2.3	−7.7 (−19.3 to 4.0)	0.19
Hematologic/inflammatory						
Hematocrit (%)	42.7 ± 0.8	0.8 ± 0.8	43.4 ± 0.8	1.7 ± 0.8	0.5 (−3.6 to 4.5)	0.8
Platelet count (×10^9 cells/L)	230 ± 10.2	15.03 ± 7.3	236 ± 10.0	14.6 ± 7.2	−5.1 (−41.6 to 31.4)	0.8
C-reactive protein (mg/L)	9.0 ± 2.5	2.0 ± 3.3	12.3 ± 2.5	3.3 ± 3.2	−9.8 (−25.3 to 5.7)	0.2
Anthropometric assessment						
Weight (kg)	77.6 ± 2.6	−2.7 ± 0.7	77.3 ± 2.6	−1.4 ± 0.7	−2.4 (−5.6 to 0.9)	0.16
Body mass index (kg/m^2)	29.8 ± 1.0	−1.0 ± 0.2	30.8 ± 1.0	−0.6 ± 0.2	−0.8 (−2.0 to 0.4)	0.19

*Mean adjusted for age, gender, duration of diabetes, and addition of new antidiabetic drugs.

the 14–30 years in the diabetes duration group. Assessment of HbA1c at baseline and at the end of the trial for each treatment group showed that, in the subgroup with longer duration of diabetes, there was a crude reduction of one percentage point in both the diacerein (9.6 ± 1.7 to 8.7 ± 1.5) and placebo (8.7 ± 1.1 to 7.7 ± 1.3) groups. In the subgroup with <14 years of diabetes duration, diacerein reduced HbA1c by one percentage point (8.7 ± 1.0 to 7.6 ± 1.3), with no appreciable change in the placebo group (8.6 ± 1.1 to 8.9 ± 1.3). Figure 2 shows that both groups of patients, independent of duration of T2DM, had HbA1c levels decreased by about one percentage point at the end of the trial; in the shorter T2DM duration subgroup, the placebo group exhibited a noticeable increase in HbA1c, while in the longer T2DM duration subgroup, there had been a reduction of approximately one percentage point, independently of gender and age. Plotting diabetes duration against HbA1C yielded a Spearman correlation coefficient of 0.42 ($P = 0.01$) for the diacerein group and 0.27 ($P = 0.12$) for the placebo group.

There were no statistically significant differences between groups in fasting glucose, HOMA-IR, and serum lipid levels; renal, hepatic, hematological, and inflammatory parameters; or anthropometric assessment (Table 2).

The results of the inflammatory markers are shown in Table 3. The diacerein group had a 50% increase in the number of participants at the lowest level of TNF-α (≤1.46 pg/mL) at the end of the trial, independently of baseline values. Adjusting for confounding factors (the same variables described in Table 2) did not change this result.

Table 4 shows a similar distribution of adverse effects between diacerein and placebo, except for a higher frequency of dark urine in the former. Five other symptoms, including diarrhea and nausea, were more often reported by participants in the diacerein group, but there was no drug-related discontinuation of treatment.

4. Discussion

This randomized controlled trial assessed the effect of diacerein (versus placebo) as an adjunctive agent in the treatment of T2DM in patients receiving antidiabetic drugs. Diacerein was able to reduce HbA1c in comparison to placebo ($P = 0.06$), but the difference became statistically

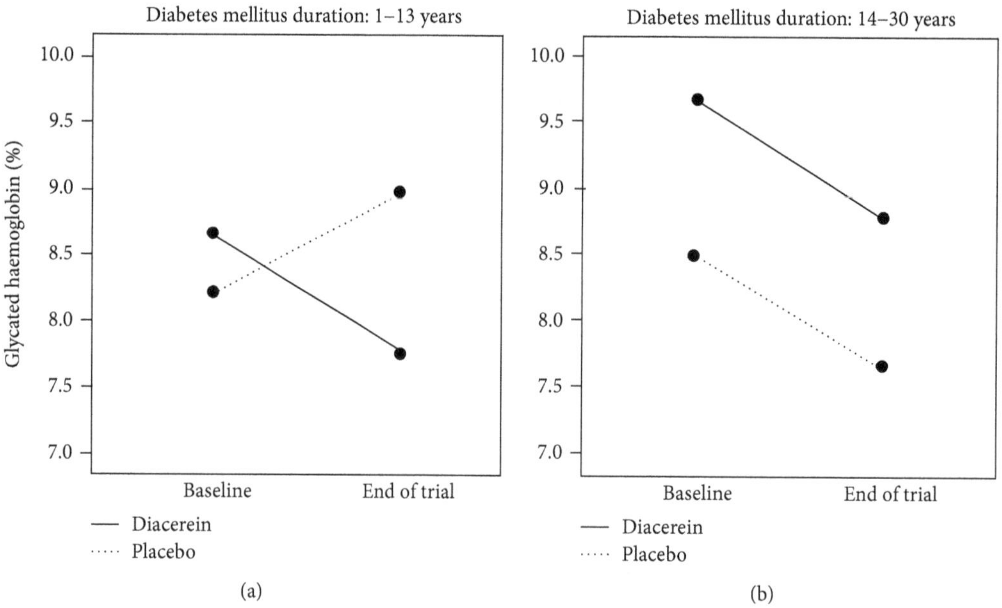

Figure 2: End-of-trial changes in HbA1c (%) in the diacerein and placebo groups, stratified by duration of diabetes < 14 (a) or ≥14 years (b), independently of age and gender.

Table 3: Effect of diacerein on inflammatory markers at end of trial.

	Diacerein ($n = 35$)	Placebo ($n = 36$)	RR (95% CI)*	P value
α − Tumor necrosis factor ≤ 1.46 (pg/mL)	23 (65.7)	14 (38.9)	1 (1.04–2.1)	0.03
Interleukin − 1β > 1.23	8 (22.9)	15 (41.7)	0.7 (0.4–1.3)	0.3
Interleukin − 6 ≤ 10.7	17 (48.6)	14 (38.9)	1.4 (0.9–2.2)	0.19
Interleukin − 8 ≤ 29.53	6 (17.1)	2 (5.6)	3.1 (0.7–14.8)	0.15
Interleukin − 10 ≤ 5.25	10 (28.6)	5 (13.9)	1.8 (0.7–4.6)	0.19
Leptin ≤ 10.3	11 (31.4)	6 (16.7)	1.4 (0.8–2.6)	0.3
Selectin ≤ 53.4	6 (17.1)	16 (44.4)	0.6 (0.3–1.2)	0.14
Adiponectin ≤ 11.8	15 (42.9)	17 (47.2)	0.8 (0.5–1.2)	0.4

Data expressed as n (%) and relative risk (95%CI). *Relative risk adjusted for baseline values of the inflammatory markers.

Table 4: Frequency of adverse events in each treatment group.

Adverse events	Diacerein ($n = 35$)	Placebo ($n = 36$)	P
Nausea	6 (17.1)	3 (8.3)	0.3
Vomiting	1 (2.9)	4 (11.1)	0.2
Diarrhea	10 (28.6)	6 (16.7)	0.2
Abdominal pain	4 (11.4)	4 (11.1)	1.0
Dark urine	21 (7.4)	8 (2.9)	0.001
Others	5 (14.3)	0	0.03

Data expressed as n (%).

significant for participants who had shorter duration of diabetes mellitus. Among participants with long-established T2DM, diacerein and placebo both reduced the HbA1c levels; therefore, there was no effect [0.05 (95% CI: −0.7 to 0.8)]. On the other hand, in participants with shorter duration of diabetes, diacerein was associated with one percentage point reduction, while in the placebo group, there was a noticeable increase in HbA1C level after controlling for age and gender. The effect toward better control of diabetes is consistent with the decrease in TNF-α level observed in the diacerein group at the end of the trial. Diacerein reduced the proportion of participants with abnormal levels comparatively to the placebo group, as detected by a 50% increase in the number of participants who migrated to the lowest percentile.

This trial was carried out in T2DM patients with long-established disease and undergoing long-term treatment with metformin, sulfonylureas, or insulin. In two previous studies [9, 10], diacerein was evaluated in small samples, among T2DM patients under the age of 60, who were drug-naïve or receiving metformin as monotherapy for diabetes. Ramos-Zavala et al. [9] evaluated the efficacy of diacerein in 40 drug-naïve patients with newly diagnosed T2DM and HbA1c levels between 7% (53 mmol/mol) and 9% (75 mmol/mol) and found a significant absolute reduction of 1.3% (14.2 mmol/mol) in HbA1c as well as in TNF-α and

IL-1β levels. Villar et al. [10] evaluated 12 patients receiving metformin as monotherapy and found a significant improvement of glycemic control, with reduction of HbA1c and glucose levels. Cardoso et al. [11] selected 84 patients aged less than 75 years, receiving full glucose-lowering treatment, who were randomized to diacerein or placebo with 48 weeks of follow-up. The diacerein group had a 0.35% reduction in HbA1c compared to the placebo group at week 24 of treatment, but this effect was attenuated to a nonsignificant difference at week 48. Participants had a median disease duration of 10 years (interquartile range: 6–18 years). The results of these trials point in the same direction, that is, a reduction in HbA1c in patients who receive diacerein. However, there are striking differences between the present trial and those of Ramos-Zavala and Cardoso, both of which selected patients who were receiving no treatment for diabetes or only monotherapy. Our trial is more similar to that of Cardoso et al. [11]. However, we enrolled patients up to 79 years of age and with longer duration of diabetes and followed participants for a longer time. These differences raised the need to evaluate the effect of diacerein by taking into account the duration of diabetes, which was done in an exploratory analysis.

The reduction in HbA1c levels was not followed by a reduction in HOMA-IR levels, suggesting that the effect of diacerein may have been on insulin secretion. Studies have shown that T2DM is an inflammatory disease. Adipose tissue appears to play a central role in the induction of inflammation, leading to the production of proinflammatory cytokines, particularly TNF-α and IL-1β. These cytokines induce β-cell dysfunction, with subsequent apoptosis and insulin deficiency [4]. However, few controlled studies have tested drugs that play a role in the inhibition of proinflammatory cytokines and their receptors in patients with T2DM. Drugs with anti-inflammatory action may be more effective in the early stages of the disease, when functional impairment of pancreatic β-cells is less severe, with a better chance of regaining their function, thus contributing to the main effect of lowering HbA1c levels among those with a shorter duration of diabetes. Malaguti et al. [13], in an experimental study, tested diacerein in nonobese diabetic mice aiming to investigate anti-inflammatory properties and their potential effects on type 1 diabetes. The results showed that diacerein, via modulation of proinflammatory cytokines (IL-1β and TNF-α), interferes with the onset of type 1 diabetes and may alter the incidence of autoimmune diabetes in treated animals. These findings are consistent with the reduced TNF-α observed in this study of T2DM patients. Although autoimmune mediators are not typical of this condition, inflammation may potentially lead to β-cell apoptosis. Another experimental study in obese mice suggests that diacerein may be a potential alternative treatment to reverse or improve clinical features of obesity-related T2DM and insulin resistance [14].

The present study has some limitations that should be noted. The size of the sample and the relatively short duration of the intervention, considering the long-standing nature of T2DM, precluded assessment of the long-term efficacy and safety of diacerein. In addition, our findings do not allow us to draw any conclusion about the effects of diacerein among patients with poor metabolic control, since patients with HbA1c ≥ 11.0% (97 mmol/mol) were excluded. Finally, the effect on the subgroup with shorter duration of diabetes should be viewed with caution, as this was a post hoc analysis.

In conclusion, diacerein therapy in patients with long-established T2DM and long-term use of glucose-lowering agents improves metabolic control as measured by HbA1c level and has a favorable impact on the inflammatory profile. Thus, the use of diacerein may be beneficial in counteracting the adverse consequences of diabetes. However, further studies with a larger sample size, including participants exposed to diacerein with shorter and longer duration of diabetes, are needed to confirm these findings.

Disclosure

The sponsors had no involvement in the design and conduct of the study, including the objectives and collection, analysis, and interpretation of the data, or in the preparation, review, or approval of the manuscript.

Conflicts of Interest

The authors declare that there is no conflict of interest regarding the publication of this article.

Acknowledgments

The authors acknowledge Dr. F. D. Fuchs from the School of Medicine, Universidade Federal do Rio Grande do Sul, for manuscript revision and suggestions. This work was supported by the National Council of Research (CNPq; Process no.: 480451/2012-5) and by a research funding of Hospital de Clínicas de Porto Alegre (GPPG: FIPE-HCPA; no.: 12-0482), Porto Alegre, Brazil.

References

[1] N. Esser, S. Legrand-Poels, J. Piette, A. J. Scheen, and N. Paquot, "Inflammation as a link between obesity, metabolic syndrome and type 2 diabetes," *Diabetes Research and Clinical Practice*, vol. 105, no. 2, pp. 141–150, 2014.

[2] B. Gustafson, "Adipose tissue, inflammation and atherosclerosis," *Journal of Atherosclerosis and Thrombosis*, vol. 17, no. 4, pp. 332–341, 2010.

[3] X. Wang, W. Bao, J. Liu et al., "Inflammatory markers and risk of type 2 diabetes: a systematic review and meta-analysis," *Diabetes Care*, vol. 36, no. 1, pp. 166–175, 2013.

[4] M. Y. Donath and S. E. Shoelson, "Type 2 diabetes as an inflammatory disease," *Nature Reviews Immunology*, vol. 11, no. 2, pp. 98–107, 2011.

[5] G. S. Hotamisligil, "Inflammation and metabolic disorders," *Nature*, vol. 444, no. 7121, pp. 860–867, 2006.

[6] R. P. Robertson, J. Harmon, P. O. Tran, and V. Poitout, "β-Cell glucose toxicity, lipotoxicity, and chronic oxidative stress in type 2 diabetes," *Diabetes*, vol. 53, Supplement 1, pp. S119–S124, 2004.

[7] N. Esser, N. Paquot, and A. J. Scheen, "Anti-inflammatory agents to treat or prevent type 2 diabetes, metabolic syndrome and cardiovascular disease," *Expert Opinion on Investigational Drugs*, vol. 24, no. 3, pp. 283–307, 2015.

[8] A. J. Scheen, N. Esser, and N. Paquot, "Antidiabetic agents: potential anti-inflammatory activity beyond glucose control," *Diabetes & Metabolism*, vol. 41, no. 3, pp. 183–194, 2015.

[9] M. G. Ramos-Zavala, M. Gonzalez-Ortiz, E. Martinez-Abundis, J. A. Robles-Cervantes, R. Gonzalez-Lopez, and N. J. Santiago-Hernandez, "Effect of diacerein on insulin secretion and metabolic control in drug-naïve patients with type 2 diabetes," *Diabetes Care*, vol. 34, no. 7, pp. 1591–1594, 2011.

[10] M. M. Villar, E. Martínez-Abundis, R. O. Preciado-Márquez, and M. González-Ortiz, "Effect of diacerein as an add-on to metformin in patients with type 2 diabetes mellitus and inadequate glycemic control," *Archives of Endocrinology and Metabolism*, vol. 61, no. 2, pp. 188–192, 2017.

[11] C. R. L. Cardoso, N. C. Leite, F. O. Carlos, A. A. Loureiro, B. B. Viegas, and G. F. Salles, "Efficacy and safety of diacerein in patients with inadequately controlled type 2 diabetes: a randomized controlled trial," *Diabetes Care*, vol. 40, no. 10, pp. 1356–1363, 2017.

[12] F. Piovesan, G. S. Tres, L. B. Moreira, M. E. Andrades, H. K. Lisboa, and S. C. Fuchs, "Effect of diacerein on renal function and inflammatory cytokines in participants with type 2 diabetes mellitus and chronic kidney disease: a randomized controlled trial," *PLoS One*, vol. 12, no. 10, article e0186554, 2017.

[13] C. Malaguti, C. A. Vilella, K. P. Vieira, G. H. M. F. Souza, S. Hyslop, and R. de Lima Zollner, "Diacerhein downregulate proinflammatory cytokines expression and decrease the autoimmune diabetes frequency in nonobese diabetic (NOD) mice," *International Immunopharmacology*, vol. 8, no. 6, pp. 782–791, 2008.

[14] N. Tobar, A. G. Oliveira, D. Guadagnini et al., "Diacerhein improves glucose tolerance and insulin sensitivity in mice on a high-fat diet," *Endocrinology*, vol. 152, no. 11, pp. 4080–4093, 2011.

8

Physical Activity Patterns and Risk of Type 2 Diabetes and Metabolic Syndrome in Middle-Aged and Elderly Northern Chinese Adults

Qian Wang,[1,2,3] **Xu Zhang**,[1,2,3] **Li Fang**,[1,2,3] **Qingbo Guan**,[1,2,3] **Ling Gao**,[2,3,4] **and Qiu Li**[1,2,3]

[1]*Department of Endocrinology, Shandong Provincial Hospital Affiliated to Shandong University, Jinan, Shandong, China*
[2]*Shandong Clinical Medical Center of Endocrinology and Metabolism, Jinan, Shandong, China*
[3]*Institute of Endocrinology and Metabolism, Shandong Academy of Clinical Medicine, Jinan, Shandong, China*
[4]*Scientific Center, Shandong Provincial Hospital Affiliated to Shandong University, Jinan, Shandong, China*

Correspondence should be addressed to Ling Gao; gaoling1@medmail.com.cn and Qiu Li; liqiu10@163.com

Academic Editor: Maria Pia Francescato

The main aim of this study is to quantitatively describe the status of physical activity and evaluate its levels in a rural population and to investigate the association between the quantifiable physical activity and type 2 diabetes and metabolic syndrome. In total, 2076 participants aged over 40 years were included in a cross-sectional analysis. Physical activity status and the contributions of different types of activity were evaluated. The association between social behaviors and physical activities was analyzed. In addition, the impact of physical activities on type 2 diabetes mellitus and metabolic syndrome was also analyzed by logistic regression. Approximately half of the total activity in rural areas consisted of work-related activity (49.3%) followed by commuting (30.2%) and recreational activity (20.5%). In rural areas, the prevalence of physical activity levels was 28.6% for low levels, 47.3% for moderate levels, and 24.1% for high levels. Educational level showed a significant negative association with the physical activity level. Lower physical activity shows a strong and significant association with type 2 diabetes and metabolic syndrome. In conclusion, insufficient physical activity among rural people over 40 years old increases the risk of type 2 diabetes and metabolic syndrome. Population-wide and individualized guidelines for physical activities especially recreational physical activities should be developed.

1. Introduction

Insufficient physical activity (PA) is now an important topic in healthcare education, especially in the context of non-communicable diseases (NCDs) because of the high risk for cardiovascular and metabolic diseases [1]. The absence of PA is also considered an urgent public health problem worldwide [2–4]. Previous research showed that insufficient PA is already a global public health concern and is increasing rapidly especially in low-income countries.

The prevalence and incidence of diabetes mellitus (DM) and metabolic syndrome (MS) are increasing rapidly worldwide, including in China. In China, the prevalence of DM and MS was 11.6% and 33.9%, respectively, in 2010 [5, 6]. Similarly, the development of DM in rural areas of China has sharply increased from less than 1% in 1980 to 10.3% in 2010 [5, 7]. In addition, type 2 diabetes (T2DM) is the predominant form of DM [8]. Although urbanization is speeding up in recent years, the rural Chinese population is still very large. Prior to 2015, 44% of the population lived in rural areas of China. Therefore, the prevention and control of T2DM and MS are urgent issues in rural areas.

Although drug therapies have been shown to be effective in the treatment of these diseases, these therapies are expensive and may have side effects. In contrast, adopting a healthy lifestyle has become one of the major approaches to easing the burden of glucose and lipid metabolic disorders. In a cross-sectional population study that controlled for body mass index (BMI) and fat distribution, PA was negatively associated with the mean of the fasting and postload insulin concentrations in two populations at risk for diabetes [9]. Other studies also showed an important role of supervised exercise interventions in lowering glycemic and lipid profile [10–12]. In the recent years, it has become essential to update the reports to including updated PA data in light of the relationship between PA and NCDs and the increasing prevalence of T2DM and MS.

The human lifestyle has changed dramatically around the world as rapid economic development has occurred. Research showed that the prevalence of low PA among individuals aged 15 or older varied from 2.6% to 62.3% [1]. The available data indicated that low PA is increasing rapidly in developing countries. For the past few years, PA levels have been assessed using the Global PA Questionnaire (GPAQ) that is used for many epidemiologic studies of DM and cardiovascular outcomes worldwide [5, 13]. However, few studies in China have assessed PA quantitatively with a worldwide activity questionnaire. The main aim of this study is to describe the status of PA in a rural Chinese population and to review the epidemiological evidence regarding the association between insufficient PA and social or morbidity factors such as T2DM and MS.

2. Methods

2.1. Study Population. The data are from the REACTION study, which aimed to investigate the epidemiology of metabolic diseases in China [14]. All of the eligible participants were over 40 years old and had been living at their current residence in each community or village for at least 5 years. The study protocol was authorized by the ethics committee of Shanghai Jiao Tong University [14]. All participants signed the informed consent before the examination.

2.2. Data Collection. Data collection was performed at local health stations by a trained medical staff. A well-established questionnaire was administered by trained interviewers through a face-to-face survey. A current smoker was defined as someone who smoked more than 100 cigarettes in the lifetime and who was currently smoking cigarettes at the time of the survey. Current drinking was defined as alcohol intake more than once a month for the past 12 months. Weight was measured in kilograms while height was measured in centimeters. Waist circumference (WC) was measured at the umbilical level with the participants in the standing position. BMI was calculated as weight (kg) divided by squared height (m^2). Blood pressure was measured at the nondominant arm three times in succession with a 3 min interval between the measurements, which was performed in a sitting position. The three readings were then averaged for data analysis. Each participant with no history of DM underwent an oral glucose tolerance test. Blood samples were collected from all participants after an overnight fast of at least 10 hours. DM- and MS-related parameters were determined. Homeostasis model assessment-insulin resistance (HOMA-IR) was estimated as fasting insulin concentration (IU/mL) × fasting plasma glucose (mmol/L)/22.5, and homeostasis model assessment of β-cell function (HOMA-β) was evaluated as fasting insulin concentration (IU/mL) × 20/(fasting plasma glucose (mmol/L) − 3.5).

2.3. Measurement of PA. PA data were collected through a face-to-face interview by using GPAQ. GPAQ was created by the World Health Organization to monitor PA and is used to measure PA levels. The questionnaire contains 16 questions about a typical or usual week of behavior [15]. PA was divided into three domains (work, transportation, and leisure time), and the frequency (days) and duration (minutes/hours) of moderate and vigorous intensities of PA and of sedentary behavior were recorded [15]; this information can be used to convert PA data to energy expenditure. Metabolic equivalent tasks (METs) are commonly used for quantifying PA. In addition, the three domains of PA are defined as working PA, transportation PA, and leisure time PA (LTPA). One MET is defined as the basic energy cost of sitting quietly (equivalent to a caloric consumption of 1 kcal/kg/hour) [15]. A person's caloric consumption at a moderate PA level is four times as much as that at the sitting level, and the consumption at vigorous level is eight times as much as that at the sitting level. The total activity is computed as the sum of all levels of PA performed in the three domains [15]. The normal PA level of each participant was classified as low, moderate, or high. The criteria for estimating the level are listed below. High-level classification is meeting any of the following criteria: (a) at least 25 MET hours/week of activity at a vigorous level for at least three days or (b) at least 50 MET hours/week of activity with any combination of levels for seven or more days. Moderate-level classification is meeting any of the following criteria and not meeting the high-level criteria: (a) PA at a vigorous level for at least 20 minutes per day for at least three days, (b) PA at a moderate level for at least 30 minutes for at least three days, or (c) PA for at least 10 MET hours/week of any combination for at least five days. Low-level classification is not meeting any of the abovementioned criteria in this category.

2.4. Definitions of T2DM and MS. According to the Chinese guideline for T2DM [16], a person was diagnosed with T2DM if the person met one or more of the following criteria: (1) typical symptoms of T2DM and a random plasma glucose level of 11.1 mmol/L or higher, (2) a fasting plasma glucose level of 7.0 mmol/L or higher, or (3) a 2-hour plasma glucose level of 11.1 mmol/L or higher. In addition, participants diagnosed with type 1 diabetes or other types of DM were excluded. If no typical symptoms were shown, the test should be repeated on another day. MS was diagnosed if three or more of the following criteria were met [16]: (1) abdominal obesity, WC ≥ 90 cm for male participants or WC ≥ 85 cm for female participants; (2) hyperglycemia, a fasting plasma glucose level of 6.1 mmol/L or higher or a 2 h plasma glucose level of 7.8 mmol/L or higher, with a diagnosis of T2DM; (3) hypertension, blood pressure of 130/85 or higher, with a diagnosis of hypertension; (4) high triglyceride, fasting plasma triglyceride of 1.7 mmol/L or higher; or (5) high-

Table 1: General characteristics of the participants.

	Overall ($n = 2076$)	Men ($n = 980$)	Women ($n = 1096$)	$p^{\dagger}$
Age (year)	55.1 ± 8.5	56.1 ± 8.5	54.3 ± 8.4	<0.001
WC (cm)	88.6 ± 10.1	90.6 ± 9.9	86.8 ± 9.9	<0.001
BMI (kg/m^2)	25.3 ± 3.6	25.2 ± 3.6	25.5 ± 3.7	0.846
Systolic blood pressure (mmHg)	137.4 ± 20.4	140.3 ± 19.5	134.8 ± 20.7	<0.001
TG (mmol/L)	1.5 ± 1.2	1.6 ± 1.4	1.4 ± 1.1	<0.001
LDL-C (mmol/L)	2.9 ± 0.9	2.9 ± 0.9	2.9 ± 0.8	0.800
HDL-C (mmol/L)	1.4 ± 0.4	1.3 ± 0.4	1.4 ± 0.3	<0.001
TC (mmol/L)	4.9 ± 1.1	4.9 ± 1.2	4.9 ± 1.1	0.607
Fasting plasma glucose (mmol/L)	6.4 ± 2.0	6.5 ± 1.9	6.4 ± 2.1	0.175
2-Hour plasma glucose (mmol/L)	9.7 ± 4.7	10.0 ± 4.8	9.4 ± 4.6	0.013
Current smoker, %	16.3	31.2	0.9	<0.001
Former smoker, %	15.7	29.4	3.4	<0.001
Current drinker, %	18.4	36.8	1.8	<0.001
Former drinker, %	21.0	29.3	13.6	<0.001
T2DM, %	26.0	28.2	24.1	0.035
MS, %	41.2	45.7	37.2	<0.001

Data are expressed as mean ± standard deviation or as percentage. $^{\dagger}p$ were analyzed between the variables of men and women. WC: waist circumference; BMI: body mass index; HDL-C: high-density lipoprotein cholesterol; LDL-C: low-density lipoprotein cholesterol; TC: total cholesterol; TG: triglyceride; n: number of subjects.

density lipoprotein cholesterol (HDL-C), fasting plasma HDL-C lower than 1.04 mmol/L. Overweight was defined as a BMI of 24.0 to 27.9, and obesity was defined as a BMI of 28.0 or higher [16].

2.5. Definitions of High BMI, High HOMA-IR, and Low HOMA-β. The definition of high BMI was 25.0 kg/m^2 or higher and was based on the China Diabetes Guideline [17]. We close the other cut-off points at the 50th percentiles because of the lack of definitive criteria for HOMA-IR and HOMA-β for the Chinese population.

2.6. Data Analysis. PA and different types of PA were evaluated in the overall population and in the subgroups according to sex, age, BMI, WC, smoking, drinking, and education. Differences between mean values were tested using Student's t-test. The chi-squared test was used to analyze whether there were any statistically significant differences in the prevalence of the various PA levels for the different stratifications. Logistic regression models were used to analyze the association between social behaviors and PA. Adjusted odds ratios (OR) were calculated with 95% confidence intervals (95% CIs). The association between PA types and T2DM or MS was also analyzed with logistic regression. The relationships between PA levels and some related parameters such as BMI, HOMA-IR, and HOMA-β were also analyzed with logistic regression.

3. Result

3.1. Sociodemographic Characteristics. The basic characteristics of the total subject population ($n = 2076$, mean age 55.2 ± 8.5 years) are presented in Table 1. Age, WC, triglyceride, HDL-C, and 2-hour plasma glucose were significantly different between men and women ($p < 0.05$). In addition, men accounted for 47.2% of the total participants, while women account for 52.8%. Among the total subject population, the prevalence of T2DM and MS was 26.0% and 41.2%, respectively. There were significant differences in the prevalence of both T2DM ($p = 0.035$) and MS ($p < 0.001$) when the participants were grouped by sex.

3.2. PA Status and Types of PA. Total PA, working PA, LTPA, transportation PA, and the contributions of each domain are shown in Table 2. Working and transportation PAs were the major components of the total PA. Approximately half of the total activity was contributed by working PA (49.3%) followed by transportation PA (30.2%) and LTPA (20.5%). Generally, with increases in age, educational level, and WC, total PA tended to decrease. No trend in total PA was found when the participants were grouped by BMI.

3.3. Prevalence of PA Levels (Low, Moderate, and High). According to the classification criteria, the prevalence of PA levels in the overall papulation was 28.6% for low levels, 47.3% for moderate levels, and 24.1% for high levels (Table 3). The prevalence of low PA was higher in men (29.4%) than in women (27.8%), but the difference was not significant. No trends in prevalence were found when we classified the prevalence of the various PA levels by BMI. The prevalence of a high PA level decreased as the educational level increased ($p < 0.001$).

3.4. Associations between Total PA and Educational Levels, Smoking, and Drinking. As presented in Table 4, the logistic regression model showed a significant negative association between the educational level and PA levels (low and moderate levels versus a high level) after adjusting for

TABLE 2: The physical activity levels in different domains of the participants grouped by different factors.

Variables	Total (MET h/wk)	Working (MET h/wk)	Transportation (MET h/wk)	LTPA (MET h/wk)
Total	62.49	30.80	18.87	12.82
Sex				
Male	61.06	29.22	17.85	13.99
Female	63.78	32.21	19.80	11.77
Age				
40–49	67.88	31.45	19.89	16.54
50–59	67.19	35.04	21.52	10.65
60–69	52.36	25.85	15.20	11.32
70+	51.02	21.96	13.19	15.87
BMI				
−24	66.49	36.17	18.84	11.49
24–28	58.34	25.61	18.73	14.00
28+	63.42	31.24	19.24	12.93
WC				
Female < 85 Male < 90	67.63	35.46	18.09	14.08
Female ≥ 85 Male ≥ 90	58.87	27.51	19.44	11.93
Education				
Illiteracy	71.03	37.60	20.03	13.40
Primary school	67.90	41.45	14.67	11.77
Junior high school	80.23	44.65	22.08	13.50
Senior high school	47.68	16.96	18.46	12.26
College or above	33.88	0.64	19.28	14.02

MET: metabolic equivalent task; WC: waist circumference; BMI: body mass index; LTPA: leisure time physical activity.

age and sex. The OR (95% CI) across decreasing categories of educational levels was 1.00 (reference), 2.53 (1.49–4.30), 6.94 (4.12–11.68), 8.89 (5.13–15.40), and 8.54 (4.70–15.52) ($p < 0.001$ for trend). No significant correlation was observed between smoking or drinking and the PA level. Same results were showed in the univariate logistic regression between PA and smoking/drinking status when we stratified the population based on sex and age (Supplement Table 1).

3.5. Insufficient PA Is a High Risk Factor for T2DM, MS, and Metabolic Parameters. Furthermore, we examined whether the level of PA has a significant association with T2DM or MS (Table 5). After adjustment for age and sex, the moderate PA level showed a significant association with T2DM, MS, and WC. In addition, the low level of PA showed a significant association with MS and WC but not with T2DM. With respect to metabolic parameters, participants with higher PA exhibited lower levels of WC, diastolic blood pressure, triglyceride, and fasting plasma glucose values but higher levels of HDL-C. When we analyzed the relationship between PA levels and some metabolic parameters, PA levels only showed significant association with HOMA-IR with and without adjusting for age and sex (Table 6). We also found that PA levels could be grouped according to the presence of T2DM or MS.

4. Discussion

A few studies of urban Chinese adults were performed in recent years, while no quantitative PA study has been performed. In addition, most of these studies focused on LTPA. However, among Chinese adults, the participation in LTPA was rather low in the early 2000s, while nonleisure time activities, including activities related to housework, commuting, or work, were the main sources of daily PA. In this study, men were generally shown to spend less time in working PAs than women. The results of this study also showed that working PA is the major component of total PA for our participants. These results were consistent with those in many developing countries where working PA, in contrast to LTPA, contributes to half or more of the overall PA [18, 19]. The existence of less industrialization and fewer lifestyle changes and the greater engagement in vigorous-intensity activities such as agricultural work in the rural areas of developing areas might also be factors that determine the contribution of different types of PA.

In our research, 28.6% of the population had a low PA level (Table 3). Among several studies, the proportion varies from 35.4% in one study [20] to 49.2% in another [21], depending on the different social conditions and the different approaches for selecting levels. A review demonstrated that

Table 3: Prevalence of physical activity levels.

Variables	Low (%)	Moderate (%)	High (%)
Total	28.6	47.3	24.1
Sex			
Male	29.4	47.2	23.4
Female	27.8	47.3	24.9
p	0.60	0.99	0.41
Age			
40–49	31.8	41.7	26.5
50–59	29.3	44.7	26.0
60–69	26.1	53.5	20.4
70+	18.5	63.9	17.6
p	0.016	<0.001	0.017
BMI			
−24	26.7	47.9	25.4
24–28	30.9	47.1	22.0
28+	27.4	46.3	26.2
p	0.14	0.86	0.15
WC			
Female < 85 Male < 90	27.5	45.4	27.1
Female ≥ 85 Male ≥ 90	29.3	48.6	22.1
p	0.36	0.16	0.009
Education			
Illiteracy	26.5	46.3	27.2
Primary school	32.7	35.9	31.3
Junior high school	24.0	44.5	31.5
Senior high school	31.0	53.7	15.7
College or above	27.7	63.6	8.6
p	0.018	<0.001	<0.001

WC: waist circumference; BMI: body mass index.

Table 4: The association between social behaviors and physical activity (high level versus the other levels).

Social behavior	OR (95% CI)	*p*
Sex	0.73 (0.54–1.005)	0.053
Age (per 10 years)	0.65 (0.57–0.75)	<0.001
Nonsmoker	1	
Former smoker	1.21 (0.86–1.70)	0.28
Current smoker	0.93 (0.65–1.39)	0.71
Nondrinker	1	
Former drinker	1.16 (0.87–1.55)	0.31
Current drinker	1.29 (0.91–1.82)	0.15
College or above	1	
Illiteracy	8.54 (4.70–15.52)	<0.001
Primary school	8.89 (5.13–15.40)	<0.001
Junior high school	6.94 (4.12–11.68)	<0.001
Senior high school	2.53 (1.49–4.30)	0.001

OR: odds ratios; CI: confidence interval.

PA estimates varied markedly even within a single country when studies were performed using different surveys in similar time periods [22]. In general, the results showed that older people and more highly educated people are less likely to have a high level of PA. A low PA level is more common in men than in women, which is consistent with the results of other studies [22, 23]. Because the data were based on a questionnaire, the standard of activity intensity for the questionnaire was based on relative cardiopulmonary capacities, which differ between sexes. In contrast, in our research, BMI showed no association with the PA level, which was consistent with the previous studies [24]. Few of these studies focused on the correlation between social behavior and PA levels. Educational levels had an obvious negative correlation with PA levels after adjusting for age and sex, consistent with previous studies [7, 9]. Nevertheless, smoking or drinking did not show a significant association with PA in our study. Although our research found no significant correlation between smoking or drinking and PA, we should be cautious about recommending alcohol and cigarette consumption for overall human health because a strong association between smoking or drinking and PA was found in other studies.

With their increasing incidence and prevalence, T2DM and MS are gaining increasing attention in China and the prevalence of DM and MS in adults was 11.6% and 35%, respectively, in China in 2010 [5, 6]. However, in our study, the prevalence of T2DM and MS was 26.01% and 41.23%, respectively, in 2011. The high prevalence in our study may be related to the age of participants, who were selected to be more than 40 years old. Currently, endocrinologists in China are putting more effort into prevention and they now strongly support its implementation. As recommended by the ADA, PA is one of the key components in the management of T2DM and MS. Previous studies demonstrated that regular increased PA can effectively improve blood glucose control and reduce the complications of T2DM [10, 25]. Other studies have shown that DM can benefit from even a small level of PA that is even less than the suggested minimum dose that is recommended in guidelines [26, 27]. Therefore, exercise is undoubtedly viewed as an important component in the treatment of DM [28]. Although several studies conducted in developed countries reported a negative association between PA and T2DM or MS, few quantitative studies of PA and its association with T2DM and MS have been performed in China. In view of the high prevalence of T2DM and MS in rural China and the lack of knowledge about T2DM or MS prevention, it is necessary to quantify PA and determine the association between PA and T2DM or MS. This analysis showed that PA was significantly and inversely associated with the risk of developing T2DM and MS. A significant correlation was shown even with each item of MS except for hypertension. The lack of a significant association between PA and hypertension is consistent with the early research in China [29]. With economic development and the popularity of mechanization in China, physical

Table 5: Multivariate logistic regression for PA levels and DM and MS.

	Model 1†						Model 2					
	Low			Moderate			Low			Moderate		
	OR	95% CI	p	OR	95% CI	p	OR	95% CI	p	OR	95% CI	p
Low HDL-C	1.43	1.05–1.95	0.025	1.32	0.96–1.82	0.092	1.42	1.04–1.93	0.028	1.30	0.95–1.80	0.11
High TG	1.34	1.04–1.73	0.023	1.12	0.86–1.46	0.40	1.33	1.03–1.71	0.028	1.11	0.85–1.45	0.44
High plasma glucose	1.35	1.08–1.69	0.01	1.28	1.02–1.62	0.034	1.40	1.12–1.74	0.003	1.31	1.04–1.65	0.020
Hypertension	1.22	0.97–1.55	0.093	0.97	0.77–1.24	0.83	1.29	1.02–1.62	0.032	1.01	0.80–1.28	0.94
High WC	1.37	1.10–1.72	0.006	1.27	1.01–1.60	0.044	1.36	1.09–1.70	0.007	1.26	1.00–1.58	0.049
The presence of MS	1.60	1.27–2.02	<0.001	1.37	1.08–1.74	0.009	1.63	1.29–2.05	<0.001	1.38	1.09–1.75	0.007
The presence of T2DM	1.34	1.03–1.75	0.031	1.34	1.02–1.76	0.035	1.46	1.13–1.90	0.005	1.38	1.05–1.81	0.02

†Adjusted age and sex. Model 1 and model 2 are all reference with the high level of the PA level. HDL-C: high-density lipoprotein cholesterol; WC: waist circumference; TG: triglyceride; MS: metabolic syndrome; T2DM: type 2 diabetes; OR: odds ratios; CI: confidence interval.

Table 6: Multivariate logistic regression for PA levels and BMI, HOMA-IR, and HOMA-β.

	Model 1†						Model 2					
	Low			Moderate			Low			Moderate		
	OR	95% CI	p	OR	95% CI	p	OR	95% CI	p	OR	95% CI	p
High BMI	1.01	0.79–1.28	0.958	1.07	0.86–1.33	0.533	1.01	0.80–1.29	0.91	1.02	0.82–1.27	0.84
High HOMA-IR	1.35	1.06–1.72	0.014	1.33	1.07–1.65	0.011	1.36	1.06–1.72	0.014	1.33	1.07–1.65	0.011
Low HOMA-β	0.83	0.65–1.07	0.14	0.83	0.66–1.04	0.095	0.86	0.68–1.09	0.23	0.92	0.74–1.14	0.44

†Adjusted age and sex. Model 1 and model 2 are all reference with the high level of the PA level. OR: odds ratios; CI: confidence interval; BMI: body mass index; HOMA-IR: homeostasis model assessment-insulin resistance; HOMA-β: homeostasis model assessment of β-cell function.

labor may be decreasing. In addition, in view of the smaller proportion of LTPA relative to the overall PA, it is urgent to popularize and emphasize the importance of PA to rural people. Considering the growing burden of metabolic diseases in our country, promoting LTPA should be a strategy implemented at the national, community, and individual levels to combat the growing prevalence of metabolic diseases. BMI used to be one of the criteria for MS. The latest guidelines in China removed BMI as a criterion for MS based on the characteristics of the Chinese population. In fact, according to the DM guideline in China [16], Chinese people are less obese and the tendency for body fat to accumulate in the abdominal cavity is higher in Chinese people than in Caucasians, making it more likely for Chinese people to develop abdominal obesity. Even within people with normal body weight (BMI < 25 kg/m^2), 14% reported a severe accumulation of intra-abdominal fat [30]. This finding may explain the nonsignificant association between PA levels and BMI. Based on our results, insufficient PA is a risk factor for insulin resistance. This finding implies that insufficient PA may increase the prevalence of diabetes by increasing insulin resistance. In addition, given our limited data, we did not delve into the mechanisms underlying insulin resistance. WHO recommends at least 150 min of moderate activity or at least 75 minutes of vigorous-intensity aerobic physical activity throughout a week. Participants in studies met the recommendation lowered not only risk of mortality but also risk of cardiovascular diseases [31, 32]. More research could be conducted to determine the association between long-term physical activity intervention and DM or MS in the future.

The main strength of the study is that it is a large population-based study performed in a rural region. The diagnosis of T2DM and MS in our study was strictly based on the criteria in the guideline for T2DM and MS in China. In addition, the quantification of PA was based on GPAQ, which has been widely used in recent studies in developing countries.

A few limitations still apply to our study. The population included in our study was from the REACTION study [14]. One of the eligibility criteria for enrollment was being aged 40–75 years, which makes the population relatively old. As a result, obesity may be more common in the population in our study than in the whole adult population; thus, our research may not reflect the exact relationship between the PA level and metabolic diseases in the adult population. Although a variety of confounders were considered, unknown residual confounding factors cannot be excluded. However, an accurate measurement of daily energy expenditure by the doubly labelled water method or motion sensors is still challenging in large population studies because these assessments are expensive and cumbersome. Since T2DM results from chronic low-grade inflammation and preexisting insulin resistance, a cohort study may be more acceptable for demonstrating the close relationship between insufficient PA and T2DM. To probe further relationships, more indexes of prediabetes, such as hsCRP, should be tested in the further research.

5. Conclusions

In summary, insufficient PA is highly prevalent among the rural population over 40 years old, which increases the risk of T2DM and MS. Population-wide and individualized guidelines for PA, especially recreational physical activities, should be developed.

Abbreviations

PA:	Physical activity
NCDs:	Noncommunicable diseases
DM:	Diabetes mellitus
T2DM:	Type 2 diabetes
MS:	Metabolic syndrome
WC:	Waist circumference
BMI:	Body mass index
HDL-C:	High-density lipoprotein cholesterol
METs:	Metabolic equivalent tasks
GPAQ:	Global PA Questionnaire
LTPA:	Leisure time PA
OR:	Odds ratios
95% CIs:	95% confidence intervals
HOMA-IR:	Homeostasis model assessment-insulin resistance
HOMA-β:	Homeostasis model assessment of β-cell function.

Consent

Written informed consent was obtained from all participants following a detailed description of the purpose of the study.

Conflicts of Interest

All authors declare that they do not have any potential conflict of interest with respect to this manuscript.

Authors' Contributions

All authors have read and approved the submission of the manuscript.

Acknowledgments

This work was supported by the National Key Research and Development Program of China (Grant nos. 2017YFC1309800 and 2017YFC0909600), the Clinical Research Fund of Chinese Medical Association (Grant no. 15010010589), the Research Fund for Public Welfare, National Health and Family Planning (Grant no. 201402005), and the Key Research and Department of Shandong Province (Grant no. 2016GSF201013). The authors thank American Journal Experts for medical editing assistance with an earlier version of the manuscript.

References

[1] T. Moholdt, U. Wisløff, T. I. Nilsen, and S. A. Slørdahl, "Physical activity and mortality in men and women with coronary heart disease: a prospective population-based cohort study in Norway (the HUNT study)," *European Journal of Cardiovascular Prevention & Rehabilitation*, vol. 15, no. 6, pp. 639–645, 2008.

[2] K. Gonzalez, J. Fuentes, and J. L. Marquez, "Physical inactivity, sedentary behavior and chronic diseases," *Korean Journal of Family Medicine*, vol. 38, no. 3, pp. 111-115, 2017.

[3] D. Vancampfort, B. Stubbs, J. Firth et al., "Physical activity correlates among 24,230 people with depression across 46 low- and middle-income countries," *Journal of Affective Disorders*, vol. 221, pp. 81–88, 2017.

[4] J. Paulsen, A. Askim, R. M. Mohus et al., "Associations of obesity and lifestyle with the risk and mortality of bloodstream infection in a general population: a 15-year follow-up of 64 027 individuals in the HUNT study," *International Journal of Epidemiology*, vol. 46, no. 5, pp. 1573–1581, 2017.

[5] Y. Xu, L. Wang, J. He et al., "Prevalence and control of diabetes in Chinese adults," *Journal of the American Medical Association*, vol. 310, no. 9, pp. 948-959, 2013.

[6] J. Lu, L. Wang, M. Li et al., "Metabolic syndrome among adults in China: the 2010 China noncommunicable disease surveillance," *The Journal of Clinical Endocrinology and Metabolism*, vol. 102, no. 2, pp. 507–515, 2017.

[7] "A mass survey of diabetes mellitus in a population of 300,000 in 14 provinces and municipalities in China (author's transl)," *Zhonghua nei ke za zhi*, vol. 20, no. 11, pp. 678–683, 1981.

[8] J. Weng, L. Ji, W. Jia et al., "Standards of care for type 2 diabetes in China," *Diabetes/metabolism Research and Reviews*, vol. 32, no. 5, pp. 442–458, 2016.

[9] A. M. Kriska, M. A. Pereira, R. L. Hanson et al., "Association of physical activity and serum insulin concentrations in two populations at high risk for type 2 diabetes but differing by BMI," *Diabetes Care*, vol. 24, no. 7, pp. 1175–1180, 2001.

[10] D. Umpierre, P. A. Ribeiro, C. K. Kramer et al., "Physical activity advice only or structured exercise training and association with HbA1c levels in type 2 diabetes: a systematic review and meta-analysis," *Journal of the American Medical Association*, vol. 305, no. 17, pp. 1790–1799, 2011.

[11] D. Umpierre, P. A. Ribeiro, B. D. Schaan, and J. P. Ribeiro, "Volume of supervised exercise training impacts glycaemic control in patients with type 2 diabetes: a systematic review with meta-regression analysis," *Diabetologia*, vol. 56, no. 2, pp. 242–251, 2013.

[12] S. Balducci, S. Zanuso, P. Cardelli et al., "Effect of high- versus low-intensity supervised aerobic and resistance training on modifiable cardiovascular risk factors in type 2 diabetes; the Italian Diabetes and Exercise Study (IDES)," *PLoS One*, vol. 7, no. 11, article e49297, 2012.

[13] P. C. Hallal, L. B. Andersen, F. C. Bull, R. Guthold, W. Haskell, and U. Ekelund, "Global physical activity levels: surveillance progress, pitfalls, and prospects," *The Lancet*, vol. 380, no. 9838, pp. 247–257, 2012.

[14] G. Ning, "Risk Evaluation of cAncers in Chinese diabeTic Individuals: a lONgitudinal (REACTION) study," *Journal of Diabetes*, vol. 4, no. 2, pp. 172-173, 2012.

[15] T. B. F. Armstrong, "Development of the World Health Organization Global Physical Activity Questionnaire (GPAQ)," *Journal of Public Health*, vol. 14, no. 2, pp. 66–70, 2006.

[16] Chinese Diabetes Society, *China Guideline for Type 2 Diabetes*, Beijing university medical press, 2014.

[17] Chinese Diabetes Society, *China Guideline for Type 2 Diabetes (2004)*, Peking University medical press, 2004.

[18] O. T. Trinh, N. D. Nguyen, M. J. Dibley, P. Phongsavan, and A. E. Bauman, "The prevalence and correlates of physical inactivity among adults in Ho Chi Minh City," *BMC Public Health*, vol. 8, no. 1, p. 204, 2008.

[19] A. Bauman, F. Bull, T. Chey et al., "The International Prevalence Study on Physical Activity: results from 20 countries," *International Journal of Behavioral Nutrition and Physical Activity*, vol. 6, no. 1, p. 21, 2009.

[20] M. Moniruzzaman, M. Mostafa Zaman, M. S. Islalm, H. A. M. N. Ahasan, H. Kabir, and R. Yasmin, "Physical activity levels in Bangladeshi adults: results from STEPS survey 2010," *Public Health*, vol. 137, pp. 131–138, 2016.

[21] A. Razzaque, L. Nahar, M. Abu Haider Mohammad Golam, K. Z. Ahsan, M. S. Islam, and M. Yunus, "Sociodemographic differentials of selected noncommunicable diseases risk factors among adults in Matlab, Bangladesh: findings from a WHO STEPS survey," *Asia Pacific Journal of Public Health*, vol. 23, no. 2, pp. 183–191, 2011.

[22] R. Macniven, A. Bauman, and M. Abouzeid, "A review of population-based prevalence studies of physical activity in adults in the Asia-Pacific region," *BMC Public Health*, vol. 12, no. 1, p. 41, 2012.

[23] R. Guthold, T. Ono, K. L. Strong, S. Chatterji, and A. Morabia, "Worldwide variability in physical inactivity a 51-country survey," *American Journal of Preventive Medicine*, vol. 34, no. 6, pp. 486–494, 2008.

[24] D. E. Laaksonen, J. Lindstrom, T. A. Lakka et al., "Physical activity in the prevention of type 2 diabetes: the Finnish diabetes prevention study," *Diabetes*, vol. 54, no. 1, pp. 158–165, 2005.

[25] R. J. A. M. Sigal and P. Colby, "Clinical practice guidelines for the prevention and management of diabetes in Canada: physical activity and diabetes," *Canadian Journal of Diabetes*, vol. 37, Supplement 1, pp. S40–44, 2013.

[26] H. Arem, S. C. Moore, A. Patel et al., "Leisure time physical activity and mortality: a detailed pooled analysis of the dose-response relationship," *JAMA Internal Medicine*, vol. 175, no. 6, pp. 959–967, 2015.

[27] C. P. Wen, J. P. Wai, M. K. Tsai et al., "Minimum amount of physical activity for reduced mortality and extended life expectancy: a prospective cohort study," *The Lancet*, vol. 378, no. 9798, pp. 1244–1253, 2011.

[28] M. J. Armstrong and R. J. Sigal, "Exercise as medicine: key concepts in discussing physical activity with patients who have type 2 diabetes," *Canadian Journal of Diabetes*, vol. 39, Supplement 5, pp. S129–S133, 2015.

[29] G. Ma, D. Luan, Y. Li et al., "Physical activity level and its association with metabolic syndrome among an employed population in China," *Obesity Reviews*, vol. 9, no. s1, pp. 113–118, 2008.

[30] W. P. Jia, J. X. Lu, K. S. Xiang, Y. Q. Bao, H. J. Lu, and L. Chen, "Prediction of abdominal visceral obesity from body mass index, waist circumference and waist-hip ratio in Chinese adults: receiver operating characteristic curves analysis," *Biomedical and Environmental Sciences*, vol. 16, no. 3, pp. 206–211, 2003.

[31] S. A. Lear, W. Hu, S. Rangarajan et al., "The effect of physical activity on mortality and cardiovascular disease in 130 000 people from 17 high-income, middle-income, and low-income countries: the PURE study," *The Lancet*, vol. 390, no. 10113, pp. 2643–2654, 2017.

[32] I. M. Lee, E. J. Shiroma, F. Lobelo, P. Puska, S. N. Blair, and P. T. Katzmarzyk, "Effect of physical inactivity on major non-communicable diseases worldwide: an analysis of burden of disease and life expectancy," *The Lancet*, vol. 380, no. 9838, pp. 219–229, 2012.

9

Remote Lifestyle Coaching Plus a Connected Glucose Meter with Certified Diabetes Educator Support Improves Glucose and Weight Loss for People with Type 2 Diabetes

Jennifer B. Bollyky,[1,2] Dena Bravata,[1,3] Jason Yang,[4] Mark Williamson,[5] and Jennifer Schneider[1,3]

[1]Livongo Health, Mountain View, CA, USA
[2]Stanford University, Hospital & Clinics, Stanford, CA, USA
[3]Center for Primary Care and Outcomes Research, Stanford University, Stanford, CA, USA
[4]Biomedical Informatics, Stanford University, Stanford, CA, USA
[5]Restore Health, Palo Alto, CA, USA

Correspondence should be addressed to Jennifer B. Bollyky; jbollyky@livongo.com

Academic Editor: Patrizio Tatti

Background. Connected health devices with lifestyle coaching can provide real-time support for people with type 2 diabetes (T2D). However, the intensity of lifestyle coaching needed to achieve outcomes is unknown. *Methods.* Livongo provides connected, two-way messaging glucose meters, unlimited blood glucose (BG) test strips, and access to certified diabetes educators. We evaluated the incremental effects of adding lifestyle coaching on BG, estimated HbA1c, and weight. We randomized 330 eligible adults (T2D, HbA1c > 7.5%, BMI ≥ 25) to receive no further intervention ($n = 75$), a connected scale ($n = 115$), scale plus lightweight coaching ($n = 73$), or scale plus intense coaching ($n = 67$) for 12 weeks. We evaluated the change in outcomes using ANOVA. *Results.* Livongo participation alone resulted in improved BG control (mean HbA1c declined: 8.5% to 7.5%, $p = 0.01$). Mean weight loss and additional BG decreases were higher in the intensive compared with the lightweight coaching and scale-only groups (weight change (lb): −6.4, −4.1, and −1.1, resp., $p = 0.01$; BG change (mg/dL): −19.4, −11.3, and −2.9, resp., $p = 0.02$). The estimated 12-week program costs were 5.5 times more for intensive than lightweight coaching. *Conclusion.* Livongo participation significantly improves BG control in people with T2D. Additional lifestyle coaching may be a cost-effective intervention to achieve further glucose control and weight loss.

1. Background

In the USA, 1 in 11 people have diabetes, costing the healthcare system over $150 billion annually [1–3]. For these patients, maintaining blood glucose in the normal range (80–180 mg/dL) [4] is a critical part of reducing emergency department visits, hospitalizations, renal failure, and other costly complications of diabetes [5, 6]. Wirelessly connected glucose meters combined with certified diabetes educator (CDE) support for managing daily fluctuations in blood glucose (e.g., Livongo for diabetes program) have demonstrated sustained improvement in glucose control by reducing HbA1c by 0.9% for up to 12 months [7]. However, not all patients achieve goal glucose control with this type of support alone and many patients with T2D find weight loss in the setting of insulin and other glucose-lowering medications to be difficult.

Lifestyle coaching through the National Diabetes Prevention Program is increasingly recommended to help patients with prediabetes and/or metabolic syndrome change their diets, increase physical activity, improve coping skills, and adopt other key behaviors associated with metabolic improvements and long-term outcomes [8, 9]. To our knowledge, there has been no published evaluation of effects of lifestyle coaching for people diagnosed with type 2 diabetes in the setting of a connected glucose meter and CDE support.

Large healthcare provider systems such as Sutter Health and the Veterans Health Administration (VHA) have made enormous investments in coaching and other educational programs for patients with diabetes. The VHA, for example, has grown its telehealth and remote patient monitoring from an initial program of 2000 patients in 2003 to over 150,000 in 2012 [10]. Patients with diabetes represent the largest population of veterans served through these programs, accounting for 48% of telehealth/remote monitoring visits per year. The annual cost to deploy these programs is $1600 per patient per year—which represents a considerable investment but one that is associated with a 20% reduction in hospital admissions related to diabetes [10] and is much lower than historical alternatives (e.g., over $13,000 per patient per year for traditional home-based care).

Increasingly, self-insured employers are investing in similar programs for their employees with diabetes [11]. Highly customized programs that are able to personalize outreach to target populations, match the intensity of support to the need of the employees, and optimize individuals' blood glucose readings and overall metabolic control are more likely to be cost-effective than with intensive programs deployed to a broad population.

We evaluated the effects of adding lifestyle modification coaching for a population of people with type 2 diabetes enrolled in a program supported by connected glucose meters and CDEs who had not yet achieved their glycemic control and weight goals. We hypothesized that intensive lifestyle coaching would be associated with greater improvements in glycemic control and weight loss than either lightweight coaching, scale-only or no further intervention. Secondarily, we investigated which patient characteristics are associated with the greatest engagement with the lifestyle coaching program.

2. Methods

2.1. Interventions

2.1.1. Livongo Diabetes Program. The Livongo for the diabetes program offers participants (1) a connected two-way messaging device that measures blood glucose, centrally stores the glucose data and other contextual data (e.g., time of day, relationship to a meal, insulin dose, and carbohydrates eaten), and delivers relevant messages back to the patient; (2) unlimited glucose test strips; and (3) access to a team of CDEs who are available to answer patient questions, help with goal setting, and provide immediate support in the setting of extreme glucose excursions. The Livongo program was provided to participants by their employer or health plan at no cost to the participant.

Algorithmic-driven messages are sent through the Livongo meter in response to each BG reading. For example, if the BG value is <50 mg/dL, the message on the BG meter could read "Your reading is very low, drink 4 oz of juice or take 4 glucose tabs and check BG again in 15 minutes". If the BG value is >400 mg/dL, the message could read "Drink a glass of water, take medication as prescribed and check BG again in 30 minutes". When a patient has a BG value of >400 mg/dL or <50 mg/dL or when the BG value is outside the specific threshold the patient sets, an alert is sent to a Livongo CDE who then contacts the patient to ensure the patient's safety and discuss an appropriate action based on the BG value. Twenty-seven percent of Livongo patients have been contacted at least once by a CDE on the basis of an alert BG value. Livongo patients can also schedule 1 : 1 telephonic sessions with CDEs for goal setting, personalized feedback, and diabetes education.

2.1.2. Restore Health Lifestyle Modification Program. The two 12-week lifestyle coaching interventions evaluated in this study were provided by Restore Health (Palo Alto, California) between May and September 2016. Lifestyle modification focused on the four key factors that drive insulin resistance: nutrition, exercise, sleep, and stress. While these topics are addressed according to the AADE7 Self-Care Behavior guidelines followed by Livongo CDEs, the Restore Health nutritional approach recommends a specific diet that is lower in carbohydrates, especially refined carbohydrates and sugar, moderate in protein, and unrestricted in healthy fats. There is no calorie restriction or macronutrient counting involved. Meals were photographed by participants and rated by Restore Health coaches using emojis they texted suggestions to provide real-time feedback to participants. Participants in the intensive coaching arm received a 60-minute onboarding call covering numerous lifestyle-related topics and goal setting and customized lessons as well as daily personalized text messages, personalized meal ratings, and activity recommendations. Participants in the lightweight coaching arm received a 20-minute onboarding call, standardized lessons and templated text message support, meal ratings, and activity recommendations.

2.1.3. Connected Scale. We provided a connected scale (BodyTrace Inc.) to participants in the three intervention arms of this study but not the control/Livongo-only group. Participants were allowed to keep the scale after the pilot program finished. For participants in the control/Livongo-only group, preintervention height and weight were obtained by self-report but no weight values were obtained at the end of the intervention period.

2.2. Study Design. 1936 adults (age ≥ 21 years) with type 2 diabetes who had been in the Livongo program (between October 1, 2014, and February 26, 2016) for at least 80 days, were overweight (BMI ≥ 25) and had not yet achieved their target glucose control (i.e., estimated HbA1c < 7.0%) were invited to participate in the study. Of these, 454 subjects agreed to participate and were randomized to one of the four intervention groups. 330 subjects provided sufficient data for analysis: (1) Livongo program with no additional support (control group, $N = 75$), (2) Livongo program plus a connected scale ($N = 115$), (3) Livongo program plus a connected scale and 12 weeks of lightweight lifestyle coaching ($N = 73$), or (4) Livongo program plus a connected scale and 12 weeks of intensive lifestyle coaching ($N = 67$).

We collected demographic data (e.g., gender and age), weight, height, and diabetes information (e.g., diabetes type, insulin use, and most recent HbA1c) from participants.

Table 1: Descriptive characteristics of the study populations.

	All participants	Livongo only	Livongo + scale	Livongo + scale + lightweight coaching	Livongo + scale + intensive coaching	ANOVA p value
N	330	75	115	73	67	
Gender, female	184 (55.8%)	45 (60%)	57 (49.6%)	38 (52.8%)	44 (65.7%)	0.14
Mean age (years)	50.3 ± 9.6	52.8 ± 11.2	49.8 ± 9.5	51.3 ± 9.8	49.9 ± 9.74	0.19
Race						
White/caucasian	212 (64.2%)	45 (60%)	73 (63.5%)	50 (68.5%)	44 (65.7%)	0.74
Hispanic/latino/mexican	3 (0.9%)	0 (0%)	2 (1.7%)	0 (0%)	1 (1.5%)	0.48
Black/african american	36 (10.9%)	9 (12%)	11 (9.6%)	10 (13.7%)	6 (9%)	0.76
Unknown race	39 (11.8%)	14 (18.7%)	18 (15.7%)	2 (2.7%)	5 (7.5%)	0.51
Insulin use						
No insulin use	189 (57.3%)	36 (48%)	57 (49.6%)	52 (71.2%)*	44 (65.7%)	**0.007**
Once/day insulin use	58 (17.6%)	14 (18.7%)	21 (18.3%)	10 (13.7%)	13 (19.4%)	0.80
More than once/day insulin use	71 (21.5%)	25 (33.3%)	27 (23.5%)	11 (15.1%)*	8 (11.9%)	**0.008**
Mean number of days in Livongo program at start of intervention	229 ± 130	217 ± 85	228 ± 143	233 ± 138	243 ± 145	0.71

*There are no statistically significant differences in these baseline characteristics among groups except that the participants randomized to the lightweight intervention were significantly less likely to be on insulin than control participants.

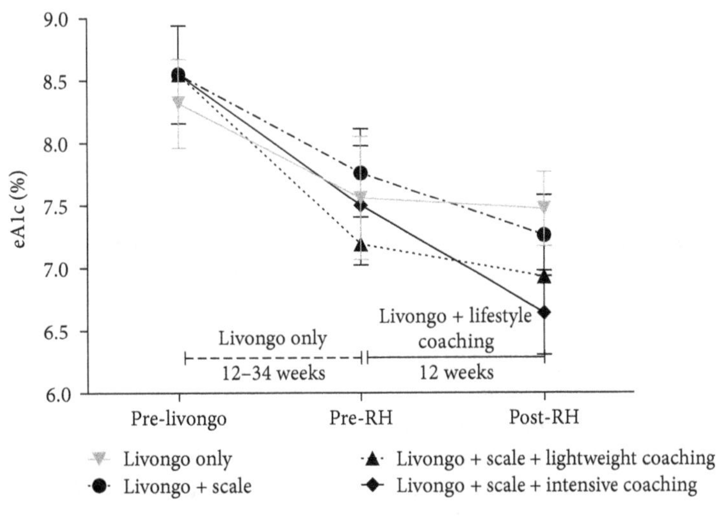

Figure 1: Estimated HbA1c (eA1c) change over time by the intervention group.

Blood glucose data were collected directly from members through their connected Livongo blood glucose meter. Weight data were collected through a connected scale for all participants who were given a scale and by self-report for participants in the control arm. All participants used the same version of the glucose meter, and no significant device or algorithmic changes were made during the study period. No specific guidelines about blood glucose testing frequency were given to participants; rather, they were instructed to follow their healthcare providers' advice. This protocol (LDR-2016) received IRB approval from Aspire Independent Review Board (Santee, CA).

2.3. Outcome Measures and Statistical Methods. We performed ANOVA to assess the extent of group assignment on the key outcomes of interest. We performed logistic regression to evaluate the characteristics of individuals with significant improvements in mean blood glucose, estimated HbA1c, and weight. We conducted all statistical analyses in R [12].

2.3.1. Estimated HbA1c. We used a linear model published from the ADAG study [13] to convert the mean blood glucose over 90 days to estimate HbA1c for participants prior to and after the intervention period. The mean blood glucose values prior to the intervention were calculated by taking the average of the blood glucose levels 30 days prior to the participant's enrollment in the study. Similarly, the blood glucose levels from the last 30 days of the study were used as the post-intervention mean blood glucose levels. When there was more than 1 blood glucose value on a given day, the average was taken to be the blood glucose for that day.

TABLE 2: Change in weight and glucose control with intervention.

Outcomes	All participants	Livongo only	Livongo + scale	Livongo + scale + lightweight RH coaching	Livongo + scale + intensive RH coaching	ANOVA p value
Weight (lb)						
N	221	NA	90	67	64	
Weight, preintervention	236 ± 52	NA	224 ± 52	246 ± 49	244 ± 55	**0.02**
Weight, postintervention	233 ± 51	NA	223 ± 50	242 ± 49	238 ± 53	**0.06**
Weight change	−3.5 ± 11.6	NA	−1.1 ± 13.7	−4.1 ± 9.4	−6.4 ± 9.7	**0.02**
BG checks per day						
N	324	75	113	71	65	
BG count, preintervention*	1.05 ± 1	1.2 ± 1.01	0.99 ± 0.85	0.95 ± 1.09	1.07 ± 1.09	0.38
BG count, postintervention**	0.86 ± 0.9	0.97 ± 0.94	0.78 ± 0.82	0.92 ± 1.06	0.8 ± 0.81	0.48
BG count change	−0.19 ± 0.82	−0.25 ± 0.74	−0.21 ± 0.85	−0.03 ± 0.8	−0.28 ± 0.85	0.26
Mean BG (mg/dL)						
N	322	75	112	71	64	
Mean BG, preintervention*	168 ± 50	172 ± 65	170 ± 43	159 ± 40	169 ± 51	0.43
Mean BG, postintervention**	158 ± 46	168 ± 51	165 ± 51	148 ± 36	146 ± 40	**0.007**
Mean BG change	−8.3 ± 44	−4.2 ± 52	−2.8 ± 47	−11.3 ± 35	−19.4 ± 35	**0.02**
Estimated HbA1c, eA1c (%)						
N	275	75	87	59	54	
eA1c, preintervention	7.5 ± 1.9	7.6 ± 2.1	7.8 ± 1.8	7.2 ± 1.6	7.5 ± 1.8	0.33
eA1c, postintervention	7.1 ± 1.4	7.5 ± 1.3	7.3 ± 1.4	6.9 ± 1.5	6.6 ± 1.3	**0.003**
eA1c, change	−0.4 ± 1.5	−0.1 ± 1.6	−0.4 ± 1.3	−0.4 ± 1.4	−0.7 ± 1.5	**0.02**

All statistically significant comparisons are indicated. *Average BG checks/day, 30 days prior to intervention. **Average BG checks/day, final 30 days of intervention.

2.3.2. Weight Data from Connected Scales. 9182 weight values were received from 230 participants. Participants who transmitted fewer than two weight values over the intervention period were excluded from analyses (number of participants removed = 8). We took several steps to assure that data received from connected scales were from the study participant and not another household member. First, transmitted weights at program initiation were compared to self-reported weights to determine a reference starting weight. Second, transmitted weight values more than 20% off of the participant's median weight were excluded (number of weights removed = 436, number of participants removed = 1). Third, if a weight change greater than 3% occurred over one day, transmitted weight values were excluded (number of weights removed = 184). Thus, a total of 8554 weight values from 221 participants were used in the analyses. Sample weight values transmitted from a single scale are shown in Supplementary Figure 1.

2.3.3. Engagement. Program engagement in the lifestyle coaching intervention groups was assessed subjectively by coaches (i.e., "engaged" or "not engaged") based on program participation, frequency of meal ratings, logged activity level, and sleep. The engagement was quantitatively assessed by the frequency of conversations recorded between coaches and participants.

Diabetes empowerment was evaluated using the Diabetes Empowerment Scale (DES), an eight-item measure of the self-efficacy of people with diabetes, prior to Livongo enrollment and during month 6 of the program [14]. A higher value indicates more positive feelings of empowerment regarding diabetes management.

3. Results

Table 1 presents the demographic data for the 330 participants. Baseline characteristics among groups were similar except that the participants randomized to the lightweight coaching intervention were significantly less likely to be on insulin than control participants ($p = 0.007$).

Figure 1 presents the change in glucose control for all participants. Livongo participation resulted in significantly improved BG control with a mean estimated HbA1c decrease from 8.5% to 7.5% ($p = 0.01$) across all groups prior to the Restore Health lifestyle modification intervention. Table 2 presents the change in the key weight and glucose control outcomes for participants in the control and intervention arms. Both coaching arms had statistically significant improvements in weight and additional mean blood glucose compared with the Livongo only and the Livongo plus scale groups. The mean weight loss was greatest in the intensive coaching group (−6.4 ± 9.7 lb) compared to the lightweight coaching (−4.1 ± 9.4 lb) and the Livongo plus scale-only groups (−1.1 ± 13.7 lb) ($p = 0.005$ for intensive coaching compared to scale-only). The additional mean improvement in blood glucose was highest in the intensive

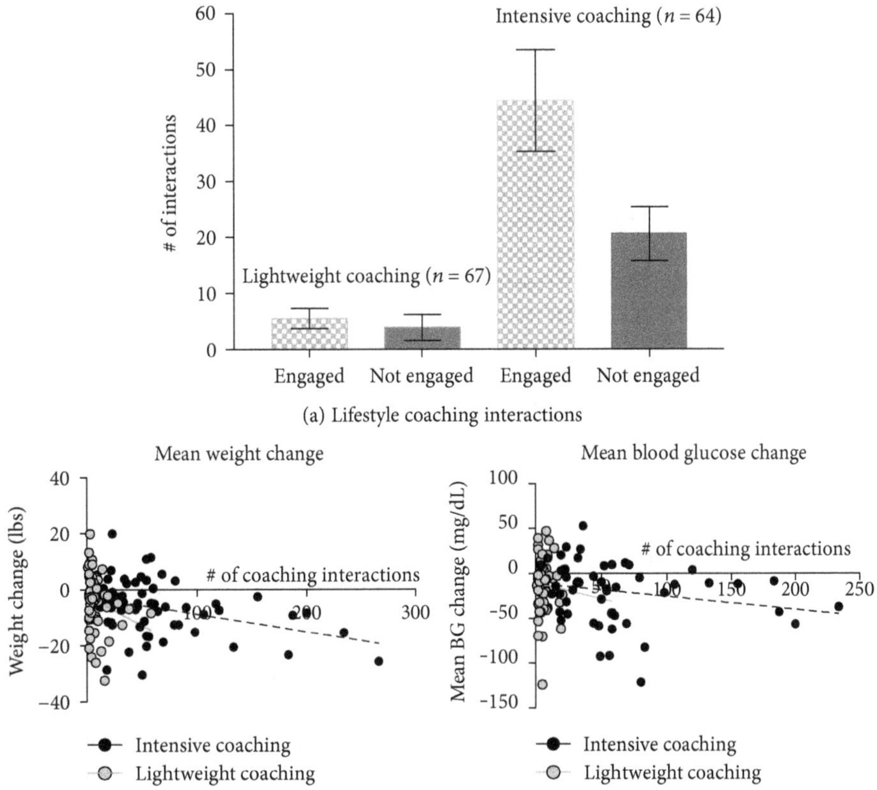

(a) Lifestyle coaching interactions

(b) Correlation between coaching interactions and outcomes

FIGURE 2: (a) Frequency of lifestyle coaching interactions correlated by engagement level and intervention arm. (b) Engagement with a Restore Health coach is correlated with weight loss and BG change.

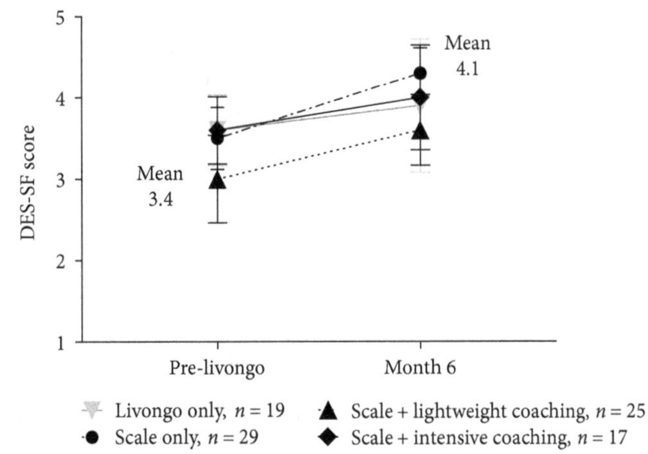

FIGURE 3: Diabetes Empowerment Scale (DES-SF). The DES-SF asks respondents on a 5-point scale how much they agree with eight statements related how they feel they are coping with diabetes (strongly disagree = 1, strongly agree = 5). Higher scores are associated with greater empowerment. Individual intervention groups did not vary significantly from each other, however the overall mean DES-SF score at registration was significantly lower than at that at 6 months after registration (0.7 difference, $p = 0.03$).

coaching group as well (-19.4 ± 34.6 mg/dL) compared to the lightweight coaching (-11.31 ± 34.7 mg/dL) and the Livongo plus scale-only (-2.8 ± 46.9 mg/dL) groups ($p = 0.02$ for intensive coaching compared to scale-only). Interestingly, there were no significant differences between the lightweight and intensive lifestyle coaching groups on any of the outcomes of interest; all statistically significant differences were between the coaching arms and the control group.

We evaluated the characteristics of those participants who had statistically significant improvements in mean blood glucose at the end of the intervention. High pre-intervention mean blood glucose was significantly associated with improved blood glucose control at the end of the intervention (177 ± 52 mg/dL versus 139 ± 26 mg/dL, $p = 0.001$). Age, gender, race/ethnicity, and insulin use were not associated with improvements in mean blood glucose.

Within each of the coaching groups, participants deemed subjectively "engaged" by Restore Health coaches had a significantly higher number of coach interactions with their Restore Health coaches and the number of coach interactions was associated with positive outcomes as shown in Figure 2. The mean number of coach interactions over the 12-week program for the intense coaching group was 44 (range 5–136) compared to 8 (range 1–32) for the lightweight coaching group. The number of coach interactions was strongly correlated with weight loss in the intensive coaching group (Pearson's $r = -0.36$, $p = 0.003$) and to a lesser degree in the lightweight group (Pearson's $r = -0.22$, $p = 0.11$), but it was not significantly correlated with a change in BG.

Diabetes empowerment as measured by the DES-SF instrument improved for all participants from a mean value of 3.4 at baseline to 4.1 at 6 months. Areas of the biggest improvement were related to participants' motivation for caring for their diabetes and positive coping strategies. No statistically significant differences between groups were noted as shown in Figure 3.

The incremental cost differences between the two coaching intervention arms were assumed to be related primarily to the coaching time as the fixed costs for the two programs were otherwise the same (i.e., lesson creation, platform for tracking progress towards goals, and connected scale). We further assumed that coaching costs were a function of estimated coach time per text (3 minutes), cost of coaching time ($0.60 per minute) based on $43,500 salary per year [15], 15% fringe benefits, and 70% work hours (40 per week) spent coaching. The mean number of text messages exchanged between coaches and participants was 44 for the intensive coaching group, 8 for the lightweight coaching group, and 0 for the scale-only group.

Based on these assumptions, the 12-week incremental costs above the Livongo program were $92 for the scale-only group, $120 for the scale plus lightweight coaching, and $240 for the scale plus intensive coaching. This translates into $84, $29, and $38 per pound lost; $31.72, $10.62, and $12.37 per mean change in 1 mg/dL of BG; and $230, $300, and $329 per 1% decrease in estimated HbA1c for the scale-only, the lightweight, and the intensive coaching intervention groups, respectively. Though the overall intervention effect size was greatest in the intensive coaching arm, lightweight coaching was more cost-effective for weight loss and change in mean BG.

Based on literature estimates of cost savings attributable to HbA1c reduction ranging from $113 to $179 per member per month [16], lifestyle coaching may be a cost-effective adjunctive therapy for reaching target glucose control for selected participants.

4. Discussion

This study has four key findings: first, participation in the Livongo Diabetes program resulted in significant improvement in blood glucose control. For many participants, this program alone is sufficient to achieve desired blood glucose control [7].

Second, among those participants who did not achieve their goal HbA1c through the Livongo program alone, weight loss and glucose control were only significantly greater in the intensive lifestyle coaching group compared to the other groups. The intensive program resulted in better, but nonstatistically significant, outcomes than lightweight coaching. Future studies should be directed to understanding the key components of the lifestyle coaching program most associated with the outcomes of interest to further reduce costs while maintaining effectiveness.

Third, those participants with the greatest improvements in glucose control at the end of the intervention had higher preintervention mean blood glucose levels. This key insight can enable risk stratification of patients entering a program like Livongo to identify the population who might require adjunctive lifestyle counseling to achieve their glucose control goals. By selectively offering lifestyle coaching to this group, the more expensive intervention can be applied to those participants likely to receive the greatest benefit from it.

Finally, all groups experienced an improvement in their sense of empowerment and well-being about managing their diabetes. We attribute this to the personalized digital and telephonic diabetes advice available to all participants through the Livongo-certified diabetes educators.

The limitations of this study include that glucose control at the end of the intervention was calculated from daily blood glucose values rather than measured by laboratory HbA1c. Notably, estimated HbA1c values have been previously demonstrated to be highly correlated with directly measured HbA1c values [13]. Additionally, the population that had the greatest improvement in glucose control may have received additional outside interventions by their primary care and other health care providers that could have contributed to this finding. We did not find significant differences in the frequency of interaction with Livongo coaches either through alerts or scheduled coaching between the groups, but other unmeasured interventions may have occurred.

Future research should be directed at understanding the key elements of the intensive lifestyle coaching program most associated with improvements in weight and glucose control so that those elements can be provided in the most cost-effective means possible to the T2D population most likely to benefit from them.

Disclosure

This was initially presented in poster format at the American Diabetes Association 77th Scientific Sessions in June 2017. (http://diabetes.diabetesjournals.org/content/diabetes/66/Supplement_1/A229.full.pdf)

Conflicts of Interest

All authors were either employees of or consultants to Livongo Health at the time of the analysis.

References

[1] A. Menke, S. Casagrande, L. Geiss, and C. C. Cowie, "Prevalence of and trends in diabetes among adults in the United States, 1988-2012," *JAMA*, vol. 314, no. 10, pp. 1021–1029, 2015.

[2] American Diabetes Association, "Economic costs of diabetes in the U.S. in 2012," *Diabetes care*, vol. 36, no. 4, pp. 1033–1046, 2013.

[3] C. W. Hunt, "Technology and diabetes self-management: an integrative review," *World Journal of Diabetes*, vol. 6, no. 2, pp. 225–233, 2015.

[4] American Diabetes Association, "Standards of medical care in diabetes—2015: summary of revisions," *Diabetes Care*, vol. 38, Supplement 1, pp. S4–S4, 2015.

[5] R. Ziegler, B. Heidtmann, D. Hilgard et al., "Frequency of SMBG correlates with HbA1c and acute complications in children and adolescents with type 1 diabetes," *Pediatric Diabetes*, vol. 12, no. 1, pp. 11–17, 2011.

[6] S. Allemann, C. Houriet, P. Diem, and C. Stettler, "Self-monitoring of blood glucose in non-insulin treated patients with type 2 diabetes: a systematic review and meta-analysis," *Current Medical Research and Opinion*, vol. 25, no. 12, pp. 2903–2913, 2009.

[7] J. Downing, J. Bollyky, and J. Schneider, "HbA1c reduction and fewer days with high and low blood glucose readings with cellular-enabled glucose meter," *Diabetes*, vol. 65, Supplement 1, 2016.

[8] Diabetes Prevention Program Research Group, "10-year follow-up of diabetes incidence and weight loss in the Diabetes Prevention Program Outcomes Study," *The Lancet*, vol. 374, no. 9702, pp. 1677–1686, 2009.

[9] The Diabetes Prevention Program (DPP) Research Group, "The diabetes prevention program (DPP): description of lifestyle intervention," *Diabetes*, vol. 25, no. 12, pp. 2165–2171, 2002.

[10] A. Darkins, P. Ryan, R. Kobb et al., "Care coordination/home telehealth: the systematic implementation of health informatics, home telehealth, and disease management to support the care of veteran patients with chronic conditions," *Telemedicine and e-Health*, vol. 14, no. 10, pp. 1118–1126, 2008.

[11] W. Su, F. Chen, T. M. Dall, W. Iacobucci, and L. Perreault, "Return on investment for digital behavioral counseling in patients with prediabetes and cardiovascular disease," *Preventing Chronic Disease*, vol. 13, article 150357, 2016.

[12] R Foundation for Statistical Computing. R Core Team, "R: a language and environment for statistical computing," 2016, https://www.R-project.org/.

[13] D. M. Nathan, J. Kuenen, R. Borg et al., "Translating the A1C assay into estimated average glucose values," *Diabetes Care*, vol. 31, no. 8, pp. 1473–1478, 2008.

[14] R. M. Anderson, M. M. Funnell, J. T. Fitzgerald, and D. G. Marrero, "The diabetes empowerment scale: a measure of psychosocial self-efficacy," *Diabetes Care*, vol. 23, no. 6, pp. 739–743, 2000.

[15] "Glassdoor.com," August 2017, https://www.glassdoor.com/Salaries/health-coach-salary-SRCH_KO0,12.htm.

[16] K. Fitch, B. S. Pyenson, and K. Iwasaki, "Medical claim cost impact of improved diabetes control for medicare and commercially insured patients with type 2 diabetes," *Journal of Managed Care & Specialty Pharmacy*, vol. 19, no. 8, pp. 609–620, 2013.

10

Retinopathy, Neuropathy, and Subsequent Cardiovascular Events in Patients with Type 2 Diabetes and Acute Coronary Syndrome in the ELIXA: The Importance of Disease Duration

Jelena P. Seferovic,[1] Rhonda Bentley-Lewis,[2] Brian Claggett,[1] Rafael Diaz,[3] Hertzel C. Gerstein,[4] Lars V. Køber,[5] Francesca C. Lawson,[6] Eldrin F. Lewis,[1] Aldo P. Maggioni,[7] John J. V. McMurray,[8] Jeffrey L. Probstfield,[9] Matthew C. Riddle,[10] Scott D. Solomon,[1] Jean-Claude Tardif,[11] and Marc A. Pfeffer[1]

[1]*Cardiovascular Division, Brigham and Women's Hospital, Harvard Medical School, Boston, MA, USA*
[2]*Massachusetts General Hospital, Harvard Medical School, Boston, MA, USA*
[3]*Estudios Clínicos Latinoamérica, Rosario, Argentina*
[4]*McMaster University, Hamilton, ON, Canada*
[5]*Rigshospitalet Copenhagen University Hospital, Copenhagen, Denmark*
[6]*Sanofi U.S., Bridgewater, NJ, USA*
[7]*Research Center of the Italian Association of Hospital Cardiologists, Florence, Italy*
[8]*British Heart Foundation Cardiovascular Research Centre, University of Glasgow, Glasgow, UK*
[9]*University of Washington Medical Center, Seattle, WA, USA*
[10]*Oregon Health and Science University, Portland, OR, USA*
[11]*Montreal Heart Institute, Université de Montréal, Montreal, Canada*

Correspondence should be addressed to Jelena P. Seferovic; jpseferovic@gmail.com

Guest Editor: João R. de Sá

Introduction. We investigated the association of diabetic retinopathy and neuropathy with increased risk of recurrent cardiovascular (CV) events in 6068 patients with type 2 diabetes mellitus (T2DM) and recent acute coronary syndrome (ACS) enrolled in the Evaluation of Lixisenatide in Acute Coronary Syndrome (ELIXA). *Methods.* History of retinopathy and neuropathy as well as duration of T2DM were self-reported at screening. Proportional hazards regression models were used to assess relationships between retinopathy, neuropathy, and recurrent CV events. *Results.* At screening, retinopathy and neuropathy were reported in 10.7% and 17.5% of patients, respectively, while 5.7% reported both. When adjusted for randomized treatment only, both retinopathy and neuropathy were associated with a primary composite outcome (CV death, nonfatal MI, stroke, or hospitalization for unstable angina) (retinopathy: HR 1.44, 95% CI 1.19–1.75; neuropathy: HR 1.33, 95% CI 1.12–1.57), CV composite (CV death, nonfatal MI, stroke, hospitalization for heart failure (HF)) (retinopathy: HR 1.57, 95% CI 1.31–1.88; neuropathy: HR 1.38, 95% CI 1.19–1.62), myocardial infarction (retinopathy: HR 1.38, 95% CI 1.08–1.76; neuropathy: HR 1.26, 95% CI 1.02–1.54), HF hospitalization (retinopathy: HR 2.03, 95% CI 1.48–2.78; neuropathy: HR 1.71, 95% CI 1.30–2.27), and all-cause mortality (retinopathy: HR 1.65, 95% CI 1.28–2.12; neuropathy: HR 1.43, 95% CI 1.14–1.78). When included in the same model, and adjusted for T2DM duration, there were no independent associations of either with CV outcomes, while T2DM duration remained strongly associated with all outcomes. Addition of demographic characteristics and CV risk factors did not further alter these relationships. *Conclusions.* In patients with T2DM and recent ACS, a history of retinopathy and/or neuropathy and longer T2DM duration could be considered clinical markers for high risk of recurrent CV events. This trial is registered with the ELIXA (Evaluation of Lixisenatide in Acute Coronary Syndrome), ClinicalTrials.gov registration number NCT01147250.

1. Introduction

Cardiovascular (CV) risk in type 2 diabetes mellitus (T2DM) was associated with disease duration and severity of hyperglycemia in many studies [1–3]. In the Framingham Heart Study, duration of T2DM significantly and positively related to the risk of coronary heart disease mortality, but not morbidity, or CV disease (CVD) morbidity or mortality [2]. The Action in Diabetes and Vascular Disease: Preterax and Diamicron Modified Release Controlled Evaluation (ADVANCE) trial, on the contrary, showed that T2DM duration was independently associated with the risk of macrovascular complications and death [3]. In a meta-analysis of five trials, intensive glycemic control led to a reduction of nonfatal myocardial infarction (MI) incidence by one-sixth, with no significant effect on the incidence of nonfatal stroke, and both CV or all-cause mortality [4].

Additionally, duration of T2DM and severity of hyperglycemia are strong and consistent risk factors for the development and progression of microvascular diabetic complications—retinopathy (DR), neuropathy (DN), and nephropathy [5–8]. For example, in the very large and diverse T2DM population in ADVANCE, T2DM duration was independently associated with the risk of DR and nephropathy [3]. In the Maastricht Study, a T2DM-enriched population-based cohort study prediabetes, T2DM, and measures of hyperglycemia were independently associated with DR and DN [9]. Improved metabolic control was associated with 25% risk reduction of microvascular composite endpoint in the United Kingdom Prospective Diabetes Study (UKPDS) [10]. Similar effect has been shown for individual complications, DR [5, 11], DN [6, 11], and nephropathy [7, 11, 12].

The association of diabetic nephropathy and increased risk of CVD has been revealed in multiple patient cohorts. Data from United States community-based study demonstrated that individuals with diabetic nephropathy were at four- and threefold higher risk for CV death and all-cause death, respectively, compared to those without [13]. In the ADVANCE study, both albuminuria and reduced estimated glomerular filtration rate (eGFR) were independently and continuously associated with the risk for CV and kidney outcomes in T2DM patients [14]. Similarly, among patients with type 1 diabetes followed for over 30 years, the development of diabetic nephropathy was associated with higher risks of CVD and renal events. However, this effect was almost entirely eliminated by adjustment for updated mean HbA1c which led to the conclusion that glycemic exposure correlates very strongly with CVD and mortality, and that this is partly mediated by hyperglycemia-induced renal disease [15]. Steno-2 study, including T2DM patients with microalbuminuria, showed that long-term intensified therapy reduced the risk of CV events, as well as diabetic nephropathy, DR, and DN [16]. Also, the risk of microalbuminuria has been shown to increase with T2DM duration [17].

Potential associations, of DR and DN with CV outcomes, whether causal or only predictive, have received less attention. We therefore investigated the association of DR and DN with increased risk of recurrent CV events, in patients with a recent acute coronary syndrome (ACS).

2. Materials and Methods

2.1. Study Design and Patients. The ELIXA (Evaluation of Lixisenatide in Acute Coronary Syndrome) was a randomized, double-blind, placebo-controlled trial designed to assess the effects of lixisenatide added to current T2DM therapy on CV morbidity and mortality in 6068 patients with a recent ACS.

We examined the primary composite (CV death, nonfatal MI, stroke, or hospitalization for unstable angina), CV composite (CV death, nonfatal MI, stroke, and hospitalization for heart failure (HF)), each of its components, and all-cause mortality. Details of the trial design, entry criteria, and the main results have been reported previously [18, 19].

For this post hoc analysis, all 6068 ELIXA participants were included. Self-reported historical data on DR and DN were collected at screening. Patients were asked to answer "yes," "no," or "unknown" on the presence of DR and/or DN. If DR was present, date of diagnosis was recorded, as well as information on photocoagulation and vitrectomy. However, these interventions were not analyzed further due to a small number of events. Presence of DN was defined as a report of either sensory/motor or autonomic neuropathy. Only "yes" responses were used to define the exposure variables for all subsequent analyses. Blood samples included in this analysis were done at screening by a central laboratory. Duration of T2DM was evaluated based on medical record review or self-report at the screening visit.

2.2. Statistical Analysis. Baseline characteristics of patients were stratified by the presence of DR and/or DN. Descriptive data are presented as the mean ± standard deviation for normally distributed variables and as median (25–75th percentile) for nonnormally distributed variables. Categorical variables are expressed as proportions and were compared by the chi-square test, while continuous variables were compared using t-tests or Wilcoxon rank-sum tests, as appropriate. Two proportional hazards regression models were used to assess the association between DR, DN, and recurrent CV events. Multivariable proportional hazards models were used to assess the association between DR, DN, and primary composite endpoint, CV composite endpoint, components, and all-cause mortality. Both DR and DN were included in the first model and adjusted for the duration of T2DM. In the second model, demographic characteristics and CV risk factors (age, sex, race, body mass index (BMI), baseline HbA1c, smoking, history of hypertension (HT), heart rate, total cholesterol, low-density lipoprotein (LDL) cholesterol, and triglycerides) were added to the previous model. Both models were adjusted for randomized study treatment. Predictors of DR and DN were determined from multivariable logistic regression model using forward stepwise selection including all variables in Table 1. Two-sided p values < 0.05 were considered significant. No adjustment was made for multiple comparisons. Analyses were performed using the Stata version 13.1 (StataCorp., College Station, TX, USA).

TABLE 1: Characteristics of all patients at baseline according to the presence of retinopathy and/or neuropathy.

Characteristic	All patients $n = 6068$	No retinopathy/ neuropathy $n = 4705$	Retinopathy and/ or neuropathy $n = 1363$	p value
Age (years)	60.3 ± 9.7	59.7 ± 9.7	62.3 ± 9.2	<0.001
Male sex (n (%))	4207 (69.3)	3379 (71.8)	828 (60.7)	<0.001
Body weight (kg)	84.9 ± 19.4	84.1 ± 18.9	87.6 ± 20.9	<0.001
Body mass index (kg/m^2)	30.2 ± 5.7	29.9 ± 5.6	31.2 ± 6.0	<0.001
Duration of T2DM (years)	7.4 (2.8, 13.6)	6.0 (2.0, 11.7)	12.4 (7.0, 20.2)	<0.001
Categories of T2DM duration (n (%))				<0.001
≤1 year	964 (15.9)	914 (19.4)	50 (3.7)	
>1–≤5 years	1294 (21.3)	1130 (24.0)	164 (12.0)	
>5–≤10 years	1359 (22.4)	1076 (22.9)	283 (20.8)	
>10 years	2451 (40.4)	1585 (33.7)	866 (63.5)	
Race (n (%))				<0.001
White	4576 (75.4)	3471 (73.8)	1105 (81.1)	
Black	221 (3.6)	171 (3.6)	50 (3.7)	
Asian	771 (12.7)	669 (14.2)	102 (7.5)	
Other	500 (8.2)	394 (8.4)	106 (7.8)	
Region (n (%))				<0.001
Africa/Near East	296 (4.9)	228 (4.8)	68 (5.0)	
Asia Pacific	703 (11.6)	615 (13.1)	88 (6.5)	
Eastern Europe	1587 (26.2)	1115 (23.7)	472 (34.6)	
North America	807 (13.3)	564 (12.0)	243 (17.8)	
South and Central America	1944 (32.0)	1600 (34.0)	344 (25.2)	
Western Europe	731 (12.0)	583 (12.4)	148 (10.9)	
Smoking status (n (%))				<0.001
Current	709 (11.7)	579 (12.3)	130 (9.5)	
Former	2746 (45.3)	2184 (46.4)	562 (41.2)	
Never	2612 (43.1)	1941 (41.3)	671 (49.2)	
Diastolic blood pressure (mmHg)	77 ± 10	77 ± 10	76.3 ± 10	<0.001
Systolic blood pressure (mmHg)	130 ± 17	129 ± 17	131 ± 17	<0.001
Heart rate (beats/min)	70 ± 10	70 ± 10	71 ± 10	0.027
Fasting plasma glucose (mg/dl)	148.3 ± 51.6	145.2 ± 49.1	159.3 ± 58.1	<0.001
Glycated hemoglobin (%)	7.7 ± 1.3	7.6 ± 1.3	8.0 ± 1.2	<0.001
Glycated hemoglobin (mmol/mol)	61 ± 14	60 ± 14	64 ± 13	<0.001
Total cholesterol (mg/dl)	153.5 ± 44.6	151.3 ± 43.5	161.1 ± 47.3	<0.001
HDL cholesterol (mg/dl)	42.9 ± 10.9	42.6 ± 10.6	44.1 ± 11.7	<0.001
LDL cholesterol (mg/dl)	78.5 ± 35.3	77.1 ± 34.7	83.4 ± 36.9	<0.001
Triglycerides (mg/dl)	137.2 (99.1, 195.6)	136.3 (100.0, 192.9)	141.6 (99.1, 208.0)	0.021
eGFR (ml/min/1.73m^2)	76 ± 21	77 ± 21	71 ± 22	<0.001
Albuminuria (n (%))				<0.001
<30 mg/g	4441 (74.3)	3579 (77.2)	862 (64.2)	
≥30–<300 mg/g	1148 (19.2)	819 (17.7)	329 (24.5)	
≥300 mg/g	389 (6.5)	237 (5.1)	152 (11.3)	
Medical history at randomization (n (%))				
Hypertension	4635 (76.4)	3463 (73.6)	1172 (86)	<0.001
Heart failure	1358 (22.4)	923 (19.6)	435 (31.9)	<0.001
Stroke	331 (5.5)	204 (4.3)	127 (9.3)	<0.001
Peripheral arterial disease	393 (6.5)	227 (4.8)	166 (12.2)	<0.001
Atrial fibrillation	366 (6.0)	247 (5.2)	119 (8.7)	<0.001
Percutaneous coronary intervention	4079 (67.2)	3263 (69.4)	816 (59.9)	<0.001
Coronary artery bypass grafting	507 (8.4)	363 (7.7)	144 (10.6)	<0.001

TABLE 1: Continued.

Characteristic	All patients $n = 6068$	No retinopathy/ neuropathy $n = 4705$	Retinopathy and/ or neuropathy $n = 1363$	p value
Qualifying ACS event (n (%))				<0.001
STEMI	2666 (44.0)	2187 (46.5)	479 (35.2)	
NSTEMI	2348 (38.7)	1817 (38.6)	531 (39.0)	
Unstable angina	1042 (17.2)	693 (14.7)	349 (25.6)	
Missing	9 (0.1)	6 (0.1)	3 (0.2)	
Antihyperglycemic therapy (n (%))				
Metformin	4243 (69.9)	3367 (71.6)	876 (64.3)	<0.001
Sulfonylureas	2266 (37.3)	1779 (37.8)	487 (35.7)	0.16
Insulin	2891 (47.6)	1948 (41.4)	943 (69.2)	<0.001
Thiazolidinediones	128 (2.1)	92 (2.0)	36 (2.6)	0.12
Alpha-glucose inhibitor	181 (3.0)	150 (3.2)	31 (2.3)	0.08
Dipeptidyl peptidase 4 inhibitor	226 (3.7)	176 (3.7)	50 (3.7)	0.90
Other	485 (8.0)	384 (8.2)	101 (7.4)	0.37

Data is presented as means ± SD, median (25–75th percentile), or percentages. HDL: high-density lipoprotein; LDL: low-density lipoprotein; MI: myocardial infarction; ACS: acute coronary syndrome; eGFR: estimated glomerular filtration rate.

3. Results

3.1. Baseline Characteristics. Demographic and clinical characteristics of the 6068 patients are shown in Table 1. In the whole population, the mean age was 60.3 years and known T2DM duration was 7.4 years. However, the reported duration of T2DM varied widely, with 15.9% of participants having known T2DM for less than 1 year, 21.3% ≤5 years, 22.4% >1–≤5 years, and 40.4% longer than10 years (Supplementary Figure 1). Of the whole population, 1363 (22.5%) reported DR and/or DN. DR was reported in 651 (10.7%) patients, DN in 1060 (17.5%) patients, and both in 348 (5.7%) patients (Figure 1). Of 651 who reported DR, 159 patients (24.4%) had prior photocoagulation, and 32 patients (4.9%) had vitrectomy.

Patients who had DR and/or DN were significantly older (mean 62.3 vs. 59.7 years) and had longer known duration of T2DM (mean 12.4 vs. 6.0 years) than those with neither complication. Smaller proportions of patients with DR and/or DN reported shorter T2DM duration of <1 year (3.7% vs 19.4%) and ≤5 years (12.0% vs. 24.0%). The distribution of T2DM duration in all patients, as well as in those with and without retinopathy and/or neuropathy, is shown in Figure 2. Participants with DR and/or DN also had higher BMI, were also more likely to be nonsmokers, and had significantly higher glycated hemoglobin, fasting plasma glucose, and total and LDL cholesterol. The subgroup with DR and/or DN also had more evidence of renal disease reflected as increased albumin-to-creatinine ratio in comparison with those without DR and/or DN. Also, they were more likely to have history of CV disease (HT, HF, stroke, peripheral arterial disease, and atrial fibrillation). Finally, patients with DR and/or DN used more frequently metformin and insulin, while other glucose-lowering agents were similarly distributed among groups (Table 1).

3.2. Retinopathy and/or Neuropathy and CV Outcomes. In univariate analysis, DR was significantly associated with primary and CV composite endpoint, all-cause and CV death, and all CV events except stroke ($p = 0.068$), while DN was associated with primary and CV composite endpoint, all-cause death, and all nonfatal CV events, but not CV death ($p = 0.08$, Table 2). When both DR and DN were included in the same model, along with T2DM duration, there were no independent associations of either with any of the outcomes, while duration of T2DM remained highly significantly associated with all outcomes (Table 2). Furthermore, the addition of demographic characteristics and CV risk factors to the previous model resulted in neither DR nor DN being associated to any of the outcomes, but identified duration of T2DM as an independent predictor of CV events, beyond DR, DN, and CV risk factors (Table 2). There were no significant interactions between DR and DN in adjusted and unadjusted models. It has previously been reported that no significant interactions were detected with respect to prespecified patient subgroups for the ELIXA

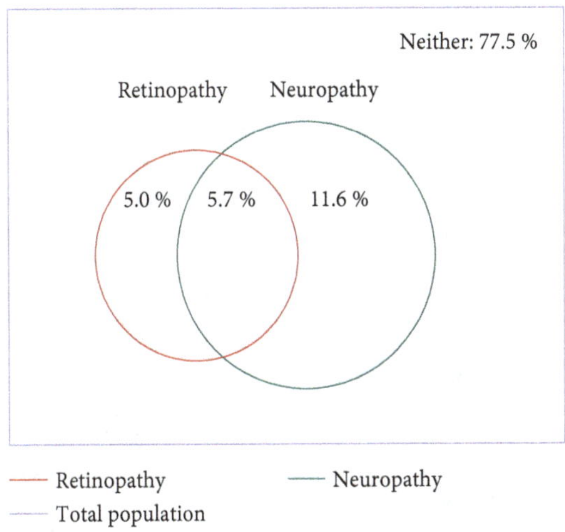

FIGURE 1: Prevalence of retinopathy and/or neuropathy.

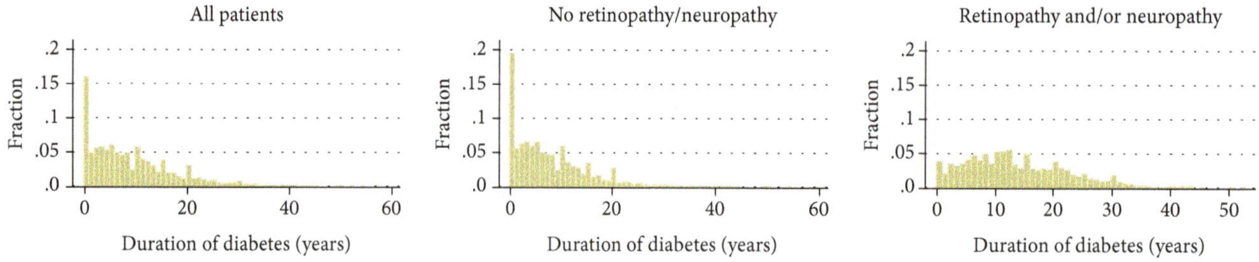

Figure 2: Distribution of T2DM duration in all patients, patients with no retinopathy/neuropathy and patients with retinopathy and/or neuropathy.

primary composite outcome, which included T2DM duration < 10 vs. >10 years [19]. In addition, no statistically significant interactions were found with respect to DR, DN, or duration of T2DM as a continuous variable.

3.3. Predictors of Retinopathy and/or Neuropathy. In both univariate and multivariate analysis, the most significant predictors of both DR and DN were duration of T2DM and insulin use (Table 3). The relationships between presence of DR and DN with duration of T2DM are shown in Supplementary Figures 2a–b. In multivariate analysis, other highly statistically significant ($p < 0.001$) predictors of DR were history of HF and stroke (Table 3) and of DN higher weight were previous percutaneous coronary intervention (PCI), total cholesterol, history of peripheral arterial disease, and previous stroke (Table 3). These models were effectively able to discriminate between patients with and without DR (area under the curve (AUC) 0.81) and DN (AUC 0.76).

4. Discussion

In this post hoc analysis of a large population selected for having a recent ACS event, together with T2DM, less than one-fourth of patients reported a history of DR, DN, or both. This was a smaller proportion than found in other studies of CV outcomes in T2DM, in which many patients had CV risk factors but not necessarily a completed event. For example, the prevalence of DR in the Trial to Reduce Cardiovascular Events with Aranesp Therapy (TREAT) study—which also relied on patient self-reports—was almost three times higher in a more severely compromised patient cohort with T2DM, chronic kidney disease, and anemia, but also twice as long T2DM duration [20]. The widely varying duration of T2DM in the ELIXA, and the inclusion of a large fraction with very short duration of T2DM, allowed our analysis to examine the relationships between duration of T2DM, presence of DR or DN, and risk of subsequent CV events.

The variability of previously reported associations between DR and/or DN and subsequent CV events could stem from variable T2DM duration and comorbidities of analyzed patient cohorts. The positive association of DR and CV events was observed in various patient cohorts [21–23]. In a recently published study with a large cohort of T2DM patients without the history of CV diseases, the risk of developing CV death, nonfatal MI, or stroke was about 40% higher in patients with DR and DN [24]. In the meta-analysis including 11,505 patients, DR was associated with 1.7-fold increased risk for CV events [25]. However, in the TREAT study, enrolling 4038 patients with T2DM, chronic kidney disease, and anemia, DR was not independently associated with a higher risk of renal or CV morbidity or death, possibly due to longer duration of T2DM and more comorbidities [20].

Our findings on DN are partially in accordance with previously published studies that revealed an association between autonomic DN and CV events [26]. Other studies have shown that DN was associated with a twofold risk increase for peripheral vascular disease [27]. In our study, we investigated the association of both DN and outcomes, but not peripheral vascular disease. Therefore, our findings on the large cohort of T2DM patients with recent ACS provide novel insight into the association between DN and recurrent CV events. These findings indicate the importance of the duration of T2DM as a traditional risk factor [28].

Consistent with prior reports, our analysis found that DR and/or DN were associated at baseline with longer T2DM duration, worse glycemic control, more insulin use, and history of prior manifest CV disease. Furthermore, both DR and DN were associated with increased risk of recurrent CV events, especially HF hospitalization. However, these associations were no longer statistically significant after adjustment for duration of T2DM, which remained a strong independent predictor of CV events [20, 29, 30]. Thus, DR and DN as well as duration of T2DM appear to be predictors of increased CV risk but, unlike diabetic nephropathy, not themselves are contributors to this risk.

While other relevant studies also adjusted clinical outcomes for the duration of T2DM—among other demographic characteristics and CV risk factors—none of them adjusted for only the known duration of the disease, which makes our findings unique. In a high-risk T2DM patient cohort used in the Veterans Affairs Diabetes Trial (VADT) (1791 subjects) [31], the duration of T2DM was significantly related to CV events. However, to the best of our knowledge, no studies included similar patient cohort, T2DM patients with recent ACS.

There are several possible explanations for the duration of T2DM being a strong independent predictor of recurrent CV events in our analysis. Longer duration of the disease may have a direct effect on progression of atherosclerotic lesions, increasing the risk of a recurrent CV event. In addition, it might be associated with autonomic DN and reduced heart rate variability, increasing the risk of CV death, which was not the case in our cohort. A long-term increase in

Table 2: Multivariable modeling.

Hazard ratio (95% CI)		Primary composite endpoint $N = 805$ events	CV composite endpoint $N = 913$ events	Cardiovascular death $N = 315$ events	Myocardial infarction $N = 531$ events	Stroke $N = 127$ events	Heart failure hospitalization $N = 249$ events	Death $N = 434$ events
Univariate**	Retinopathy	1.44 (1.19–1.75)*	1.57 (1.31–1.88)*	1.58 (1.17–2.13)*	1.38 (1.08–1.76)*	1.56 (0.97–2.51)	2.03 (1.48–2.78)*	1.65 (1.28–2.12)*
	Neuropathy	1.33 (1.12–1.57)*	1.38 (1.19–1.62)*	1.29 (0.99–1.68)	1.26 (1.02–1.54)*	1.59 (1.07–2.37)*	1.71 (1.30–2.27)*	1.43 (1.15–1.78)*
	T2DM duration (per 5 years)	1.17 (1.13–1.22) *	1.19 (1.15–1.23)*	1.22 (1.16–1.29)*	1.19 (1.14–1.25)*	1.08 (0.98–1.19)	1.30 (1.23–1.38)*	1.22 (1.17–1.28)*
Model 1**	Retinopathy	1.07 (0.86–1.32)	1.13 (0.94–1.31)	1.12 (0.80–1.56)	1.00 (0.77–1.31)	1.27 (0.74–2.16)	1.21 (0.85–1.73)	1.13 (0.85–1.50)
	Neuropathy	1.10 (0.92–1.31)	1.11 (0.94–1.31)	1.01 (0.76–1.34)	1.02 (0.82–1.28)	1.43 (0.93–2.20)	1.23 (0.90–1.66)	1.12 (0.88–1.42)
	T2DM duration (per 5 years)	1.16 (1.12–1.21)*	1.18 (1.14–1.22)*	1.21 (1.14–1.29)*	1.19 (1.14–1.25)*	1.04 (0.94–1.16)	1.28 (1.20–1.36)*	1.21 (1.15–1.27)*
Model 2**	Retinopathy	1.07 (0.86–1.33)	1.13 (0.92–1.38)	1.12 (0.80–1.57)	1.00 (0.76–1.32)	1.28 (0.75–2.19)	1.15 (0.81–1.65)	1.15 (0.87–1.53)
	Neuropathy	1.02 (0.85–1.23)	0.99 (0.84–1.18)	0.91 (0.68–1.22)	1.00 (0.78–1.24)	1.27 (0.82–1.99)	0.96 (0.70–1.31)	1.03 (0.81–1.31)
	T2DM duration (per 5 years)	1.10 (1.05–1.15)*	1.12 (1.07–1.16)*	1.14 (1.07–1.22)*	1.13 (1.08–1.20)*	0.95 (0.85–1.07)	1.21 (1.13–1.30)*	1.13 (1.07–1.19)*

Primary composite endpoint: CV death, nonfatal MI, stroke, or hospitalization for unstable angina; CV composite endpoint: CV death, nonfatal MI, stroke, hospitalization for heart failure (HF); $^{*}p \le 0.05$. Univariate: adjusted for randomized study treatment only; model 1: adjusted for retinopathy, neuropathy, T2DM duration, and randomized study treatment; model 2: model 1+ age, sex, race, BMI, baseline HbA1c, smoking, history of hypertension, heart rate, total cholesterol, LDL cholesterol, and triglycerides; $^{**}p \le 0.05$.

Table 3: Predictors of retinopathy and neuropathy multivariate models.

Parameter	Retinopathy OR (95% CI)	Retinopathy |Z| score	Neuropathy OR (95% CI)	Neuropathy |Z| score
Duration of diabetes (per 5 years)	1.48 (1.41–1.56)	14.64	1.31 (1.25–1.37)	11.52
Insulin use	2.77 (2.23–3.46)	9.13	2.19 (1.86–2.58)	9.36
Weight (per 5 kg)	—	—	1.09 (1.07–1.11)	8.83
Previous PCI	0.75 (0.61–0.91)	2.94	0.60 (0.51–0.70)	6.32
Total cholesterol (per 10 mg/dl)	—	—	1.05 (1.04–1.07)	6.23
History of PAD	—	—	1.88 (1.45–2.43)	4.82
History of HF	1.65 (1.35–2.02)	4.82	1.32 (1.12–1.56)	3.23
Previous stroke	2.06 (1.51–2.82)	4.54	1.86 (1.42–2.45)	4.45
Diastolic blood pressure (per 10 mmHg)	—	—	0.88 (0.82–0.95)	3.25
Sulphonylurea use	—	—	1.29 (1.11–1.51)	3.24
Previous CABG	0.72 (0.52–0.98)	2.11	0.66 (0.51–0.86)	3.06
Presence of hypertension	1.46 (1.11–1.91)	2.69	1.39 (1.12–1.72)	3.00
Body mass index (per 5 kg/m^2)	1.12 (1.04–1.22)	2.99	—	—
Glucose (per 10 mg/dl)	1.02 (1.0-1.04)	2.29	1.02 (1.01–1.03)	2.87
eGFR (per 10 ml/min/1.73m^2)	0.94 (0.90–0.98)	2.66	—	—
Male sex	—	—	1.25 (1.06–1.47)	2.60
HDL cholesterol (per 10 mg/dl)	1.11 (1.02–1.20)	2.53	—	—
Age (per 5 years)	—	—	1.05 (1.01–1.10)	2.20
HbA1c (per 1%)	1.09 (1.00–1.19)	1.98	—	—

Model AUC = 0.81 (retinopathy) and model AUC = 0.76 (neuropathy). HF: heart failure; PCI: percutaneous coronary intervention; eGFR: estimated glomerular filtration rate; HDL: high-density lipoprotein; CABG: coronary artery bypass grafting; HbA1c: glycated hemoglobin; PAD: peripheral artery disease.

oxidative stress in T2DM patients may cause increased risk of CV death. Also, longer exposure to hyperglycemia may simply reflect greater exposure to other, perhaps unmeasured, CV risk factors.

The major limitation of our study was the assessment of DR and DN which was based on patients' answers to self-report questionnaires. Therefore, the prevalence of both might have been underestimated. Such potential misclassification bias might have potentially weakened our results, and, therefore, the real association of DR and DN with recurrent CV events could be stronger than presented in this analysis. Another important limitation is the fact that T2DM duration was evaluated based on medical record or self-report and could therefore be underestimated, as patients often remain undiagnosed for many years. Also, having in mind that the study cohort included high-risk patients with T2DM and recent ACS, the results may not be applicable to other populations such as those without CV disease or with a less advanced stage of it. In addition, the design of this study was cross-sectional and therefore does not provide information on whether or not DR and DN developed before or after the onset of any CV disease antecedent to the qualifying ACS event. Finally, our findings should be considered post hoc and hypothesis-generating.

5. Conclusions

In a population with recent ACS together with T2DM, recurrent CV events, DR, and DN were all strongly associated with the T2DM duration. A history of either DR or DN was associated with increased risk of recurrent CV events. As these associations were eliminated by adjustment for the duration of T2DM, which remained a strong independent predictor of recurrent CV events, the link between DR and/or DN and these events is not likely to be a causal one. However, history of DR, DN, or both and longer duration of T2DM could be considered clinical markers for high risk of recurrent CV events. It is important to point out that the presence of both DN and DR is expected to positively correlate with patients' level of interaction with healthcare providers. Furthermore, it is expected that their level of healthcare provider interaction would correlate negatively with the frequency and magnitude of adverse outcomes.

Disclosure

The company, Sanofi, played no role in the design and execution of this analysis.

Conflicts of Interest

JPS has no competing interests. RBL is a consultant and research support of Sanofi and a research support and spouse/partner of Sanofi, Amgen Inc., and Novartis

Pharmaceuticals Corporation. BC has no competing interests. RD is a research support of Sanofi. HCG is an advisory panel of Sanofi, Novo Nordisk Inc., Bristol-Myers Squibb Company, Roche Pharmaceuticals, AstraZeneca Pharmaceuticals LP, GlaxoSmithKline, Bayer HealthCare, LLC, Merck, Boehringer Ingelheim Pharmaceuticals Inc., and Eli Lilly and Company; a consultant of Sanofi; and a research support of Sanofi and Eli Lilly and Company. LVK has a relationship with Sanofi and Novartis Pharmaceuticals Corporation. FL is an employee of Sanofi. EFL is a consultant and spouse/partner of Sanofi; a research support of Amgen Inc., Novartis Pharmaceuticals Corporation, and Sanofi; and a research support and spouse/partner of Sanofi. APM has a relationship with Sanofi, Oxford University, Eli Lilly and Company, and BMS. JMcM has a relationship with GlaxoSmithKline, PPD Development LP, Merck, Oxford University, Amylin Pharmaceuticals Inc., Eli Lilly and Company, Parexel, Bayer HealthCare, LLC, Abbvie, and Sanofi. JLP is an advisory panel of Sanofi, a consultant of Sanofi, and a research support of Sanofi. MCR is a consultant of Eli Lilly and Company, AstraZeneca Pharmaceuticals LP, Sanofi, Valeritas, LLC, and Elcelyx Therapeutics Inc.; a research support of AstraZeneca Pharmaceuticals LP, Eli Lilly and Company, Sanofi, and Novo Nordisk Inc.; and has a relationship with Sanofi. These dualities of interest have been reviewed and managed by Oregon Health & Science University. SDS is a consultant of Novartis Pharma AG and Amgen Inc. and a research support of Abbott Laboratories Inc., Amgen Inc., Daiichi-Sankyo Inc., Novartis Pharma AG, Theracos, Boston Scientific, NHLBI, Lone Star Heart, and Sanofi. JCT has no competing interests. MAP is a consultant of Aastrom Biosciences Inc., Abbott Laboratories Inc., Amgen Inc., FibroGen Inc., Cerenis Pharmaceuticals, Concert Pharmaceuticals, GlaxoSmithKline, Hamilton Health Sciences, Medtronic, Merck, Roche Pharmaceuticals, Servier, Teva Pharmaceuticals, and University of Oxford; a research support of Amgen Inc., Celladon, Novartis Pharma AG, and Sanofi; and has a relationship with Novartis Pharma AG.

Authors' Contributions

The presented analysis was prepared jointly by all authors. The corresponding author and coauthors had full access to the data in the study, contributed to the writing of the manuscript, and had final responsibility for the decision to submit for publication.

Acknowledgments

The ELIXA trial was supported by Sanofi.

References

[1] H. C. Gerstein, "Glucose: a continuous risk factor for cardiovascular disease," *Diabetic Medicine*, vol. 14, Supplement 3, pp. S25–S31, 1997.

[2] C. S. Fox, L. Sullivan, D'Agostino RB Sr, P. W. Wilson, and Framingham Heart Study, "The significant effect of diabetes duration on coronary heart disease mortality: the Framingham Heart Study," *Diabetes Care*, vol. 27, no. 3, pp. 704–708, 2004.

[3] for the ADVANCE Collaborative group, S. Zoungas, M. Woodward et al., "Impact of age, age at diagnosis and duration of diabetes on the risk of macrovascular and microvascular complications and death in type 2 diabetes," *Diabetologia*, vol. 57, no. 12, pp. 2465–2474, 2014.

[4] I. Tkác, "Effect of intensive glycemic control on cardiovascular outcomes and all-cause mortality in type 2 diabetes: overview and metaanalysis of five trials," *Diabetes Research and Clinical Practice*, vol. 86, Supplement 1, pp. S57–S62, 2009.

[5] T. H. Tung, S. J. Chen, F. L. Lee, J. H. Liu, C. H. Lin, and P. Chou, "A community-based study for the utility values associated with diabetic retinopathy among type 2 diabetics in Kinmen, Taiwan," *Diabetes Research and Clinical Practice*, vol. 68, no. 3, pp. 265–273, 2005.

[6] S. Tesfaye, N. Chaturvedi, S. E. Eaton et al., "Vascular risk factors and diabetic neuropathy," *The New England Journal of Medicine*, vol. 352, no. 4, pp. 341–350, 2005.

[7] S. Adler, "Structure-function relationships in diabetic nephropathy: lessons and limitations," *Kidney International. Supplement*, vol. 60, pp. S42–S45, 1997.

[8] A. I. Adler, E. J. Boyko, J. H. Ahroni, V. Stensel, R. C. Forsberg, and D. G. Smith, "Risk factors for diabetic peripheral sensory neuropathy. Results of the Seattle Prospective Diabetic Foot Study," *Diabetes Care*, vol. 20, no. 7, pp. 1162–1167, 1997.

[9] B. M. Sörensen, A. J. H. M. Houben, T. T. J. M. Berendschot et al., "Prediabetes and type 2 diabetes are associated with generalized microvascular dysfunction: the Maastricht Study," *Circulation*, vol. 134, no. 18, pp. 1339–1352, 2016.

[10] I. M. Stratton, A. I. Adler, H. A. Neil et al., "Association of glycaemia with macrovascular and microvascular complications of type 2 diabetes (UKPDS 35): prospective observational study," *BMJ*, vol. 321, no. 7258, pp. 405–412, 2000.

[11] B. Nazimek-Siewniak, D. K. Moczulski, and W. Grzeszczak, "Risk of macrovascular and microvascular complications in type 2 diabetes: results of longitudinal study design," *Journal of Diabetes and its Complications*, vol. 16, no. 4, pp. 271–276, 2002.

[12] M. A. Gall, P. Hougaard, K. Borch-Johnsen, and H. H. Parving, "Risk factors for development of incipient and overt diabetic nephropathy in patients with non-insulin dependent diabetes mellitus: prospective, observational study," *BMJ*, vol. 314, no. 7083, pp. 783–788, 1997.

[13] B. C. Astor, S. I. Hallan, E. R. Miller, E. Yeung, and J. Coresh, "Glomerular filtration rate, albuminuria, and risk of cardiovascular and all-cause mortality in the US population," *American Journal of Epidemiology*, vol. 167, no. 10, pp. 1226–1234, 2008.

[14] T. Ninomiya, V. Perkovic, B. E. de Galan et al., "Albuminuria and kidney function independently predict cardiovascular and renal outcomes in diabetes," *Journal of the American Society of Nephrology*, vol. 20, no. 8, pp. 1813–1821, 2009.

[15] I. H. de Boer, X. Gao, P. A. Cleary et al., "Albuminuria changes and cardiovascular and renal outcomes in type 1 diabetes: the DCCT/EDIC study," *Clinical Journal of the American Society of Nephrology*, vol. 11, no. 11, pp. 1969–1977, 2016.

[16] P. Gæde, P. Vedel, N. Larsen, G. V. H. Jensen, H.-H. Parving, and O. Pedersen, "Multifactorial intervention and cardiovascular disease in patients with type 2 diabetes," *The New England Journal of Medicine*, vol. 348, no. 5, pp. 383–393, 2003.

[17] V. Monhart, "Microalbuminuria. From diabetes to cardiovascular risk," *Vnitřní Lékařství*, vol. 57, pp. 293–298, 2011.

[18] R. Bentley-Lewis, D. Aguilar, M. C. Riddle et al., "Rationale, design, and baseline characteristics in Evaluation of LIXisenatide in Acute Coronary Syndrome, a long-term cardiovascular end point trial of lixisenatide versus placebo," *American Heart Journal*, vol. 169, no. 5, pp. 631–638.e7, 2015.

[19] M. A. Pfeffer, B. Claggett, R. Diaz et al., "Lixisenatide in patients with type 2 diabetes and acute coronary syndrome," *The New England Journal of Medicine*, vol. 373, no. 23, pp. 2247–2257, 2015.

[20] N. A. Bello, M. A. Pfeffer, H. Skali et al., "Retinopathy and clinical outcomes in patients with type 2 diabetes mellitus, chronic kidney disease, and anemia," *BMJ Open Diabetes Research & Care*, vol. 2, no. 1, article e000011, 2014.

[21] G. Targher, L. Bertolini, L. Zenari et al., "Diabetic retinopathy is associated with an increased incidence of cardiovascular events in type 2 diabetic patients," *Diabetic Medicine*, vol. 25, no. 1, pp. 45–50, 2008.

[22] R. Klein, A. R. Sharrett, B. E. Klein et al., "The association of atherosclerosis, vascular risk factors, and retinopathy in adults with diabetes: the atherosclerosis risk in communities study," *Ophthalmology*, vol. 109, no. 7, pp. 1225–1234, 2002.

[23] N. Cheung, S. Rogers, D. J. Couper, R. Klein, A. R. Sharrett, and T. Y. Wong, "Is diabetic retinopathy an independent risk factor for ischemic stroke?," *Stroke*, vol. 38, no. 2, pp. 398–401, 2007.

[24] J. R. W. Brownrigg, C. O. Hughes, D. Burleigh et al., "Microvascular disease and risk of cardiovascular events among individuals with type 2 diabetes: a population-level cohort study," *The Lancet Diabetes and Endocrinology*, vol. 4, no. 7, pp. 588–597, 2016.

[25] R. S. Rosenson, P. Fioretto, and P. M. Dodson, "Does microvascular disease predict macrovascular events in type 2 diabetes?," *Atherosclerosis*, vol. 218, no. 1, pp. 13–18, 2011.

[26] C. M. Forsblom, T. Sane, P. H. Groop et al., "Risk factors for mortality in type II (non-insulin-dependent) diabetes: evidence of a role for neuropathy and a protective effect of HLA-DR4," *Diabetologia*, vol. 41, no. 11, pp. 1253–1262, 1998.

[27] L. Kärvestedt, E. Mårtensson, V. Grill et al., "Peripheral sensory neuropathy associates with micro- or macroangiopathy: results from a population based study of type 2 diabetic patients in Sweden," *Diabetes Care*, vol. 32, no. 2, pp. 317–322, 2009.

[28] S. Del Prato, "Megatrials in type 2 diabetes. From excitement to frustration?," *Diabetologia*, vol. 52, no. 7, pp. 1219–1226, 2009.

[29] M. Lovestam-Adrian, C. Hansson-Lundblad, and O. Torffvit, "Sight-threatening retinopathy is associated with lower mortality in type 2 diabetic subjects: a 10-year observation study," *Diabetes Research and Clinical Practice*, vol. 77, no. 1, pp. 141–147, 2007.

[30] H. H. Parving, E. Hommel, E. Mathiesen et al., "Prevalence of microalbuminuria, arterial hypertension, retinopathy and neuropathy in patients with insulin dependent diabetes," *BMJ*, vol. 296, no. 6616, pp. 156–160, 1988.

[31] W. C. Duckworth, C. Abraira, T. E. Moritz et al., "The duration of diabetes affects the response to intensive glucose control in type 2 subjects: the VA Diabetes Trial," *Journal of Diabetes and its Complications*, vol. 25, no. 6, pp. 355–361, 2011.

11

The Effects of Tai Chi on Type 2 Diabetes Mellitus

Mengyao Chao, Chunyan Wang, Xiaosheng Dong, and Meng Ding

College of Physical Education, Shandong Normal University, 88 Wenhuadong Street, Jinan 250014, China

Correspondence should be addressed to Meng Ding; dingmengpy@aliyun.com

Academic Editor: Eusebio Chiefari

Objective. To investigate the effects of Tai chi in type 2 diabetes mellitus (type-2 DM) patients using systematic review and meta-analysis. *Methods.* Seven electronic resource databases were searched, and randomized controlled trials on the role of Tai chi in type-2 DM patients were retrieved. The meta-analysis was performed with RevMan 5.3, and research quality evaluation was conducted with the modified Jadad scale. *Results.* Fourteen studies, with 798 individuals related to the intervention of Tai chi on diabetes, were included. The results showed that, compared with nonexercise, Tai chi had the effect of lowering fasting blood glucose [MD = −1.39, 95% CI (−1.95, −0.84), $P < 0.0001$] and the subgroup effect size decreased with the increase of total exercise amount, there is no significant difference between Tai chi and other aerobic exercises [MD = −0.50, 95% CI (−1.02, 0.02), $P = 0.06$]; compared with nonexercise, Tai chi could reduce HbA1c [MD = −0.21, 95% CI (−0.61, 0.19), $P = 0.31$], and the group effect size decreased with the increase of total exercise amount. The reducing HbA1c effect of Tai chi was better than that of other aerobic exercises, but the difference was at the margin of statistical significance [MD = −0.19, 95% CI (−0.37, 0.00), $P = 0.05$]; compared with nonexercise, Tai chi had the effect of reducing 2 h postprandial blood glucose [MD = −2.07, 95% CI (−2.89, −1.26), $P = 0.0002$], there is no significant difference between Tai chi and other aerobic exercises in reducing 2 h postprandial blood glucose [MD = −0.44, 95% CI (−1.42, 0.54), $P = 0.38$]. *Conclusion.* Tai chi can effectively affect the management of blood glucose and HbA1c in type-2 DM patients. Long-term adherence to Tai chi has a better role in reducing blood glucose and HbA1c levels in type 2 DM patients.

1. Introduction

Diabetes mellitus (DM) is a chronic disease characterized by chronic hyperglycemia, which triggers the changes in lipids and proteins. There are 425 million people with diabetes in the world. There will be 629 million people with diabetes in the world in 2045 [1]. Diabetes has become the third major noncontagious disease threatening human health in modern countries, only second to cardiovascular disease and cancer [2].

According to the latest statistics, there were about 110 million adults suffering from diabetes in China, and it had rapidly become one of the countries with the medium prevalence (3%–10%) from the previous one with low prevalence (<3%) in less than 20 years [3, 4]. At present, the total cost of medical treatment due to diabetes and its complications in China was 20.86 billion yuan per year, accounting for 4.38% of the total national medical expenses, resulting in tremendous personal, family, and socioeconomic burdens [5, 6].

It is believed that the improvement of lifestyles can effectively control and prevent the occurrence of type-2 DM and its complications. The American Diabetes Association (ADA) pointed out that exercise therapy was an important part of improving lifestyle: effective exercise could prevent and control type-2 DM, playing a positive role in lowering blood glucose [7]. For example, moderate-intensity aerobic exercise and appropriate resistance exercise had an improving effect on blood glucose and blood lipid indicators of type-2 DM. Aerobic exercise could ameliorate the levels of visceral fat area and HbA1c in middle-aged and elderly obese patients with type-2 DM and improve the lipid metabolism, body composition, and cardiopulmonary function at the same time; accordingly, the blood glucose level was effectively controlled and the incidence of type-2 DM was reduced. In summary, exercise therapy has become an important part of the first level intervention of diabetes, which contributes to the management of type-2 DM patients [8].

The pathogenesis of type-2 DM is closely related to individual's physical and mental state. The traditional exercise, Tai chi, is a combination of physical activity and respiration, which combines limb movement and mind, making people enjoying physical and mental pleasure while exercising [9]. Therefore, Tai chi would play a more effective role in maintaining the body's neuroendocrine balance and controlling blood glucose. Although some researchers have done some works on the effects of Tai chi in type-2 DM patients using systematic evaluation and meta-analysis [10, 11], there are some inadequacies, including limited number of subjects and not typical enough detection indicators. In addition, as a form of physical and mental integration, whether Tai chi have more advantages beyond other aerobic exercises in the management of type-2 DM still lacks relevant merged research evidence. Accordingly, it is necessary to further confirm the effects of Tai chi on type-2 DM by including more high-quality studies. Besides, although some studies have explored the dose-response relationship between exercise and the incidence of type-2 DM using meta-analysis [12, 13], whether exercise, including Tai chi, had a dose-response relationship with blood glucose control was rarely studied. Therefore, this study also intends to preliminarily investigate the dose-response relationship between the exercise amount of Tai chi and blood glucose lowering in type-2 DM patients using meta-analysis.

2. Materials and Methods

2.1. Data Sources and Search Strategies. Electronic resource databases were searched, including PubMed, The Cochrane Library, EM base, SCI, CNKI, Wanfang Data, and VIP, and randomized controlled trials on the intervention effect of Tai chi on diabetes were retrieved. The time was all set as from the beginning to June 2016. Meanwhile, the references of the included papers were also reviewed to avoid omission. The search terms were divided into two parts: target (diabetes) search and intervention measure (Tai chi) search, and adjusted according to each database. All the searches used a combination of thematic and free search; all search strategies were determined after multiple presearch. The search strategy was mainly based on advanced search terms, including Tai chi, Taiji, Taijiquan, diabetes, type-2 diabetes mellitus, and DM.

2.2. Inclusion and Exclusion Criteria. Inclusion criteria included randomized controlled trials, published in Chinese and English language, with no restrictions on age or gender of type-2 DM; experimental group that takes Tai chi as the major intervention in the exercise of type-2 DM; the control group that does not take any exercise or other aerobic exercises (aerobic exercise except traditional sports including Tai chi and Qigong: jogging, walking, etc.) or antiresistance exercises; and patients without serious DM-related complications.

Exclusion criteria included experimental groups that used voluntary grouping principles and other nonrandomized controlled experiments; studies that did not include indicators to be discussed in this study; experimental groups that used other main exercises excluding Tai chi; and patient with DM-related complications.

2.3. Trial Inclusion and Data Extraction. During the process, two researchers (M. C. and X. D.) independently completed the trial inclusion and data extraction, and in case of disagreements, the third researcher (M. D.) would determine whether to include and extract. Data extraction information included information of the first author, publication time, published journals, title of trials, intervention measures of the experimental group and the control group, intervention time, subject number of the experimental group and the control group, whether outcome indicator was complete, whether there were subjects lost to follow-up, and basic information of patients (age, gender, sex ratio, and whether there were other complications). Diabetes indicator data included fasting blood glucose (FBG), HbA1c, and 2 h postprandial blood glucose (2hPBG); FBG was the first indicator of this study.

2.4. Trial Quality Assessments. During the data extraction process, the quality of the included studies was evaluated using modified Jadad quality scoring scale [14]. Modified Jadad quality scoring scale included the generation of random sequences, distribution methods, randomized concealment, whether blind method was adopted, and so on. There were corresponding criteria and scores for each item, 1–3 points for low-quality study and 4–7 points for high-quality study. Two raters performed the quality assessment independently (M. C. and C.W.). Disagreements were resolved by seeking the opinion of the third rater (M. D.)

2.5. Statistical Analysis. Meta-analysis was performed with Review Manager 5.3 available from Cochrane. The heterogeneity test χ^2 of the results was included. When there was statistical homogeneity between studies, it was shown in $P > 0.1$ and $I^2 < 50\%$ and a fixed-effect model was used; the heterogeneity was shown in $P < 0.1$ and $I^2 > 50\%$, and heterogeneity source analysis was performed, then subgroup analysis was conducted based on the heterogeneity. If there was no heterogeneity between subgroups, a fixed-effect model was used, while if there was heterogeneity between subgroups, the meta-analysis was performed with a random-effect model; if the heterogeneity within the group was too large, descriptive analysis was carried out.

To reveal whether there was a dose-response relationship between Tai chi with blood glucose control and HbA1c lowering in type-2 DM patients, Tai chi and nonexercise in the included studies were compared based on total exercise amount, and stratified subgroup analysis was performed in this study. Since most of the selected studies did not report Tai chi exercise intensity, the exercise intensity of all selected studies was treated as the same by default; thus, the total exercise amount could be expressed by total exercise time. According to total exercise amount, the included studies were divided into 4 subgroups, namely, small

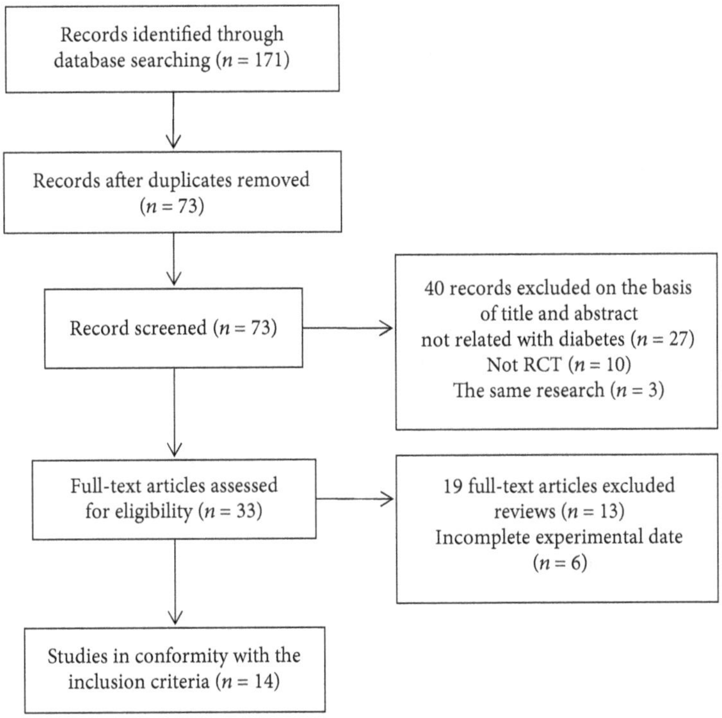

FIGURE 1: Flowchart of trial selection process.

exercise group (with exercise amount less than 1999 minutes), medium exercise group (with exercise amount of 2000–3999 minutes), large exercise group (with exercise amount of 4000–5999 minutes), and super large exercise group (with exercise amount above 6000 minutes). The total exercise amount was calculated as total exercise amount (minutes) = Tai chi exercise time (minutes) per day * Tai chi exercise days per week * total of Tai chi exercise weeks (calculated as 4 weeks per month).

3. Results

3.1. Trial Search. Databases, including PubMed, The Cochrane Library, EMbase, SCI, CNKI, Wanfang Data, and VIP, were searched, and according to the criteria of exclusion and inclusion, randomized controlled trials on the intervention of Tai chi on type-2 DM were retrieved. A total of 171 potentially relevant articles were identified by the database searches. After excluding duplicates, 73 records remained. Of these, 40 articles were removed through reading titles and abstracts and 19 were excluded after reviewing the full text against the eligibility criteria. Finally, a total of 14 trials [15–27], including 5 English ones and 9 Chinese ones, were included. One trial titled "Health Qigong Tai Ji Quan Adjuvant Therapy in Patients with Type 2 Diabetes Clinical Observational Studies" is an unpublished literature, which was retrieved from the Doctoral and Master Dissertation Library of CNKI. The study selection process is shown in Figure 1.

3.2. Characteristics of Included Studies and Quality Assessments. Fourteen studies, with 798 individuals related to the intervention of Tai chi on diabetes, were included. The average age ranged 48.0–64.0. All patients in intervention groups received Tai chi intervention while maintaining routine medication. Seven articles have adopted the 24-style (short form) Tai chi [17, 18, 22, 23, 25, 27, 28], 1 article adopted the 24-form Yang TC style [19], 1 article adopted Yang and Sun 20-form TC style [20], 1 article adopted the Lin Housheng's style [24], 1 article adopted the DaYuan's TC style [15], 1 article adopted the Yang TC style [21], and 2 articles did not report the type of Tai chi [16, 26]. The frequencies of Tai chi exercise in the included articles were from 3 to 7 times per week, and exercise durations lasted from 15 to 60 minutes across the different articles. The control groups were divided into nonexercise groups and other aerobic exercise groups. The exercise forms of other aerobic exercise groups include social dance, Qigong, and general aerobic exercise (see Table 1 for details). In the case of modified Jadad scoring, there were 6 studies with 2 points, 5 studies with 3 points, 2 studies with 5 points, and 1 study with 6 points. There were 11 low-quality trials, with an average of 2.4 points, and 3 high-quality trials, with an average of 5.3 points (see Table 2 for details).

3.3. Outcomes

3.3.1. Fasting Blood Glucose

(1) Tai Chi versus Nonexercise. Initially, the data of 11 related studies ($n = 529$) [15, 17, 23–27] was pooled, but the data heterogeneity was quite high. After subgroup analysis according to total exercise amount, it was found that the heterogeneity of 4 studies in a large exercise group was as high as 94%. Through sensitivity analysis of the data, it was speculated

Table 1: Characteristics and quality assessments of the included trials.

First author, year	Patients (total, E/C)	Age (mean (SD), E/C)	Experimental intervention	Control	Duration, sessions with supervision per week, time per session
Yan 2004	18, 10/8	51.8 (7.4)/53.1 (7.8)	Tai chi	N	24 weeks, 7, 40 min
Yu 2004	40, 20/20	50 (58)/49 (5.6)	Tai chi	N	12 weeks, 7, 60 min
Jiang 2007	36, 18/18	57.2 (4.2)/55.0 (6.2)	Tai chi	N	20 weeks, 7, 40 min
Tracey T. 2007	38, 18/20	65 (7.8)	Tai chi	N	16 weeks, 2, 60 min
Paul Lam 2008	53, 28/15	63.2 (8.6)/60.7 (12.2)	Tai chi	N	24 weeks, 2, 60 min
Ying Zhang 2008	20, 10/9	57.4 (6.2)	Tai chi	N	14 weeks, 5, 60 min
Wang 2009	54, 28/26	49.21 (11.12)/48.83 (10.54)	Tai chi	Social dancing exercise	24 weeks, 5, 30 min
Wu 2010	40, 20/20	NR	Tai chi	N	24 weeks, 3, 60 min
Shih-Chuen Chen 2010	104, 56/48	59.1 (6.2)/57.4 (5.8)	Tai chi	Aerobic exercise	12 weeks, 3, 60 min
Li X. 2013	60, 30/30	57.3 (10.3)	Tai chi	N	8 weeks, 7, 45 min
Li Z. 2013	87, 43/44	54.21 (9.47)/52.69 (8.37)	Tai chi	N	12 weeks, 7, 30 min
Sununta 2013	64, 32/32	NR	Tai chi	N	12 weeks, 5, 30 min
Tang 2014	28, 14/14	61.40 (5.08)/61.53 (6.23)	Tai chi	N	24 weeks, 5, 15 min
Tang 2014	29, 15/14	62.73 (7.17)/61.53 (6.23)	Tai chi	N	24 weeks, 5, 30 min
Tang 2014	27, 13/14	59.40 (6.68)/61.53 (6.23)	Tai chi	N	24 weeks, 5, 45 min
Zhang 2015	100, 50/50	55.36 (2.78)/61.53 (6.23)	Tai chi	N	4 weeks, 7, 30 min

E: experimental group; C: control group; N: nonexercise; NR: not reported; min: minute; SD: standard deviation.

that the data of Yu 2004 was the main source of heterogeneity in this subgroup. Accordingly, the data of this study was excluded, and the data of the other 3 studies was pooled. Finally, the data of 10 studies ($n = 489$) was pooled, and the results showed that, compared with nonexercise, Tai chi had an effect of lowering FBG and that the difference was statistically significant [MD = −1.39, 95% CI (−1.95, −0.84), $P < 0.0001$]. Within 6000-minute exercise amount, the subgroup pooled effect size decreased with the increase of total exercise amount, and only one study was included above 6000 minutes, its effect size was close to the group of 4000–5999 minutes and the difference was not statistically significant (see Figure 2).

(2) Tai Chi versus Other Aerobic Exercises. As shown in Figure 3, 7 related studies ($n = 342$) [18, 21, 22, 25] allowed for data pooling. After data pooling using a random-effect model, the results suggested that, compared with other aerobic exercises, Tai chi did not show a better role in lowering FBG, and the difference was not statistically significant [MD = −0.21, 95% CI (−0.61, 0.19), $P = 0.31$].

3.3.2. HbA1c

(1) Tai Chi versus Nonexercise. Initially, the data of 9 studies ($n = 356$) [15, 16, 24, 25] was pooled, but the data heterogeneity was quite high. After subgroup analysis according to total exercise amount, it was found that the heterogeneity was mainly from the large exercise group. After sensitivity analysis, it was speculated that the data of Jiang 2007 and Wu 2010 was the main source of heterogeneity. Accordingly, the data of these two studies was excluded, and data pooling was reperformed. Finally, data pooling was carried out for 7 studies ($n = 293$), and the results showed that HbA1c in the Tai chi group was lower than that in the control group, with statistically significant difference [MD = −0.73, 95% CI (−0.95, −0.52), $P = 0.03$]. The grouping effect size of HbA1c decreased with the increase of total exercise amount (see Figure 4).

(2) Tai Chi versus Other Aerobic Exercises. As shown in Figure 5, 7 related studies ($n = 372$) [19, 21, 22, 25] allowed for data pooling. After data pooling using a random-effect model, the results suggested that, compared with other aerobic exercises, Tai chi had a better effect of reducing HbA1c and that the difference was statistically significant [MD = −0.19, 95% CI (−0.37, 0.00), $P = 0.05$]. However, the statistical significance was at the margin.

3.3.3. Two-Hour Postprandial Blood Glucose

(1) Tai Chi versus Nonexercise. As shown in Figure 6, 5 related studies ($n = 162$) [15, 26] allowed for data pooling. After data pooling using a random-effect model, the results

Table 2: The quality evaluation of the methodology.

Inclusion research	Randomization	Concealment of allocation	Double blinding	Withdrawals and dropouts	Jadad score
Yan 2004	Yes	No	No	No	2
Yu 2004	Yes	No	No	No	2
Jiang 2007	Yes	No	No	No	2
Tracey T. 2007	Yes	No	Double blind	Yes	5
Paul Lam 2008	Yes	Computer generation	Double blind	Yes	6
Ying Zhang 2008	Yes	No	No	Yes	3
Wang 2009	Yes	No	No	Yes	3
Wu 2010	Yes	No	No	No	2
Shih-Chuen Chen 2010	Yes	No	No	Yes	3
Li X. 2013	Yes	No	No	No	2
Li Z. 2013	Yes	No	No	Yes	3
Sununta 2013	Yes	No	Double blind	Yes	5
Tang 2014	Yes	No	No	Yes	3
Zhang 2015	Yes	No	No	No	2

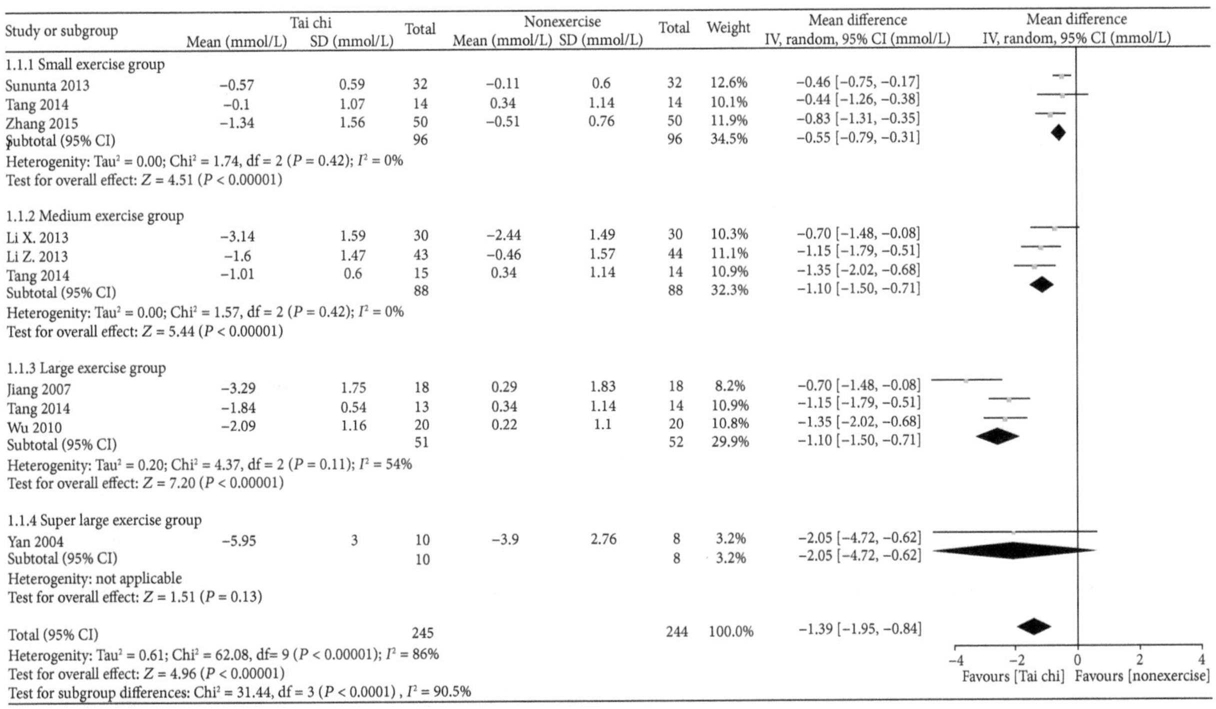

Figure 2: The meta-analysis for comparing FBG between Tai chi and the nonexercise. CI: confidence interval; SD: standard deviation.

suggested that the 2hPBG in the Tai chi group was lower than that in the nonexercise group and that the difference was statistically significant [MD = −2.07, 95% CI (−2.89, −1.26), $P = 0.0002$].

(2) Tai Chi versus Other Aerobic Exercises. As shown in Figure 7, for 3 related studies ($n = 84$), after data pooling using a random-effect model, the results showed that there was no statistically significant difference in 2hPBG between the Tai chi group and the other aerobic exercise group [MD = −0.44, 95% CI (−1.42, 0.54), $P = 0.38$].

3.4. Publication Bias Evaluation

3.4.1. Publication Bias Evaluation between Tai Chi and Nonexercise.

In this study, funnel plot analysis was performed on the indicator, FBG, in the Tai chi group and the nonexercise group. A total of 11 studies, with 529 subjects, were included. The results showed that the distribution of included studies on both sides of the funnel plot was asymmetric, indicating that there might be potential publication bias in the comparison of Tai chi and nonexercise.

Study or subgroup	Tai chi Mean (mmol/L)	Tai chi SD (mmol/L)	Total	Other aerobic exercise Mean (mmol/L)	Other aerobic exercise SD (mmol/L)	Total	Weight	Mean difference IV, random, 95% CI (mmol/L)
2.1.1 FBG								
Li Z. 2013	−1.61	1.46	43	−1.29	1.66	48	15.0%	−0.32 [−0.96, 0.32]
Shih-Chuen Chen 2010	−0.35	1.15	50	−0.21	1.03	44	18.9%	−0.14 [−0.58, 0.30]
Tang 2014	−0.1	1.07	14	−0.69	1.01	14	12.8%	0.59 [−0.18, 1.36]
Tang 2014	−1.01	0.6	15	−0.69	1.01	14	15.6%	−0.32 [−0.93, 0.29]
Tang 2014	−1.48	0.54	13	−0.69	1.01	14	15.7%	−0.79 [−1.40, − 0.18]
Wang 2009	−0.58	1.05	28	−0.86	1.71	26	18.2%	0.28 [−0.20, 0.76]
Ying Zhang 2008	−2.3	1.67	10	−0.08	2.39	9	3.8%	−2.22 [−4.09, −0.35]
Subtotal (95% CI)			173			169	100.0%	−0.21 [−0.61, 0.19]
Heterogeneity: Tau² = 0.17; Chi² = 16.25, df = 6 (P = 0.01); I² = 63%								
Test for overall effect: Z = 1.02 (P = 0.31)								
Total (95% CI)			173			169	100.0%	−0.21 [−0.61, 0.19]
Heterogeneity: Tau² = 0.17; Chi² = 16.25, df = 6 (P = 0.01); I² = 63%								
Test for overall effect: Z = 1.02 (P = 0.31)								
Test for subgroup differences: not applicable								

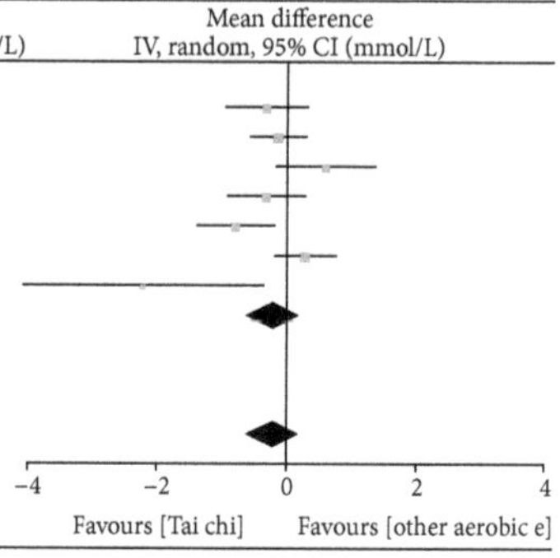

Figure 3: The meta-analysis for comparing FBG between Tai chi and other aerobic exercises. CI: confidence interval; SD: standard deviation.

Study or subgroup	Tai chi Mean (%)	Tai chi SD (%)	Total	Nonexercise Mean (%)	Nonexercise SD (%)	Total	Weight	Mean difference IV, random, 95% CI (%)
1.2.1 Small exercise group								
Sununta 2013	−1.07	1.03	32	−0.26	1.25	32	9.6%	−0.81 [−1.37, −0.25]
Tang 2014	−0.25	0.38	14	0.28	0.37	14	19.2%	−0.53 [−0.81, −0.25]
Subtotal (95% CI)			46			46	28.9%	−0.59 [−0.83, −0.34]
Heterogeneity: Tau² = 0.00; Chi² = 0.77, df = 1 (P = 0.38); I² = 0%								
Test for overall effect: Z = 4.61 (P < 0.00001)								
1.2.2 Medium exercise group								
Li Z. 2013	−1.72	1.46	43	−0.82	1.47	44	8.5%	−0.90 [−1.52, −0.28]
Tang 2014	−0.09	0.35	15	0.28	0.37	14	19.9%	−0.37 [−0.63, −0.11]
Subtotal (95% CI)			58			58	28.4%	−0.56 [−1.06, −0.06]
Heterogeneity: Tau² = 0.08; Chi² = 2.41, df = 1 (P = 0.12); I² = 58%								
Test for overall effect: Z = 2.20 (P = 0.03)								
1.2.3 Large exercise group								
Tang3 2014	−0.66	0.37	13	0.28	0.37	14	19.1%	−0.81 [−1.37, −0.25]
Yu 2004	−1.2	0.52	20	−0.3	0.27	20	20.1%	−0.53 [−0.81, −0.25]
Subtotal (95% CI)			33			34	39.3%	−0.59 [−0.83, −0.34]
Heterogeneity: Tau² = 0.00; Chi² = 0.04, df = 1 (P = 0.84); I² = 0%								
Test for overall effect: Z = 9.52 (P < 0.00001)								
1.2.4 Super large exercise group								
Yan 2004	−3.1	1.15	10	−1.9	1.17	8	3.5%	−1.20 [−2.28, −0.12]
Subtotal (95% CI)			10			8	3.5%	−1.20 [−2.28, −0.12]
Heterogeneity: not applicable								
Test for overall effect: Z = 2.18 (P = 0.03)								
Total (95% CI)			147			146	100.0%	−0.73 [−0.95, −0.52]
Heterogeneity: Tau² = 0.04; Chi² = 14.04, df = 6 (P = 0.03); I² = 57%								
Test for overall effect: Z = 6.69 (P < 0.00001)								
Test for subgroup differences: Chi² = 5.75, df = 3 (P = 0.12), I² = 47.8%								

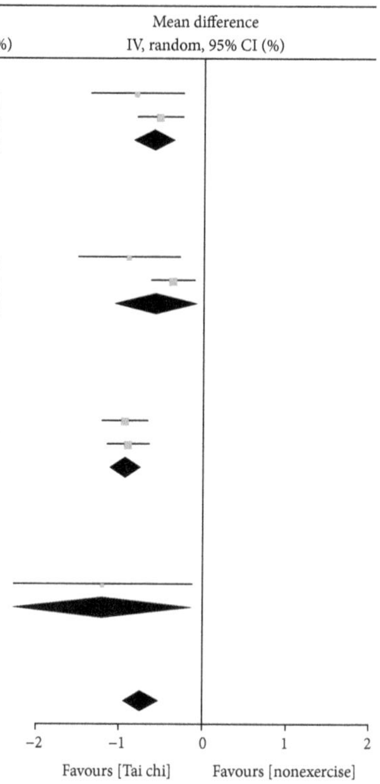

Figure 4: The meta-analysis for comparing HbA1c between Tai chi and the nonexercise. CI: confidence interval; SD: standard deviation.

Study or subgroup	Tai chi Mean (%)	Tai chi SD (%)	Total	Other aerobic exercise Mean (%)	Other aerobic exercise SD (%)	Total	Weight	Mean difference IV, random, 95% CI (%)
2.2.1 HbalC								
Li Z. 2013	−1.72	1.46	43	−1.34	1.47	48	6.9%	−0.38 [−0.98, 0.22]
Shih-Chuen Chen 2010	−0.6	1.62	50	−0.3	2.24	44	4.4%	−0.30 [−1.10, 0.50]
Tang 2014	−0.25	0.38	14	−0.1	0.3	20	17.6%	−0.15 [−0.39, 0.09]
Tang 2014	−0.09	0.35	15	−0.1	0.3	20	18.3%	0.01 [−0.21, 0.23]
Tang 2014	−0.66	0.37	13	−0.1	0.3	20	17.5%	−0.56 [−0.80, −0.32]
Tracey Tsang 2007	−0.07	0.4	17	0.12	0.3	14	17.2%	−0.19 [−0.44, 0.06]
Wang 2009	−1.03	0.38	28	−1.08	0.46	26	18.1%	0.05 [−0.18, 0.28]
Subtotal (95% CI)			180			192	100.0%	−0.19 [−0.37, 0.00]
Heterogeneity: Tau² =0.04; Chi² = 16.93, df = 6 (P = 0.010); I² = 65%								
Test for overall effect: Z = 1.96 (P = 0.05)								
Total (95% CI)			180			192	100.0%	−0.19 [−0.37, 0.00]
Heterogeneity: Tau² =0.04; Chi² = 16.93, df = 6 (P = 0.010); I² = 65%								
Test for overall effect: Z = 1.96 (P = 0.05)								
Test for subgroup differences: not applicable								

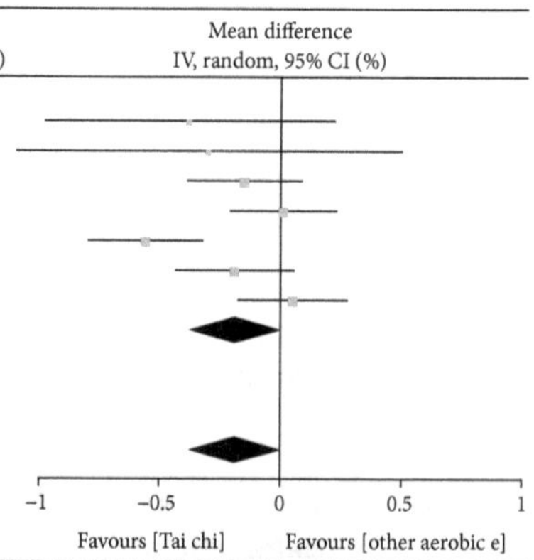

Figure 5: The meta-analysis for comparing HbA1c between Tai chi and other aerobic exercises. CI: confidence interval; SD: standard deviation.

Study or subgroup	Tai chi Mean (mmol/L)	Tai chi SD (mmol/L)	Total	Nonexercise Mean (mmol/L)	Nonexercise SD (mmol/L)	Total	Weight	Mean difference IV, random, 95% CI (mmol/L)
1.3.1 2 hPBG								
Li X. 2013	−6.25	3.2	30	−4.82	3.45	30	23.4%	−1.43 [−3.11, 0.25]
Tang 2014	−1.86	2.94	14	−0.15	2.24	14	17.7%	−1.71 [−3.65, 0.23]
Tang 2014	−2.54	2.35	15	−0.15	2.24	14	23.8%	−2.39 [−4.06, −0.72]
Tang 2014	−2.65	1.57	13	−0.15	2.24	14	31.5%	−2.50 [−3.95, −1.05]
Yan 2014	−7.1	4.76	10	−4.9	4.49	8	3.6%	−2.20 [−6.49, 2.09]
Subtotal (95% CI)			82			80	100.0%	−2.07 [−2.89, −1.26]
Heterogeneity: Tau² = 0.00; Chi² = 1.17, df = 4 (P = 0.88); I² = 0%								
Test for overall effect: Z = 4.99 (P < 0.00001)								
Total (95% CI)			82			80	100.0%	−2.07 [−2.89, −1.26]
Heterogeneity: Tau² = 0.00; Chi² = 1.17, df = 4 (P = 0.88); I² = 0%								
Test for overall effect: Z = 4.99 (P < 0.00001)								
Test for subgroup diffrences: not applicable								

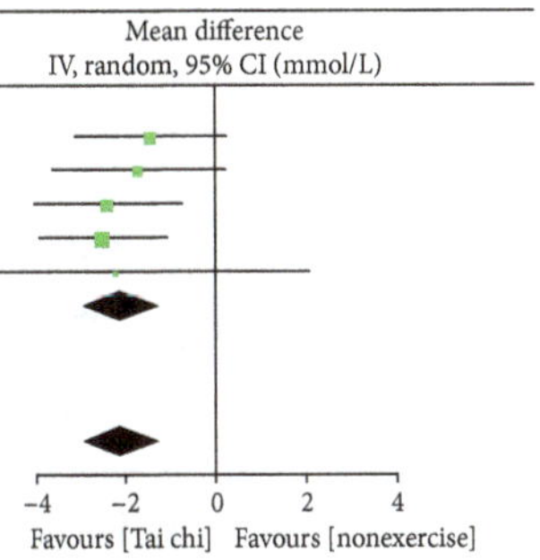

Figure 6: The meta-analysis for comparing 2hPBG between Tai chi and the nonexercise. CI: confidence interval; SD: standard deviation.

Study or subgroup	Tai chi Mean (mmol/L)	Tai chi SD (mmol/L)	Total	Other aerobic exercise Mean (mmol/L)	Other aerobic exercise SD (mmol/L)	Total	Weight	Mean difference IV, random, 95% CI (mmol/L)
2.3.1 2hPBG								
Tang 2014	−1.86	2.94	14	−1.98	2.36	14	24.7%	0.12 [−1.85, 2.09]
Tang 2014	−2.54	2.35	15	−1.98	2.36	14	32.7%	−0.56 [−2.28, 1.16]
Tang 2014	−2.65	1.57	13	−1.98	2.36	14	42.6%	−0.67 [−,17, 0.83]
Subtotal (95% CI)			42			42	100.0%	−0.44 [−1.42, 0.54]
Heterogeneity: Tau² = 0.00; Chi² = 0.42, df = 2 (P = 0.81); I² = 0%								
Test for overall effect: Z = 0.88 (P = 0.38)								
Total (95% CI)			42			42	100.0%	−0.44 [−1.42, 0.54]
Heterogeneity: Tau² = 0.00; Chi² = 0.42, df = 2 (P = 0.81); I² = 0%								
Test for overall effect: Z = 0.88 (P = 0.38)								
Test for subgroup differences: not applicable								

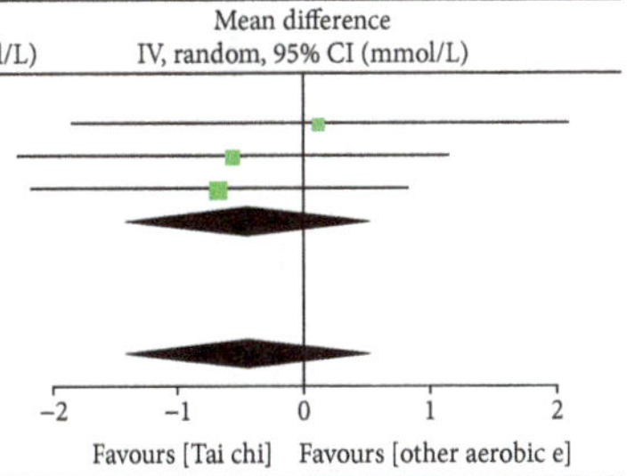

Figure 7: The meta-analysis for comparing 2hPBG between Tai chi and other aerobic exercises. CI: confidence interval; SD: standard deviation.

3.4.2. Publication Bias Evaluation between Tai Chi and Other Aerobic Exercises. Funnel plot analysis was performed on the indicator, FBG, in the Tai chi group and the other aerobic exercise group. A total of 7 studies, with 342 subjects, were included. The results showed that the distribution of included studies on both sides of the funnel plot was asymmetric, indicating that there might be potential publication bias in the comparison of Tai chi and other aerobic exercises.

4. Discussion

Tai chi is one of the unique traditional exercises in China. In the practice of Tai chi, it is required to be concentrated, move slowly, and be tranquil in movement. The intensity is not so high, and adequate physical and mental relaxation can be achieved. Thus, Tai chi is fit for older people with weaker constitution and chronic diseases, which is a moderate general movement. Theoretically, Tai chi should be a suitable exercise for type-2 DM patients. However, there were contradictions in published systematic review and meta-analysis. Zhang Yeting and others included 4 studies and systematically reviewed the effect of Tai chi in type-2 DM patients before and after exercise; the results showed that there was a significant decrease of blood glucose level in type-2 DM patients after Tai chi exercise, indicating the effect of Tai chi on diabetes, while two meta-analysis researches published in 2013 and 2015 [10, 11] considered that there was still no sufficient evidence to confirm the blood glucose lowering effect of Tai chi in type-2 DM patients.

However, according to the results of this study, compared with nonexercise, Tai chi had significant decreasing effect on FBG, HbA1c, and 2hPBG among type-2 DM patients, indicating that Tai chi had a positive effect for diabetics. Theoretically, as a regular small- and medium-intensity aerobic exercise, Tai chi can promote the metabolism of cells and tissues, promote blood back-flowing to the heart, improve body's utilization of glucose, increase target cell reactivity, improve body's glucose tolerance, prevent the composition of HbA1c, and accelerate the combination of hemoglobin and oxygen. Therefore, the blood glucose can be further controlled, thereby reducing the levels of FBG, HbA1c, and 2hPBG.

From the results of this study, compared with other aerobic exercise, including running, walking, and dancing, Tai chi did not show a better effect on blood glucose control in type-2 DM patients, which was consistent with the results published by Lee et al. However, in the case of reducing HbA1c, this study showed that Tai chi had some advantages over other aerobic exercise, but the difference was at the margin of statistical significance ($P = 0.05$). Relevant studies, including our previous study, have found that mind-body exercises had the effect of reducing HbA1c in type-2 DM patients. One study showed that walking combined with meditation exercise had a better effect on HbA1c regulation than simple walking [29]; the results of our previous meta-analysis also showed that, compared with other aerobic exercise, Qigong exercise had more advantages in downregulating HbA1c level of type-2 DM patients [30]. Therefore, we considered that Tai chi as an exercise with the combination of movement and meditation could suppress sympathetic activation, thus can improve glycemic control as neutrally mediated vasoconstriction, and in the meanwhile reduce glucose delivery and uptake in skeletal muscle [31].

At present, there were few studies on whether there was dose-response relationship between physical exercise, including Tai chi, with FBG and HbA1c control in type-2 DM patients. However, a recent study showed that there was curvilinear dose-response relationship between HbA1c and total exercise amount, higher exercise amount was associated with lower HbA1c level [32]. According to the results of this study, for both FBG and HbA1c, higher exercise amount subgroup corresponded to lower effect size in a certain range. Therefore, we believed that there was a certain dose-response relationship between Tai chi with FBG and HbA1c control in type-2 DM patients, while the authenticity needs to be verified by more rigorous clinical trials or meta-analysis.

According to meta-analysis and the included studies, total Tai chi exercise amount of 4000–5999 minutes could result in better blood glucose and HbA1c control. For type-2 DM patients, to regulate blood glucose and HbA1c levels, Tai chi exercise of 80–120 minutes per week for more than one year or 160–240 minutes per week for more than a half year was recommended. This recommended Tai chi exercise amount was basically the same as the 150-minute moderate-intensity exercise per week mentioned in most current clinical practice guidelines [33].

There are limitations to this study that must be considered. Firstly, due to limited conditions, only PubMed, The Cochrane Library, EM base, SCI, CNKI, Wan Fang Data, and VIP were searched, and there might be omissions; secondly, the quality of included papers was low, the random distribution method and blind method was not described, some trials failed to indicate whether there was missing subject, only indicating random distribution, and the modified Jadad score of most trials was 2; thirdly, the heterogeneity of included studies was quite large, only random-effect model could be adopted, which had certain impact on the results; fourthly, there was a large possibility of publication bias among included trials.

5. Conclusion

Tai chi can effectively affect the management of blood glucose and HbA1c in type-2 DM patients. Long-term adherence to Tai chi has a better role in reducing blood glucose and HbA1c levels in type-2 DM patients.

Conflicts of Interest

The authors declare that there is no conflict of interest regarding the publication of this paper.

References

[1] Federation ID, "IDF DIABETES ATLAS eighth edition 2017," 2017, http://www.diabetesatlas.org/.

[2] WHO, "Diabetes," http://www.who.int/mediacentre/factsheets/fs312/en/.

[3] Y. Xu, L. Wang, J. He et al., "Prevalence and control of diabetes in Chinese adults," *Journal of the American Medical Association*, vol. 310, no. 9, pp. 948–959, 2013.

[4] L. Wang, P. Gao, M. Zhang et al., "Prevalence and ethnic pattern of diabetes and prediabetes in China in 2013," *Journal of the American Medical Association*, vol. 317, no. 24, pp. 2515–2523, 2017.

[5] R. C. W. Ma, K. Y. Tsoi, W. H. Tam, and C. K. C. Wong, "Developmental origins of type 2 diabetes: a perspective from China," *European Journal of Clinical Nutrition*, vol. 71, no. 7, pp. 870–880, 2017.

[6] Y. Huang, P. Vemer, J. Zhu, M. J. Postma, and W. Chen, "Economic burden in Chinese patients with diabetes mellitus using electronic insurance claims data," *PLoS One*, vol. 11, no. 8, article e0159297, 2016.

[7] Association AD, "Cardiovascular disease and risk management: standards of medical care in diabetes-2018," *Diabetes Care*, vol. 41, Supplement 1, pp. S86–S104, 2018.

[8] M. J. Armstrong and R. J. Sigal, "Exercise as medicine: key concepts in discussing physical activity with patients who have type 2 diabetes," *Canadian Journal of Diabetes*, vol. 39, Supplement 5, pp. S129–S133, 2015.

[9] W. C. Wang, A. L. Zhang, B. Rasmussen et al., "The effect of tai chi on psychosocial well-being: a systematic review of randomized controlled trials," *Journal of Acupuncture and Meridian Studies*, vol. 2, no. 3, pp. 171–181, 2009.

[10] M. S. Lee, J. H. Jun, H. J. Lim, and H. S. Lim, "A systematic review and meta-analysis of tai chi for treating type 2 diabetes," *Maturitas*, vol. 80, no. 1, pp. 14–23, 2015.

[11] J. H. Yan, W. J. Gu, and L. Pan, "Lack of evidence on tai chi-related effects in patients with type 2 diabetes mellitus: a meta-analysis," *Experimental and Clinical Endocrinology & Diabetes*, vol. 121, no. 5, pp. 266–271, 2013.

[12] A. Wahid, N. Manek, M. Nichols et al., "Quantifying the association between physical activity and cardiovascular disease and diabetes: a systematic review and meta-analysis," *Journal of the American Heart Association*, vol. 5, no. 9, p. e002495, 2016.

[13] A. D. Smith, A. Crippa, J. Woodcock, and S. Brage, "Physical activity and incident type 2 diabetes mellitus: a systematic review and dose-response meta-analysis of prospective cohort studies," *Diabetologia*, vol. 59, no. 12, pp. 2527–2545, 2016.

[14] A. R. Jadad, R. A. Moore, D. Carroll et al., "Assessing the quality of reports of randomized clinical trials: is blinding necessary?," *Controlled Clinical Trials*, vol. 17, no. 1, pp. 1–12, 1996.

[15] C. X. Yan Ju, R. Shilao, M. ZhenYing, Y. Jianyu, and L. Zhen, "The source of hypoglycemic _ tai chi exercise on blood glucose in patients with type 2 diabetes mellitus effect observation, Guangming," *Journal of Chinese Medicine*, vol. 19, no. 3, pp. 16-17, 2004.

[16] Y. Yang, "Effects and mechanism of physical exercise on type II diabetes mellitus associated with hypertension," *Journal of Shenyang Institute of Physical Education*, vol. 23, no. 3, pp. 444-445, 2004.

[17] J. Rongkang, "The influence of Taijiquan on the mellitus II patients' lipid constituents and insulin-resistance Wushu," *Science*, vol. 4, no. 10, pp. 35-36, 2007.

[18] Y. Zhang and F. H. Fu, "Effects of 14-week Tai Ji Quan exercise on metabolic control in women with type 2 diabetes," *The American Journal of Chinese Medicine*, vol. 36, no. 4, pp. 647–654, 2008.

[19] T. Tsang, R. Orr, P. Lam, E. Comino, and M. F. Singh, "Effects of tai chi on glucose homeostasis and insulin sensitivity in

older adults with type 2 diabetes: a randomised double-blind sham-exercise-controlled trial," *Age and Ageing*, vol. 37, no. 1, pp. 64–71, 2008.

[20] P. Lam, S. M. Dennis, T. H. Diamond, and N. Zwar, "Improving glycaemic and BP control in type 2 diabetes the effectiveness of tai chi," *Australian Family Physician*, vol. 37, no. 10, pp. 884–887, 2008.

[21] W. A. N. G. P. HQ, L. I. Guangting, and L. I. A. N. G. Renrui, "Evaluation of varying aerobics interferential effects on type 2 *diabetes* patients in community," *China Medical Herald*, vol. 6, no. 9, pp. 34-35, 2009.

[22] S.-C. Chen, K.-C. Ueng, S.-H. Lee, K.-T. Sun, and M.-C. Lee, "Effect of T'ai chi exercise on biochemical profiles and oxidative stress indicators in obese patients with type 2 diabetes," *The Journal of Alternative and Complementary Medicine*, vol. 16, no. 11, pp. 1153–1159, 2010.

[23] W. Fan Se-f, B. Yan, X. Jian-wu, and J. Ru-han, "Tai chi for the treatment of type 2 diabetes," *Chinese Journal of Physical Medicine and Rehabilitation*, vol. 32, no. 3, pp. 205–207, 2010.

[24] S. Youngwanichsetha, S. Phumdoung, and T. Ingkathawornwong, "The effects of tai chi qigong exercise on plasma glucose levels and health status of postpartum Thai women with type 2 diabetes," *Focus on Alternative and Complementary Therapies*, vol. 18, no. 4, pp. 182–187, 2013.

[25] Q. L. LI Zhibin, Z. Lei, and L. Hengliang, "Study on advantages of treating type 2 diabetes mellitus with Baduanjin for aerobic exercise Liaoning," *Journal of Traditional Chinese Medicine*, vol. 09, no. 40, pp. 1858–1860, 2013.

[26] L. Xiaobing, "Effect of Taijiquan exercise on oxidative stress and inflammation in elderly patients with type 2 diabetes," *Chinese Journal of Gerontology*, vol. 21, pp. 5465-5466, 2013.

[27] Z. Hui, "Analysis of the effect of Taijiquan on blood sugar in type 2 diabetic patients," *Contemporary Medicine Forum*, vol. 13, no. 18, pp. 4-5, 2015.

[28] T. Yuanbo, "Health Qigong Tai Ji Quan adjuvant therapy in patients with type 2 diabetes clinical observational studies," *Nanjing University of Chinese Medicine (NJUCM).*, vol. 2, p. 35, 2014.

[29] A. Gainey, T. Himathongkam, H. Tanaka, and D. Suksom, "Effects of buddhist walking meditation on glycemic control and vascular function in patients with type 2 diabetes," *Complementary Therapies in Medicine*, vol. 26, pp. 92–97, 2016.

[30] W. C. Ding Meng, D. Xiaosheng, and Y. Xiangrenhttps://www.hindawi.com/journals/ecam/2018/8182938/.

[31] M. Paul-Labrador, D. Polk, J. H. Dwyer et al., "Effects of a randomized controlled trial of transcendental meditation on components of the metabolic syndrome in subjects with coronary heart disease," *Archives of Internal Medicine*, vol. 166, no. 11, pp. 1218–1224, 2006.

[32] J. L. Gay, D. M. Buchner, and M. D. Schmidt, "Dose-response association of physical activity with HbA1c: intensity and bout length," *Preventive Medicine*, vol. 86, pp. 58–63, 2016.

[33] P. R. Conlin, J. Colburn, D. Aron, R. M. Pries, M. P. Tschanz, and L. Pogach, "Synopsis of the 2017 U.S. Department of Veterans Affairs/U.S. Department of Defense clinical practice guideline: management of type 2 diabetes mellitus," *Annals of Internal Medicine*, vol. 167, no. 9, pp. 655–663, 2017.

12

PTPN2 Downregulation is Associated with Albuminuria and Vitamin D Receptor Deficiency in Type 2 Diabetes Mellitus

Li Zheng,[1] Wei Zhang,[1] Aimei Li,[1] Yan Liu,[1] Bin Yi,[1] Farid Nakhoul,[2] and Hao Zhang[1]

[1]*Department of Nephrology, The Third Xiangya Hospital of Central South University, 138 Tongzipo Road, Changsha, Hunan, China*
[2]*Diabetic Nephropathy Lab, Baruch Padeh Poriya Medical Center Affiliated to the Faculty of Medicine in Galilee, 15208 Lower Galilee, Israel*

Correspondence should be addressed to Hao Zhang; zhanghaoliaoqing@163.com

Academic Editor: Monika A. Niewczas

Objective. Inflammation plays a major role in albuminuria in type 2 diabetes mellitus (T2DM). Our previous studies have shown that the expression of vitamin D receptor (VDR) is downregulated in T2DM which is closely associated with the severity of albuminuria. In this study, we investigated the expression of anti-inflammatory cytokine protein tyrosine phosphatase nonreceptor type 2 (PTPN2) in T2DM and explored its relationship to albuminuria and VDR. *Methods.* 101 T2DM patients were divided into three groups based on urinary albumin-to-creatinine ratio (uACR): normal albuminuria (uACR < 30 mg/g, $n = 29$), microalbuminuria (30 mg/g $\leq$ uACR < 300 mg/g, $n = 34$), and macroalbuminuria (uACR ≥ 300 mg/g, $n = 38$). Thirty healthy individuals were included as controls. Serum was analyzed for PTPN2 and IL-6 expression, and peripheral blood mononuclear cells (PBMCs) were analyzed for PTPN2 and VDR expression. THP-1 cells were incubated with high glucose and further treated with or without paricalcitol, a vitamin D analog. The levels of PTPN2, VDR, IL-6, TNFα, and MCP-1 were analyzed. In addition, anti-inflammatory activities of PTPN2 were further explored in THP-1 cells stimulated with high glucose after PTPN2 silencing or overexpression. *Results.* PTPN2 expression was downregulated in T2DM with the lowest level observed in macroalbuminuria patients. PTPN2 level positively correlated with VDR but negatively correlated with uACR and IL-6. When stimulated with high glucose, there was an increase in inflammatory factors and a decrease in PTPN2 expression. Treatment with paricalcitol reversed these effects. However, paricalcitol failed to exert anti-inflammatory effects in the setting of PTPN2 knockdown. Thus, low levels of PTPN2 aggravated glucose-stimulated inflammation, while high levels of PTPN2 reduced it. *Conclusion.* PTPN2, an anti-inflammatory factor regulated by VDR, was reduced in T2DM CKD stages 1-2. Taken together, our results suggest that therapeutic strategies that enhance PTPN2 may be beneficial for controlling inflammation in T2DM.

1. Introduction

Diabetes mellitus (DM) is a prevalent metabolic disease that adversely affects the length and quality of life. Approximately 387 million suffer from DM worldwide [1]. Long-standing diabetes mellitus may finally lead to diabetic kidney disease and even end-stage renal disease [2] and significantly increased mortality [3]. Therefore, there is an urgent need to identify novel therapeutic targets for DM.

The pathogenesis of diabetes mellitus is not entirely clear, but growing evidence has shown that inflammation plays a vital role in the disease development [4–6]. Vitamin D receptor (VDR), a member of the nuclear receptor superfamily, is an important anti-inflammatory mediator that has been studied widely in the pathogenesis of diabetic kidney disease. Patients with diabetes mellitus have varying degrees of vitamin D deficiency [7] which is associated with renal inflammation [8]. Active vitamin D analogs have potent anti-inflammatory properties and have been shown to reduce urine albuminuria *in vivo* [9–11] and *in vitro* [12–14]. The biological effects of vitamin D are mediated by VDR, a ligand-inducible transcription factor that can regulate expression of a gene network [15].

One of the genes closely associated with VDR is PTPN2 [16]. PTPN2, also known as T cell protein tyrosine phosphatase (TCPTP), is an intracellular tyrosine-specific phosphatase that is expressed ubiquitously in epithelial cells, fibroblasts, and endothelial cells and is abundant in hematopoietic and lymphoid cells [17]. PTPN2 has two variants, a 48 kDa form in the endoplasmic reticulum and a 45 kDa form in the nucleus. The nuclear variant translocates to the cytoplasm in response to proinflammatory stimuli. PTPN2 has been implicated in the regulation of insulin signaling and glucose homeostasis [18, 19] and is also associated with chronic inflammatory and autoimmune diseases such as rheumatoid arthritis (RA) [20], Crohn's disease [21], periodontitis [22], and type 1 diabetes mellitus (T1DM) [23]. In humans, PTPN2 shows a negative association with inflammatory disease [21, 24]. It was found that cultured macrophages from *Ptpn2*$^{-/-}$ mice were hypersensitive to LPS and that decreased expression of PTPN2 enhanced the secretion of monocyte chemoattractant protein (MCP-1) and interleukin 6 (IL-6) [25, 26].

The role of PTPN2 in T2DM and its relationship to VDR have not been explored. Recently, the Diabetes Autoimmunity Study in the Young (DAISY) reported an interaction between a PTPN2 variant PTPN2 rs1893217 and a functional VDR variant VDR rs2228570 which is associated with progression of T1DM [27]. The anti-inflammatory role of VDR is widely recognized, but the exact mechanism of its action is not clear. Based on the findings that VDR interacts with PTPN2, we hypothesized that VDR may mediate anti-inflammatory effects by regulating PTPN2 which may be responsible for reducing inflammatory responses associated with diabetic kidney disease which in turn postpone the progression of diabetic kidney disease. We investigated the expression of PTPN2 in T2DM and its correlation with the severity of diabetic kidney disease, VDR, and inflammatory factors MCP-1, IL-6, and TNFα. We also verified the anti-inflammatory effects of PTPN2 in THP-1 cells in the presence of high glucose.

2. Materials and Methods

2.1. Recruitment of T2DM Patients and Healthy Controls. According to the World Health Organization (WHO) 1999 standard [28], we recruited 101 T2DM patients from the Departments of Nephrology and Endocrinology at the Third Xiangya Hospital, Central South University, China, from 2014 to 2015. Patients with the following conditions were excluded: T1DM, secondary diabetes, diabetic acute complications (such as diabetic ketoacidosis and hypertonic coma), estimated glomerular filtration rate (eGFR) < 60 mL/min/1.73 m^2, infection, and severe cardiovascular and cerebrovascular diseases 3–6 months before recruitment. We also recruited 30 age- and gender-matched healthy adults as controls (NC). The clinical parameters of each study subject were collected and analyzed. Qualified T2DM patients were divided into three groups based on their spot urinary albumin-to-creatinine ratio (uACR): the normal albuminuria group (normo, uACR < 30 mg/g; $n = 29$), the microalbuminuria group (micro, 30 mg/g ≤ uACR < 300 mg/g; $n = 34$), and the macroalbuminuria group (macro, uACR ≥ 300 mg/g; $n = 38$). The study was carried out in accordance with the Declaration of Helsinki (2013) of the World Medical Association. Written informed consent was obtained from all study participants, and the study protocol was approved by the Ethics Committee of the Third Xiangya Hospital of Central South University (Changsha, China).

2.2. Sample Collection. Peripheral venous blood samples were collected from all 131 participants, including 101 T2DM patients and 30 healthy controls, after overnight fasting (at least 8 hours). PBMCs, including monocytes, lymphocytes, and other leukocytes, were isolated by Percoll continuous density gradient separation from the blood samples as previously described [29]. Serum biochemical indices were measured by automatic biochemical analyzers (Hitachi 7600). Spot morning urine samples were collected from the 101 T2DM patients, centrifuged, and stored at −20°C for further analyses. uACR was calculated as urinary albumin concentration divided by urinary creatinine concentration.

2.3. Cell Culture, Treatment, and Transfection. Human acute monocytic leukemia cells (THP-1) were purchased from the Cell Biology Department of Central South University. Cells were cultured in RPMI 1640 medium (Hyclone, New York, USA) supplemented with 10% fetal bovine serum (FBS), 100 μg/mL streptomycin, and 100 U/mL penicillin (Life Technologies, New York, USA) at 37°C in a humidified atmosphere of 5% CO_2 and 95% air.

Cells were seeded into 12-well culture plates for 24 h and then incubated with or without paricalcitol (0.2 ng/mL) for 6 h. Cells were further stimulated with high glucose (30 mmol/L) for 48 h. For transfection experiments, cells were seeded into 12-well culture plates in complete medium without penicillin or streptomycin for 24 h. Cells were transfected with either siRNA against PTPN2 or with scrambled control siRNA using Lipofectamine 2000 (Life Technologies, New York, USA) according to the manufacturer's instructions. Six hours after transfection, the culture medium was replaced with fresh medium and cells were divided into five groups: siCtrl group, siCtrl + HG group (high glucose 30 mmol/L for 48 h), siCtrl + HG + PTPN2 group (recombined human PTPN2 50 ng/mL for 24 h), HG + siPTPN2 group, and HG + siPTPN2 + pari group (paricalcitol 0.2 ng/mL).

2.4. Western Blot. Cells were lysed with buffer containing 20 mM Tris-HCl (pH 7.4), 4% sodium dodecyl sulfate, and 10% glycerol. Lysates were boiled at 100°C for 10 minutes. Protein concentration was determined with the BCA Protein Assay Kit (Pierce, USA). For Western blot analysis, protein samples were separated on a 10% SDS-PAGE gel and transferred to polyvinylidene difluoride membranes (Millipore, Bedford, USA). Membranes were incubated with specific primary antibodies against PTPN2 (Abcam, 1 : 1000, Cambridge, UK), VDR (Santa Cruz, 1 : 200, Dallas, USA), and GAPDH (Abcam, 1 : 10000, Cambridge, UK) overnight at 4°C. Horseradish peroxidase- (HRP-) labeled secondary antibodies were added for 1 h at room temperature. Signal was developed using ECL Plus Western Blotting Detection Reagents (Advansta, Menlo Park, CA, USA) and X-ray film (Kodak, Rochester, NY, USA). Bands were quantified using ImageJ software.

2.5. Real-Time PCR. Total RNA was isolated from THP-1 cells using Trizol (Thermo, New York, USA) reagent according to the manufacturer's instruction. First-strand cDNAs were synthesized from 2 μg of total RNA in a 20 μL reaction using the Revert Aid First Strand cDNA Synthesis Kit. Specific primers used were PTPN2 (forward: 5′-ATCGAGCGG GAGTTCGA-3′; reverse: 5′-TCTGGAAACTTGGCCACT C-3′), VDR (forward: 5′-AGTGCAGAGGAAGCGGGAGA TG-3′; reverse: 5′-CTGGCAGAAGTCGGAGTAGGTG-3′), MCP-1 (forward: 5′-CTCAGCCAGATGCAATCAAT-3′; reverse: 5′-GCTTCTTTGGGACACTTGCT-3′), IL-6 (forward: 5′-CCCCTGACCCAACCACA-3′; reverse: 5′-TGCC GAAGAGCCCTCA-3′), TNFα (forward: 5′-AGCTCCAGT GGCTGAACCG-3′; reverse: 5′-TGGTAGGAGACGGCGA TGC-3′), and GAPDH (forward: 5′-CAGCCTCAAGATCA TCAGCAA-3′; reverse: 5′-TGTGGTCATGAGTCCTTCC A-3′) and were designed based on the gene sequences and synthesized by Generay Biotech. Real-time reverse transcription- (RT-) PCR quantification for individual target mRNA expression was performed with the CFX96 Real-Time Detection System (Bio-Rad, Hercules, CA, USA) using a Takara SYBR green real-time PCR kit (Takara, Japan). The amount of specific mRNA in each sample was calculated from the standard curve and normalized GAPDH mRNA. The comparative $2^{-\Delta\Delta CT}$ method was used for quantification and statistical analysis.

2.6. ELISA. Serum levels of PTPN2 and IL-6 in T2DM patients and levels of MCP-1, IL-6, and TNFα in cell culture supernatant were determined with ELISA kits (R&D, Minnesota, USA).

2.7. Statistical Analysis. All data were analyzed using SPSS 19.0 statistical software and presented as mean ± SD (standard derivation). Difference between the two groups was tested using t-test. Differences among 3 or more groups were tested by one-way ANOVA. Spearman correlation and stepwise multiple linear regression analyses were used to determine the correlations between PTPN2 and uACR, VDR, or other variables. In particular, because the value of uACR is nonnormally distributed, its value was used for performing Ln transformation in correlation analysis. $P < 0.05$ was considered statistically significant.

3. Results

3.1. Clinical and Biochemical Data of the Study Participants. To investigate the correlation between PTPN2 in PBMCs and the severity of albuminuria, we minimized the variables in the study subjects by selecting patients and healthy individuals with comparable parameters (Table 1). There were no statistical differences in age, gender, BMI, hemoglobin, or calcium levels among all the four groups. Moreover, no difference in the duration of disease, serum albumin (ALB), HbA1c, and total cholesterol (TC) was observed in the three T2DM groups. However, compared to the NC group, the T2DM groups had dramatically higher levels of fasting blood glucose (FBG), eGFR, uACR, and IL-6 and a lower level of serum albumin (ALB) and VDR mRNA. We observed increased triglyceride (TG), eGFR, uACR, and IL-6 and decreased 25(OH)D, and VDR mRNA in the macro group was particularly prominent.

3.2. PTPN2 Is Downregulated in Serum and PBMCs Isolated from T2DM Patients and Is Inversely Correlated with the Severity of Albuminuria. We first analyzed the PTPN2 level in the serum of all subjects. Expression levels of PTPN2 decreased with an increase in uACR (Figure 1(a)). We next used Spearman correlation analysis to study the relationship between serum PTPN2 levels and uACR in T2DM patients, an indicator for the severity of albuminuria. As shown in Figure 1(a), serum PTPN2 protein ($n = 101$, including all the three diabetic groups) levels were inversely correlated with uACR in these patients ($r = -0.4199$, $P < 0.001$). After adjusting the potential confounding factors (FBG, SBP, DBP, ALB, TG, TC, 25(OH)D, eGFR, and IL-6), multiple stepwise regression analysis showed that PTPN2 protein ($\beta = -0.398$, $P < 0.001$) remained inversely associated with the uACR levels, an indication of increased risk of kidney malfunction. PTPN2 mRNA showed a positive correlation with both VDR mRNA ($\beta = 0.577$, $P = 0.022$) and 25(OH)D ($\beta = 0.185$, $P < 0.001$). Diabetic kidney disease is a microvascular disease with low-grade chronic inflammation [30]. We showed that the level of IL-6 was significantly higher in T2DM patients than in the healthy controls, and Spearman correlation analysis revealed that PTPN2 negatively correlated with IL-6 ($r = -0.2014$, $P = 0.043$) (Figure 1(b)).

To analyze the correlation between PTPN2 and VDR, we measured PTPN2 and VDR mRNA levels in PBMCs isolated from all subjects. Protein samples from ten subjects from each group were randomly selected for Western blotting. Both protein and mRNA levels of PTPN2 and VDR in PBMCs derived from the normo, micro, and macro groups were significantly lower when compared to the NC group (Figures 2(a) and 2(b)). Among the three diabetic groups, the normo group had the highest levels of both PTPN2 and VDR, whereas the macro group had the lowest levels (Figures 2(a) and 2(b)). Spearman correlation analysis showed that PTPN2 mRNA ($n = 101$) levels were positively correlated with VDR mRNA levels ($r = 0.6033$, $P<0.001$) (Figure 2(b)) but inversely correlated with uACR ($r = -0.2972$, $P<0.001$) (Figure 2(c)) in these patients. Taken together, these results indicate that reduced PTPN2 expression is independently associated with the degree of albuminuria and VDR level in T2DM patients.

Table 1: Clinical parameters ($\bar{X} \pm S$) of study participants.

Subjects	NC	Normo	Micro	Macro
n	30	29	34	38
Gender, M/F	14/16	16/13	19/15	25/13
Age, y	52.34 ± 16.82	53.92 ± 11.92	51.82 ± 13.53	52.42 ± 18.13
BMI, kg/m^2	23.01 ± 3.92	23.73 ± 4.02	24.52 ± 3.89	23.27 ± 3.15
Duration of disease, y	—	6.92 ± 5.79	7.39 ± 6.28	8.11 ± 6.23
SBP, mmHg	123.3 ± 11.7	126.8 ± 12.3	$132.8 \pm 16.8^{*}$	$148.6 \pm 19.2^{*\#}$
DBP, mmHg	72.8 ± 9.7	73.8 ± 11.9	$84.2 \pm 10.4^{*\#}$	$85.9 \pm 13.3^{*\#}$
ALB, g/L	46.68 ± 4.98	$40.23 \pm 5.18^{*}$	$39.43 \pm 6.92^{*}$	$38.23 \pm 7.90^{*}$
Hb, g/L	135.8 ± 15.9	138.5 ± 14.8	136.6 ± 15.2	127.3 ± 21.6
TG, mmol/L	2.11 ± 2.09	2.03 ± 1.83	2.21 ± 2.05	$2.98 \pm 2.82^{*\#\triangle}$
TC, mmol/L	4.37 ± 1.03	4.73 ± 2.85	4.88 ± 2.05	$5.07 \pm 2.85^{*}$
FBG, mmol/L	5.03 ± 1.64	$8.01 \pm 2.66^{*}$	$8.49 \pm 2.38^{*}$	$8.20 \pm 2.55^{*}$
HbA1c, %	—	8.49 ± 2.03	8.99 ± 2.58	9.23 ± 1.98
Calcium, mmol/L	2.33 ± 0.19	2.12 ± 0.18	2.11 ± 0.14	2.29 ± 0.12
25(OH)D, ng/mL	21.72 ± 3.92	19.63 ± 3.72	18.76 ± 7.92	$14.20 \pm 6.86^{*\#\triangle}$
IL-6, pg/mL	47.82 ± 39.77	$136.50 \pm 129.60^{*}$	$327.39 \pm 318.36^{**\#}$	$370.39 \pm 328.53^{**\#}$
eGFR, mL/min	112.24 ± 12.84	118.63 ± 29.83	113.53 ± 31.84	$82.63 \pm 23.62^{*\#\triangle}$
uACR, μg/mg	8.98 ± 3.62	$13.80 \pm 7.35^{*}$	$138.52 \pm 96.31^{*\#}$	$1263.11 \pm 787.77^{**\#\#\triangle\triangle}$
VDR mRNA in PBMC	1.24 ± 0.62	$0.82 \pm 0.52^{*}$	$0.62 \pm 0.56^{*\#}$	$0.39 \pm 0.36^{*\#\triangle}$

M: male; F: female; —: no data. Results are expressed as mean ± SD or ratio. Compared with the NC group, $^{*}P < 0.05$, $^{**}P < 0.01$; compared with the normo group, $^{\#}P < 0.05$, $^{\#\#}P < 0.01$; compared with the micro group, $^{\triangle}P < 0.05$, $^{\triangle\triangle}P < 0.01$.

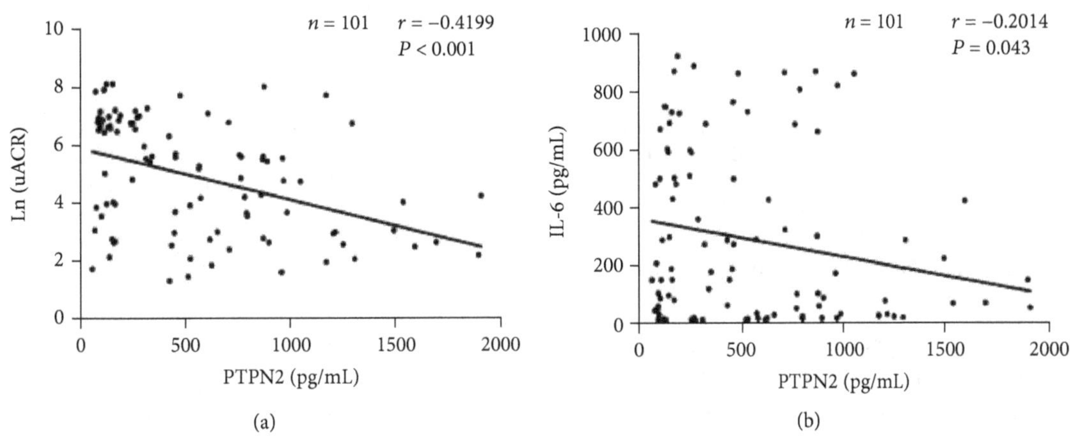

Figure 1: PTPN2 expression in serum is downregulated in T2DM and inversely correlated with uACR and IL-6. (a) PTPN2 protein levels in NC ($n = 30$), normo ($n = 29$), micro ($n = 34$), and macro ($n = 38$) groups were quantified by ELISA. Scatterplot shows an inverse relationship between PTPN2 protein levels and uACR ($n = 101$; $r = -0.4199$; $P < 0.001$). (b) Scatterplot showing an inverse relationship between PTPN2 and IL-6 in protein levels ($n = 101$; $r = -0.2014$; $P = 0.043$). Data represents mean ± SD.

3.3. High Glucose Increased Inflammatory Factors and Decreased PTPN2 Expression and These Changes Were Reversed by VDR Induction. Cultured THP-1 cells stimulated with glucose produced a significant inflammatory response (Figure 3(d)) which was accompanied by a decreased PTPN2 at both protein and mRNA levels. But VDR expression did not change significantly (Figures 3(a) and 3(b)). Under the stimulation of high glucose, intervention with paricalcitol significantly upregulated VDR and PTPN2 expression (Figures 3(a) and 3(b)) and reduced the level of inflammatory cytokines (Figure 3(d)). These data indicate that inflammation can change the expression of PTPN2 and its expression is regulated by VDR.

3.4. PTPN2 Has Anti-Inflammatory Activities and the Anti-Inflammatory Activity of VDR Is Partially Dependent on PTPN2. Knockdown of PTPN2 (Figures 4(a)–4(c)) further elevated the protein and mRNA levels of inflammatory cytokines by high-glucose treatment in THP-1 cells (Figure 4(d) and Table 2). Moreover, paricalcitol failed to

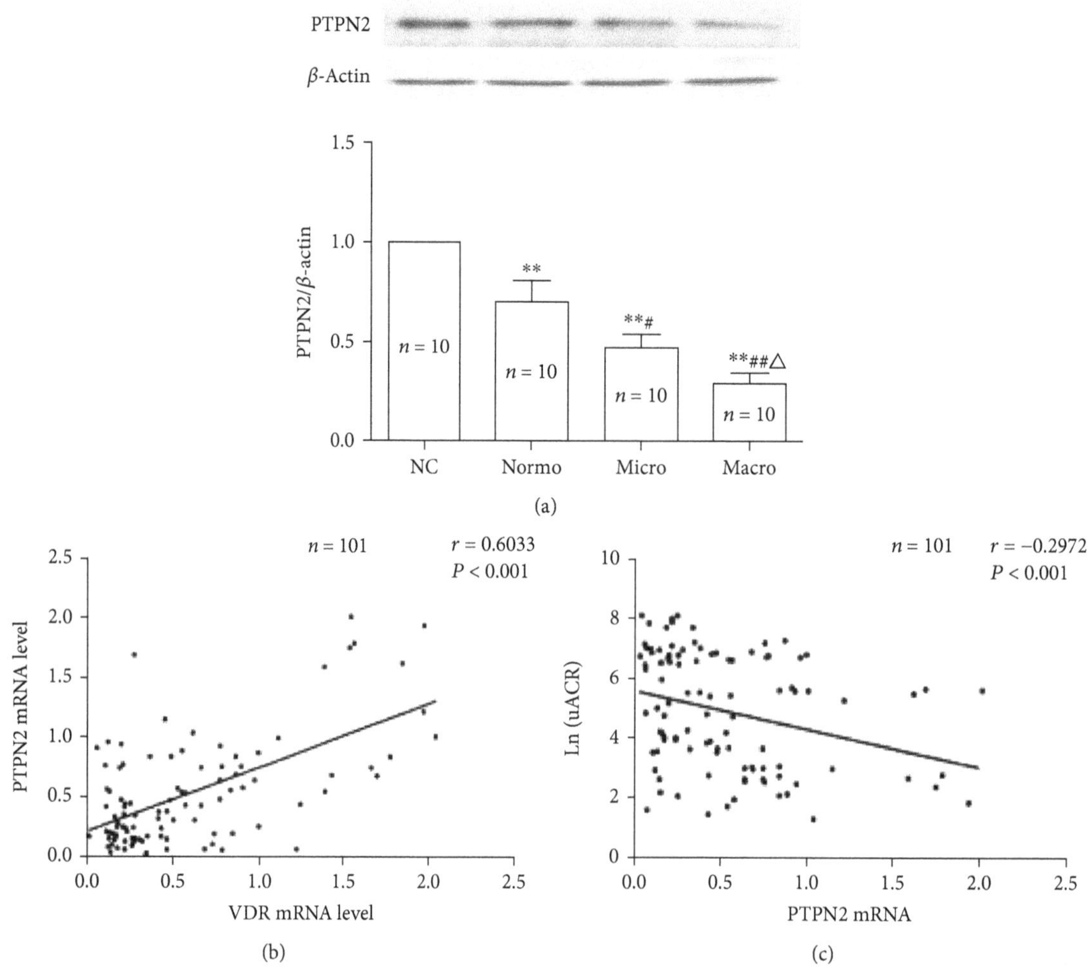

FIGURE 2: PTPN2 expression in PBMCs is downregulated in T2DM and positively correlated with VDR. (a) PTPN2 protein levels determined by Western blot ($n = 10$ in each group, age- and gender-matched); β-actin was used as loading controls. (b) PTPN2 mRNA levels in NC ($n = 30$), normo ($n = 29$), micro ($n = 34$), and macro ($n = 38$) groups were quantified by real-time RT-qPCR. Scatterplot showing a positive relationship between PTPN2 mRNA levels and VDR mRNA level ($n = 101$; $r = 0.6033$; $P < 0.001$). (c) Scatterplot showing inverse relationship between PTPN2 mRNA levels and uACR level ($n = 101$; $r = -0.2972$; $P < 0.001$). Data represents mean ± SD versus NC ($^{**}P < 0.01$), versus normo ($^{\#}P < 0.05$, $^{\#\#}P < 0.01$), and versus micro ($^{\triangle}P < 0.05$).

exert its anti-inflammatory effect when PTPN2 was knocked down. Next, we treated the cells with recombined human PTPN2 to upregulate its expression. We found that PTPN2 suppressed the expression of MCP-1, IL6, and TNFα mediated by HG. All these results demonstrated that PTPN2 has anti-inflammatory activities and the anti-inflammatory utility of VDR is partially dependent on PTPN2.

4. Discussion

In this report, we investigated the relationship between VDR and PTPN2 expression and between PTPN2 and the severity of albuminuria and inflammation in T2DM. First, we showed that PTPN2 expression in serum and PBMCs was much lower in T2DM patients than in healthy adults. In contrast, elevated serum levels of IL-6 were observed in T2DM. PTPN2 was negatively correlated with uACR and IL-6. Our previous studies showed that VDR expression in renal biopsy tissues and PBMCs was significantly downregulated in T2DM patients [31]. Our current results showed a similar profile for PTPN2 in T2DM patients and that PTPN2 was positively correlated with VDR. Multiple stepwise regression analysis and correlation analysis demonstrated that a reduction of PTPN2 is associated with lower VDR and higher uACR, a major indicator for assessing the development of diabetic kidney disease. Our study has limitations. Due to the difficulty in obtaining renal biopsies from T2DM patients, we could not demonstrate the expression of PTPN2 in renal tissues or analyze the correlation between PTPN2 expression in renal tissues and the severity of albuminuria and inflammation. Moreover, the correlation between PTPN2 in PBMCs and the severity of albuminuria was calculated in a cross-sectional study. Also, the number of PBMCs used in this study was small. Thus, future prospective longitudinal studies focused on larger sample quantity are needed to further confirm these observations.

The role of inflammation in the pathogenesis of T2DM and its associated complications is now well established

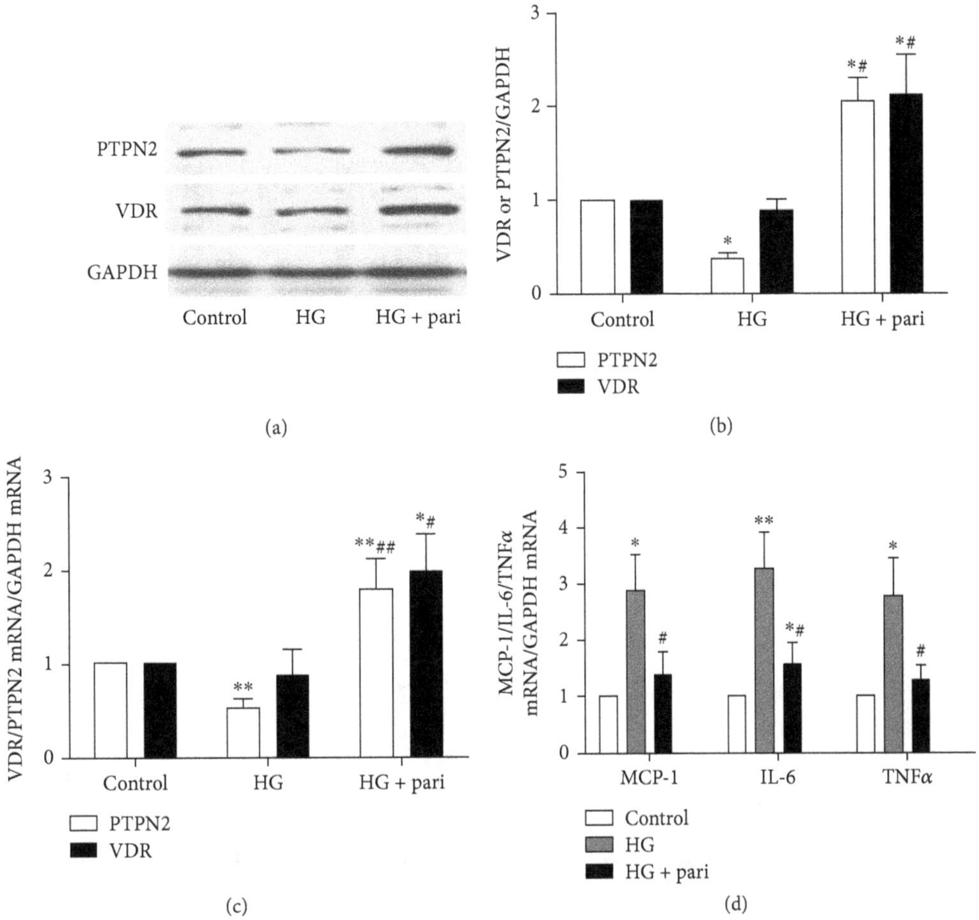

FIGURE 3: High glucose downregulated PTPN2 in THP-1 cells, and this is reversed by increasing VDR level. THP-1 cells were stimulated with high glucose (30 mmol/L) for 48 hours (HG). Cells were pretreated with paricalcitol (0.2 ng/mL) (HG + pari) for 6 hours before HG. (a, b) PTPN2 and VDR protein levels as determined by Western blot; GAPDH was used as a loading control. (c) PTPN2 and VDR mRNA levels as quantified by real-time RT-qPCR. (d) ELISA for inflammatory cytokines MCP-1, IL-6, and TNFα. Experiments were repeated three times, and data represent mean ± SD versus control ($^*P < 0.05$, $^{**}P < 0.01$) and versus HG ($^\#P < 0.05$, $^{\#\#}P < 0.01$).

[30, 32, 33]. PTPN2 is involved in T1DM, modulates pancreatic β-cell apoptosis [34], controls $CD4^+$ T cell differentiation, and limits intestinal inflammation [35]. At present, there are many reports of PTPN2-knockout mouse model to study diabetes. The phenotype of PTPN2-knockout mice varies according to its background. PTPN2-knockout C57BL/6 mice have a normal lifespan but showed a reduction in obesity symptoms and increased insulin sensitivity [36], but PTPN2-knockout BALB/C mice exhibited a significant systemic inflammatory response, and a large amount of IL-12, IFNγ, and TNFα infiltrated in the spleen and nonlymphoid tissues [25, 37]. Pancreas-specific-PTPN2-knockout mice exhibited impaired glucose tolerance during normal dietary feeding and remarkable impaired glucose tolerance and decreased insulin secretion during high-fat diets [38]. It was reported that deficiency of PTPN2 in the pancreas aggravated apoptosis induced by IL-1β and IFNγ and also promoted IFNγ-induced phosphorylation of STAT1-inducing β-cell death [39]. These findings suggest that PTPN2 is an important regulator of diabetes and inflammation. This is the first report, to our knowledge, linking PTPN2 expression levels to inflammation in T2DM. Here, we showed a significant decrease in PTPN2 expression in serum and PBMCs from T2DM patients, with the lowest level seen in the macro group. TNFα, IL-6, and MCP-1 are important inflammatory mediators that are upregulated in T2DM patients [30]. Our results are in agreement with these observations. Furthermore, we showed that PTPN2 is inversely proportional to IL-6 but positively associated with anti-inflammatory VDR. Our *in vitro* experiments demonstrated that exogenous PTPN2 downregulated these inflammatory markers. Deficiency of PTPN2 further aggravated inflammation induced by high glucose. This confirms the anti-inflammatory properties of PTPN2. Taken together, our data showed that high blood glucose can downregulate PTPN2 and inflammation may play an important role in it. In contrast, several *in vivo* studies show that the expression of PTPN2 increased in epithelial cells like HK2 with the stimulation of high glucose [21, 40, 41]. These discrepancies may be due to difference in cell types that express PTPN2 and how they regulate inflammation. Constitutive expression of PTPN2 was stronger in THP-1 monocytes than in other epithelial cells, so it may

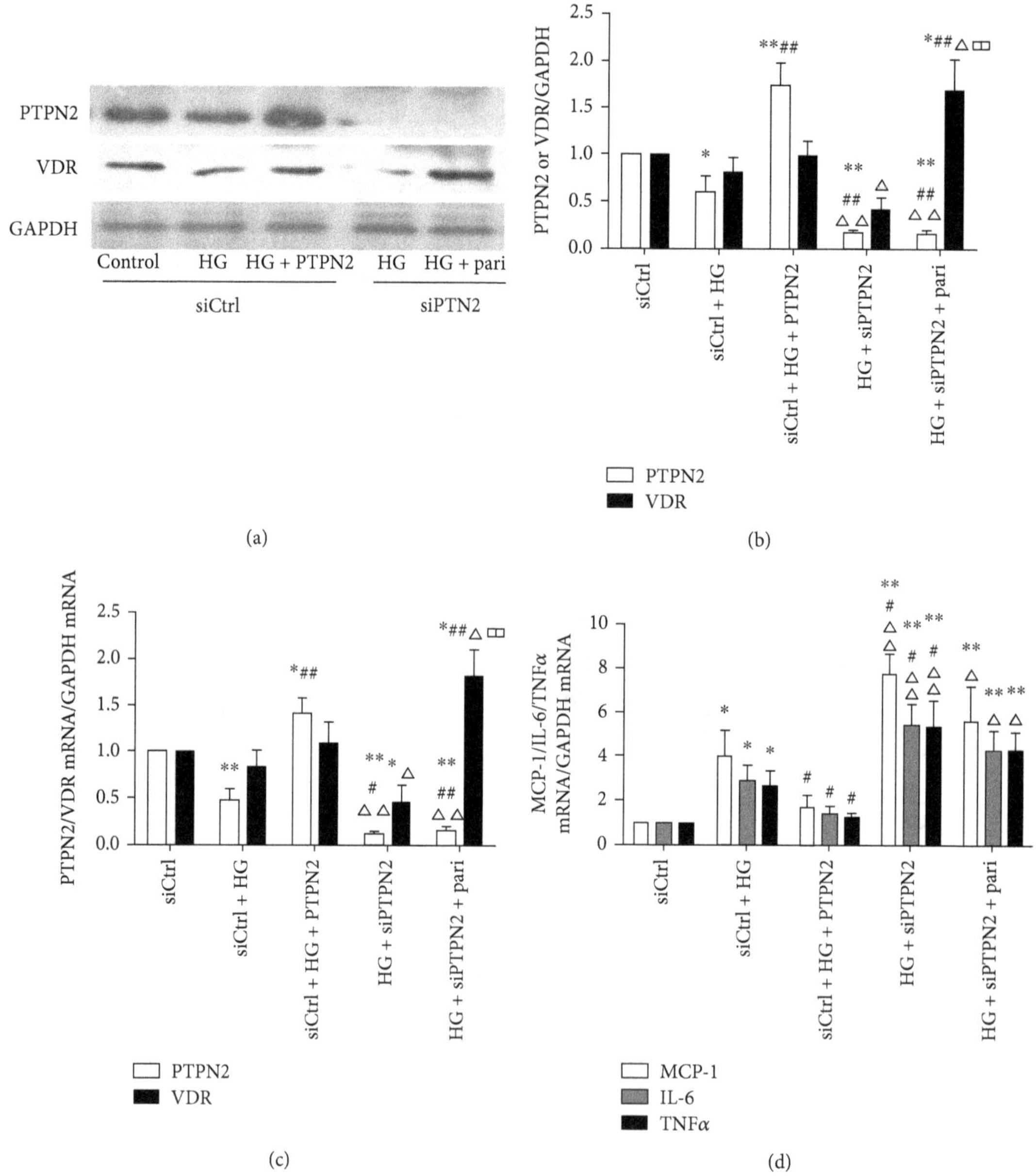

FIGURE 4: PTPN2 inhibits inflammatory factors induced by high glucose in THP-1 cells. siCtrl and siPTPN2 THP-1 cells were stimulated with high glucose (30 mmol/L) for 48 hours and then treated with or without paricalcitol (0.2 ng/mL for 6 hours) or recombined human PTPN2 (50 ng/mL for 24 hours). (a, b) PTPN2 and VDR protein levels were determined by Western blot; GAPDH was used as a loading control. (c) PTPN2 and VDR mRNA levels were quantified by real-time RT-PCR. (d) Real-time RT-PCR of inflammatory cytokines MCP-1, IL-6, and TNFα. Experiments were repeated three times, and data represent mean ± SD versus siCtrl ($^{*}P < 0.05$, $^{**}P < 0.01$), versus siCtrl + HG ($^{\#}P < 0.05$, $^{\#\#}P < 0.01$), versus siCtrl + HG + PTPN2 ($^{\triangle}P < 0.05$, $^{\triangle\triangle}P < 0.01$), and versus HG + siPTPN2 ($^{\square\square}P < 0.01$).

TABLE 2: ELISA of inflammatory cytokines stimulated with high glucose after PTPN2 silencing.

Subjects	siCtrl	siCtrl + HG	siCtrl + HG + PTPN2	HG + siPTPN2	HG + siPTPN2 + pari
MCP-1 (pg/mL)	91.5 ± 39.1	252.9 ± 96.9**	148.3 ± 80.6$^{\#}$	403.8 ± 168.7$^{**\#\Delta\Delta}$	369.2 ± 87.5$^{*\Delta\Delta}$
IL-6 (pg/mL)	3.26 ± 1.58	15.9 ± 4.86**	9.04 ± 4.99$^{*\#}$	25.9 ± 9.15$^{**\#\#\Delta\Delta}$	24.6 ± 11.4$^{**\Delta\Delta}$
TNFα (pg/mL)	7.66 ± 4.32	26.3 ± 11.5**	14.2 ± 4.22$^{*\#}$	43.7 ± 18.9$^{**\#\Delta\Delta}$	35.0 ± 20.2$^{**\Delta\Delta}$

Results are expressed as mean ± SD or ratio. Compared with the siCtrl group: $^{*}P < 0.05$, $^{**}P < 0.01$; compared with the siCtrl + HG group: $^{\#}P < 0.05$, $^{\#\#}P < 0.01$; compared with the siCtrl + HG + PTPN2 group: $^{\Delta\Delta}P < 0.01$.

be consumed at first and then increase synthesis after an ongoing stimulation. Of course, this bold hypothesis needs to be confirmed by more experiments.

Vitamin D-VDR signaling is associated with a strong anti-inflammatory activity. Activated VDR can reduce the expression of TNFα by inhibiting p65 nuclear translocation and NF-κB activation [42]. The Diabetes Autoimmunity Study in the Young (DAISY) reported an interaction between sequence variants at PTPN2 and VDR as being associated with the risk of T1DM progression in children with islet autoantibodies [27]. Such an interaction is mechanistically consistent with the presence of vitamin D-responsive elements (VDREs) across the PTPN2 locus and the observation that PTPN2 expression in lymphoblastoid cell lines is upregulated when exposed to the VDR ligand calcitriol [43]. Our study showed that anti-inflammatory effects of VDR were suppressed in PTPN2-deficient cells. Therefore, it is conceivable that when the levels of inflammatory factors are elevated in T2DM, PTPN2 expression is downregulated in immunocytes but upregulated in epithelial cells (as seen in other studies) and acts synergistically with VDR to attenuate the inflammation and protect against renal injury. Further studies are needed to test this hypothesis.

The mechanism of interaction between PTPN2 and VDR in T2DM is not entirely clear. Future studies should be carried out to test the anti-inflammatory effects of PTPN2 on T2DM in the laboratory. This strategy is both promising and challenging.

Conflicts of Interest

The authors declare no conflict of interest.

Acknowledgments

The study was funded by the National Natural Science Foundation of China (no. 81470961), the Natural Science Foundation of Hunan Province (no. 2015JJ4082), and the New Xiangya Talent Project of the Third Xiangya Hospital of Central South University (no. 20150313).

References

[1] Z. Aziz, P. Absetz, J. Oldroyd, N. P. Pronk, and B. Oldenburg, "A systematic review of real-world diabetes prevention programs: learnings from the last 15 years," *Implementation Science*, vol. 10, no. 1, p. 172, 2015.

[2] Y. Xu, L. Wang, J. He et al., "Prevalence and control of diabetes in Chinese adults," *JAMA*, vol. 310, no. 9, pp. 948–959, 2013.

[3] M. Afkarian, M. C. Sachs, B. Kestenbaum et al., "Kidney disease and increased mortality risk in type 2 diabetes," *Journal of the American Society of Nephrology*, vol. 24, no. 2, pp. 302–308, 2013.

[4] J. F. Navarro-Gonzalez and C. Mora-Fernandez, "The role of inflammatory cytokines in diabetic nephropathy," *Journal of the American Society of Nephrology*, vol. 19, no. 3, pp. 433–442, 2008.

[5] P. Du, B. Fan, H. Han et al., "NOD2 promotes renal injury by exacerbating inflammation and podocyte insulin resistance in diabetic nephropathy," *Kidney International*, vol. 84, no. 2, pp. 265–276, 2013.

[6] A. Festa, R. D'agostino Jr, G. Howard, L. Mykkänen, R. P. Tracy, and S. M. Haffner, "Inflammation and microalbuminuria in nondiabetic and type 2 diabetic subjects: the Insulin Resistance Atherosclerosis Study," *Kidney International*, vol. 58, no. 4, pp. 1703–1710, 2000.

[7] M. Herrmann, D. R. Sullivan, A. S. Veillard et al., "Serum 25-hydroxyvitamin D: a predictor of macrovascular and microvascular complications in patients with type 2 diabetes," *Diabetes Care*, vol. 38, no. 3, pp. 521–528, 2015.

[8] D. Zehnder, M. Quinkler, K. S. Eardley et al., "Reduction of the vitamin D hormonal system in kidney disease is associated with increased renal inflammation," *Kidney International*, vol. 74, no. 10, pp. 1343–1353, 2008.

[9] J. Guo, Z. Ma, Q. Ma et al., "1, 25(OH)(2)D(3) inhibits hepatocellular carcinoma development through reducing secretion of inflammatory cytokines from immunocytes," *Current Medicinal Chemistry*, vol. 20, no. 33, pp. 4131–4141, 2013.

[10] H. Korf, M. Wenes, B. Stijlemans et al., "1,25-Dihydroxyvitamin D_3 curtails the inflammatory and T cell stimulatory capacity of macrophages through an IL-10-dependent mechanism," *Immunobiology*, vol. 217, no. 12, pp. 1292–1300, 2012.

[11] X. Feng, C. Lv, F. Wang, K. Gan, M. Zhang, and W. Tan, "Modulatory effect of 1,25-dihydroxyvitamin D3 on IL1β-induced RANKL, OPG, TNFα, and IL-6 expression in human rheumatoid synoviocyte MH7A," *Clinical & Developmental Immunology*, vol. 2013, article 160123, 8 pages, 2013.

[12] O. Erbas, V. Solmaz, D. Aksoy, A. Yavasoglu, M. Sagcan, and D. Taskiran, "Cholecalciferol (vitamin D 3) improves cognitive dysfunction and reduces inflammation in a rat fatty liver model of metabolic syndrome," *Life Sciences*, vol. 103, no. 2, pp. 68–72, 2014.

[13] M. Z. Adzemovic, M. Zeitelhofer, S. Hochmeister, S. A. Gustafsson, and M. Jagodic, "Efficacy of vitamin D in treating multiple sclerosis-like neuroinflammation depends on developmental stage," *Experimental Neurology*, vol. 249, pp. 39–48, 2013.

[14] S. S. Yilmaz, D. Hizli, E. Yilmaz, O. G. Eryilmaz, F. Hizli, and H. Haltas, "Effect of vitamin D on postoperative adhesion formation in a rat uterine horn adhesion model," *The Journal of Reproductive Medicine*, vol. 58, no. 11-12, pp. 511–516, 2013.

[15] J. Ahn, S. Park, B. Zuniga, A. Bera, C. S. Song, and B. Chatterjee, "Vitamin D in prostate cancer," *Vitamins and Hormones*, vol. 100, pp. 321–355, 2016.

[16] J. A. Ellis, K. J. Scurrah, Y. R. Li et al., "Epistasis amongst PTPN2 and genes of the vitamin D pathway contributes to risk of juvenile idiopathic arthritis," *The Journal of Steroid Biochemistry and Molecular Biology*, vol. 145, pp. 113–120, 2015.

[17] K. M. Doody, A. Bourdeau, and M. L. Tremblay, "T-cell protein tyrosine phosphatase is a key regulator in immune cell signaling: lessons from the knockout mouse model and implications in human disease," *Immunological Reviews*, vol. 228, no. 1, pp. 325–341, 2009.

[18] S. Galic, M. Klingler-Hoffmann, M. T. Fodero-Tavoletti et al., "Regulation of insulin receptor signaling by the protein tyrosine phosphatase TCPTP," *Molecular and Cellular Biology*, vol. 23, no. 6, pp. 2096–2108, 2003.

[19] A. Fukushima, K. Loh, S. Galic et al., "T-cell protein tyrosine phosphatase attenuates STAT3 and insulin signaling in the

liver to regulate gluconeogenesis," *Diabetes*, vol. 59, no. 8, pp. 1906–1914, 2010.

[20] J. E. Cobb, D. Plant, E. Flynn et al., "Identification of the tyrosine-protein phosphatase non-receptor type 2 as a rheumatoid arthritis susceptibility locus in Europeans," *PLoS One*, vol. 8, no. 6, article e66456, 2013.

[21] M. Scharl, D. F. McCole, A. Weber et al., "Protein tyrosine phosphatase N2 regulates TNFα-induced signalling and cytokine secretion in human intestinal epithelial cells," *Gut*, vol. 60, no. 2, pp. 189–197, 2011.

[22] Q. Wang, P. Zhang, R. Aprecio et al., "Comparison of experimental diabetic periodontitis induced by Porphyromonas gingivalis in mice," *Journal of Diabetes Research*, vol. 2016, Article ID 4840203, 10 pages, 2016.

[23] R. C. Sharp, M. Abdulrahim, E. S. Naser, and S. A. Naser, "Genetic variations of PTPN2 and PTPN22: role in the pathogenesis of type 1 diabetes and Crohn's disease," *Frontiers in Cellular and Infection Microbiology*, vol. 5, 2015.

[24] P. D. Simoncic, A. Lee-Loy, D. L. Barber, M. L. Tremblay, and C. J. McGlade, "The T cell protein tyrosine phosphatase is a negative regulator of Janus family kinases 1 and 3," *Current Biology*, vol. 12, no. 6, pp. 446–453, 2002.

[25] K. M. Heinonen, F. P. Nestel, E. W. Newell et al., "T-cell protein tyrosine phosphatase deletion results in progressive systemic inflammatory disease," *Blood*, vol. 103, no. 9, pp. 3457–3464, 2004.

[26] M. Scharl, P. Hruz, and D. F. McCole, "Protein tyrosine phosphatase non-receptor type 2 regulates IFN-γ-induced cytokine signaling in THP-1 monocytes," *Inflammatory Bowel Diseases*, vol. 16, no. 12, pp. 2055–2064, 2010.

[27] B. Frederiksen, E. Liu, J. Romanos et al., "Investigation of the vitamin D receptor gene (VDR) and its interaction with protein tyrosine phosphatase, non-receptor type 2 gene (PTPN2) on risk of islet autoimmunity and type 1 diabetes: the Diabetes Autoimmunity Study in the Young (DAISY)," *The Journal of Steroid Biochemistry and Molecular Biology*, vol. 133, pp. 51–57, 2013.

[28] K. G. M. M. Alberti, P. Z. Zimmet, and WHO Consultation, "Definition, diagnosis and classification of diabetes mellitus and its complications. Part 1: diagnosis and classification of diabetes mellitus provisional report of a WHO consultation," *Diabetic Medicine*, vol. 15, no. 7, pp. 539–553, 1998.

[29] A. J. Ulmer, W. Scholz, M. Ernst, E. Brandt, and H. D. Flad, "Isolation and subfractionation of human peripheral blood mononuclear cells (PBMC) by density gradient centrifugation on Percoll," *Immunobiology*, vol. 166, no. 3, pp. 238–250, 1984.

[30] M. Y. Donath, "Targeting inflammation in the treatment of type 2 diabetes: time to start," *Nature Reviews Drug Discovery*, vol. 13, no. 6, pp. 465–476, 2014.

[31] B. Yi, J. Huang, W. Zhang et al., "Vitamin D receptor downregulation is associated with severity of albuminuria in type 2 diabetes patients," *The Journal of Clinical Endocrinology and Metabolism*, vol. 101, no. 11, pp. 4395–4404, 2016.

[32] T. Jourdan, G. Godlewski, R. Cinar et al., "Activation of the Nlrp 3 inflammasome in infiltrating macrophages by endocannabinoids mediates beta cell loss in type 2 diabetes," *Nature Medicine*, vol. 19, no. 9, pp. 1132–1140, 2013.

[33] C. Y. Westwell-Roper, J. A. Ehses, and C. B. Verchere, "Resident macrophages mediate islet amyloid polypeptide–induced islet IL-1β production and β-cell dysfunction," *Diabetes*, vol. 63, no. 5, pp. 1698–1711, 2014.

[34] I. Santin, F. Moore, M. L. Colli et al., "PTPN2, a candidate gene for type 1 diabetes, modulates pancreatic β-cell apoptosis via regulation of the BH3-only protein Bim," *Diabetes*, vol. 60, no. 12, pp. 3279–3288, 2011.

[35] M. R. Spalinger, S. Kasper, C. Chassard et al., "PTPN2 controls differentiation of $CD4^+$ T cells and limits intestinal inflammation and intestinal dysbiosis," *Mucosal Immunology*, vol. 8, no. 4, pp. 918–929, 2015.

[36] L. D. Klaman, O. Boss, O. D. Peroni et al., "Increased energy expenditure, decreased adiposity, and tissue-specific insulin sensitivity in protein-tyrosine phosphatase 1B-deficient mice," *Molecular and Cellular Biology*, vol. 20, no. 15, pp. 5479–5489, 2000.

[37] F. Wiede, S. H. Chew, C. van Vliet et al., "Strain-dependent differences in bone development, myeloid hyperplasia, morbidity and mortality in Ptpn2-deficient mice," *PLoS One*, vol. 7, no. 5, article e36703, 2012.

[38] Y. Xi, S. Liu, A. Bettaieb et al., "Pancreatic T cell protein-tyrosine phosphatase deficiency affects beta cell function in mice," *Diabetologia*, vol. 58, no. 1, pp. 122–131, 2015.

[39] F. Moore, M. L. Colli, M. Cnop et al., "PTPN2, a candidate gene for type 1 diabetes, modulates interferon-gamma-induced pancreatic beta-cell apoptosis," *Diabetes*, vol. 58, no. 6, pp. 1283–1291, 2009.

[40] M. Scharl, G. Paul, A. Weber et al., "Protection of epithelial barrier function by the Crohn's disease associated gene protein tyrosine phosphatase N2," *Gastroenterology*, vol. 137, no. 6, pp. 2030–2040.e5, 2009.

[41] B. Aradi, M. Kato, M. Filkova et al., "Protein tyrosine phosphatase nonreceptor type 2: an important regulator of interleukin-6 production in rheumatoid arthritis synovial fibroblasts," *Arthritis & Rhematology*, vol. 67, no. 10, pp. 2624–2633, 2015.

[42] Y. Chen, J. Zhang, X. Ge, J. Du, D. K. Deb, and Y. C. Li, "Vitamin D receptor inhibits nuclear factor κB activation by interacting with IκB kinase β protein," *The Journal of Biological Chemistry*, vol. 288, no. 27, pp. 19450–19458, 2013.

[43] S. V. Ramagopalan, A. Heger, A. J. Berlanga et al., "A ChIP-seq defined genome-wide map of vitamin D receptor binding: associations with disease and evolution," *Genome Research*, vol. 20, no. 10, pp. 1352–1360, 2010.

13

The Relationship between Frequently used Glucose-Lowering Agents and Gut Microbiota in Type 2 Diabetes Mellitus

You Lv, Xue Zhao, Weiying Guo, Ying Gao, Shuo Yang, Zhuo Li, and Guixia Wang

Department of Endocrinology and Metabolism, The First Hospital of Jilin University, Changchun, Jilin, China

Correspondence should be addressed to Zhuo Li; noble_zhuo@yahoo.ca and Guixia Wang; gwang168@jlu.edu.cn

Academic Editor: Peter Bolli

Metabolic diseases, especially diabetes mellitus, have become global health issues. The etiology of diabetes mellitus can be attributed to genetic and/or environmental factors. Current evidence suggests the association of gut microbiota with metabolic diseases. However, the effects of glucose-lowering agents on gut microbiota are poorly understood. Several studies revealed that these agents affect the composition and diversity of gut microbiota and consequently improve glucose metabolism and energy balance. Possible underlying mechanisms include affecting gene expression, lowering levels of inflammatory cytokines, and regulating the production of short-chain fatty acids. In addition, gut microbiota may alleviate adverse effects caused by glucose-lowering agents, and this can be especially beneficial in diabetic patients who experience severe gastrointestinal side effects and have to discontinue these agents. In conclusion, gut microbiota may provide a novel viewpoint for the treatment of patients with diabetes mellitus.

1. Introduction

Over the past few decades, metabolic diseases such as type 2 diabetes mellitus (T2DM), obesity, dyslipidemia, and cardiovascular diseases have become major public health issues all over the world. Accordingly, an increasing amount of research has been conducted to further investigate the pathogenesis, phenotypes, and treatments of such diseases. One of the most common metabolic disorders is T2DM, which is characterized by chronic hyperglycemia that can be attributed to genetic and/or environmental factors. Recently, the role played by gut microbiota in T2DM has gained increasing attention, with several studies investigating the composition and function of gut microbiota in T2DM [1].

It was found that, for a standard-weight male, the ratio of bacterial cells to human cells is approximately 1 : 3, with an uncertainty of 25% and a variation of 53% [2]. Several studies reported an association between gut microbiota and metabolic diseases [3–9], with some studies presenting the differences between gut microbiota in T2DM patients and healthy individuals [3, 10]. For example, Qin et al. [11] reported that many opportunistic pathogens, such as *Bacteroides caccae*, *Clostridium hathewayi*, *Clostridium ramosum*, *Clostridium symbiosum*, *Eggerthella lenta*, and *Escherichia coli*, are enriched in T2DM patients. In addition, Karlsson et al. [12] reported an increase in *Lactobacillus* spp. (*Lactobacillus gasseri* JV-V03, *Lactobacillus gasseri* SJ-9E-US, *Lactobacillus gasseri* 202-4, and *Lactobacillus salivarius* ACS-116-V-Col5a) and a decrease in *Clostridium* spp. (*Clostridium beijerinckii* NCIMB 8052, *Clostridium* sp. 7_2_43FAA, *Clostridium botulinum* B str. Eklund 17B, *Clostridium botulinum* E3 str. Alaska E43, and *Clostridium thermocellum* DSM 1313) in T2DM patients. Treatment with metformin affects gut microbiota, and thus, it might be an important confounder in the above studies. Gut microbiota were found to control body weight after bariatric surgery, regulate plasma glucose and insulin levels, maintain the intestinal epithelial barrier integrity, and lower the levels of inflammatory cytokines [13–16]. Moreover, some probiotic supplements exhibit beneficial metabolic properties [15–17]. All this information suggests that gut microbiota may be involved in the etiology of diabetes mellitus.

Short-chain fatty acids (SCFAs) including acetate (C2), propionate (C3), butyrate (C4), and valerate (C5) are

Table 1: Glucose-lowering agents and associated gut microbiota alterations.

Glucose-lowering agent		Gut microbiota alteration		Research subjects
		Increased abundance	Decreased abundance	
Biguanides	Metformin	*Escherichia* [1, 12, 24] *Shigella* [12] *Klebsiella* [12] *Salmonella* [12] *Adlercreutzia* [30] *Clostridium cocleatum* [43] *Akkermansia muciniphila* [24, 43, 44] *Bifidobacterium adolescentis* [24]	*Intestinibacter* [1, 24] *Clostridium* [12] *Eubacterium* [12]	T2DM patients [1, 24, 30] Old women with T2DM [12] HFD-fed mice [43, 44]
α-Glucosidase inhibitors	Acarbose	*Bifidobacterium longum* [23, 55] *Lactobacillus gasseri* [23] *Lactobacillus* [58] *Dialister* [58]	*Bacteroides plebeius* [23] *Bacteroides dorei/vulgatus* [23] *Clostridium bolteae* [23] *Butyricicoccus* [58] *Phascolarctobacterium* [58] *Ruminococcus* [58]	T2DM patients [23, 55] Prediabetic patients [58]
PPAR-γ partial agonist (Chinese medicine)	Danshensu Bingpian Zhi	*Akkermansia muciniphila* [67]	*Helicobacter marmotae* [67]	HFD-fed mice [67]
DPP-4 inhibitor	Vildagliptin	*Bacteroidetes* [68]	*Prevotellaceae* [68] *Ruminococcaceae* [68]	HFD/STZ SD rats [68]
	Sitagliptin	*Roseburia* [13] *Bifdobacterium* [13]	*Blautia* [13]	HF/HC-STZ SD rats [13]

T2DM: type 2 diabetes mellitus; HFD: high-fat diet; PPAR-γ: peroxisome proliferator-activated receptor γ; DPP-4: dipeptidyl peptidase-4; STZ: streptozotocin; HF/HC: high fat/high carbohydrate; SD rats: Sprague Dawley rats.

produced by anaerobic bacteria through the fermentation of nondigestible dietary polysaccharides in the colon [18–20]. Some researchers suggested that a common form of gut microbiota alteration in T2DM is the reduction in butyrate-producing bacteria [11, 21]. Sodium butyrate was found to lower plasma glucose and lipid levels, improve insulin resistance, and reduce gluconeogenesis in diabetic rats [22]. Thus, SCFAs might have a promising role in the prevention and treatment of diabetes mellitus.

Currently available therapeutic options for T2DM, especially glucose-lowering agents, target different pathophysiologic processes. A large body of evidence suggests that gut microbiota and SCFAs exhibit positive effects on glucose-lowering agents in T2DM. Glucose-lowering agents can influence the composition of gut microbiota [23, 24] and affect the production of SCFAs, thereby leading to significant beneficial effects [1, 25, 26]. Moreover, adverse effects of glucose-lowering agents may be improved by altered gut microbiota [27, 28]. This review summarizes current information on the relationship between frequently used glucose-lowering agents and gut microbiota (Table 1) to better understand the role of the intestinal microenvironment in the treatment of diabetes mellitus.

2. Metformin and Gut Microbiota

2.1. Metformin Mechanism of Action and Side Effects. Metformin is a biguanide that reduces hepatic glucose production, increases glucose uptake by peripheral tissues, and activates AMP-dependent protein kinase (AMPK). Metformin is actively transported into cells by organic cation transporters (OCT) [29, 30]. The mechanism of action of metformin is not yet fully understood. In an experimental study on mice with alanine knock-in mutations in both acetyl-CoA carboxylase (Acc) 1 (Ser79) and Acc2 (Ser212), treatment with metformin reduced hepatic lipogenesis and lipid accumulation via activating AMPK and inhibited both Acc1 and Acc2, thereby increasing insulin sensitivity [31]. Duca et al. [32] found that metformin could activate duodenal mucosal AMPK and attenuate hepatic glucose production in a rat model of high-fat diet (HFD). In addition, Miller et al. [33] found that metformin lowers the fasting glucose level by inhibiting glucagon-stimulated cyclic adenosine monophosphate production, which leads to reduced protein kinase A activity and glucagon-stimulated glucose output. Metformin was also found to alter intestinal microbiota [34].

Currently, metformin is the first-line treatment for T2DM and is recommended by the American Diabetes Association and the European Association for the Study of Diabetes with proven efficacy, safety, and low cost [35]. It can lower plasma glucose and insulin levels, improve lipid profiles, and promote modest weight loss. An extended-release formulation of metformin that has fewer gastrointestinal (GI) side effects, for example, diarrhea, anorexia, nausea, and metallic taste, is also available [21, 29]. About 30% of the patients treated with metformin report suffering from GI adverse effects [1]. In a previous clinical study in which 360 T2DM patients were administered a new prescription of metformin for 3 months, about 88% of the participants reported single or multiple GI symptoms, including diarrhea, heartburn, and nausea [36]. Possible underlying mechanisms for metformin adverse effects include stimulation of intestinal serotonin secretion, changes in incretin and glucose metabolism, bile salt malabsorption, and high intestinal metformin concentrations after oral administration [37]. Since OCT1 is involved in the absorption of metformin from the intestinal lumen, its inhibition results in increased metformin intolerance [37]. Recent data illustrated that delayed-release metformin performs its action predominantly in the intestine, so it is considered to be safe for T2DM patients with renal impairment [38].

2.2. The Effect of Metformin on Gut Microbiota in T2DM. Metformin has pleiotropic effects. It accumulates mainly in the intestine, where its concentration is nearly 300 times higher than its plasma concentration [39]. Thus, the intestine is the major site of metformin exposure and is responsible for its glucose-lowering effect [38]. In 1984, Bonora et al. [40] found that intravenous administration of metformin did not improve glucose metabolism compared to oral administration, which suggests the importance of the intestine in the regulation of glucose metabolism by metformin. Metformin was found to increase the life span of *Caenorhabditis elegans* cocultured with *Escherichia coli* by altering microbial folate and methionine metabolism [41], which suggests that the effects of metformin on aging in nematodes are microbiota dependent. Recently, the relationship between metformin and the gut has been comprehensively reviewed [21]; researchers indicated that metformin can affect the gut microenvironment by modulating glucose uptake and utilization, increasing glucagon-like peptide-1 (GLP-1) and bile acid levels and altering gut microbiota. In conclusion, the interaction between metformin and gut microbiota may contribute to the pleiotropic effects of metformin.

A large body of evidence confirms the effects of metformin on intestinal microbiota. The abundance of *Akkermansia muciniphila* was found to be decreased in obesity and diabetes [9], while higher baseline levels were associated with improvements in the cardiometabolic parameters of obesity [11, 42]. Experimental studies revealed that the abundances of *Akkermansia muciniphila* [43, 44] and *Clostridium cocleatum* [43] increased significantly in HFD-fed mice after metformin treatment. The higher abundance of *Akkermansia muciniphila* was involved in maintaining mucin layer integrity [45, 46], and the changes in gut microbiota were attributed to SCFA-producing bacteria in human and animal guts [45, 46]. It is suggested that the effects of metformin on the abundance of these species may indirectly contribute to its modulatory effects on glucose metabolism and other metabolic processes. These results suggest that the therapeutic effect of metformin might be partially mediated by the intestinal tract.

Forslund et al. [1] found that metformin-treated T2DM patients exhibited decreased abundances of *Intestinibacter* spp. and increased abundances of *Escherichia* spp. However, the latter was only found in Danish and Swedish populations. In a cross-sectional study that recruited 145 European old women with T2DM, impaired glucose tolerance, or normal glucose tolerance, patients treated with metformin showed different gut microbial composition than those who were not treated with metformin [12]. Napolitano et al. also evaluated T2DM with and without metformin monotherapy to characterize the gut-based mechanisms of metformin, and their results showed that *Adlercreutzia* spp. were significantly elevated in fecal samples of metformin-treated patients [30]. Wu et al. [24] found that the altered microbiota mainly belonged to the phyla γ-Proteobacteria and Firmicutes. They found an increase in *Escherichia* spp. and a decrease in *Intestinibacter* spp., as well as a significant increase in fecal propionate and butyrate concentrations in the metformin group. A possible underlying mechanism for metformin-microbiota interaction is regulating the expression of genes encoding for metalloproteins in gut bacteria. These results demonstrate the influence of metformin on gut microbial diversity and the role of the intestine in the glucose-lowering effect of metformin.

Unfortunately, alteration of gut microbiota by metformin may contribute to its GI intolerance [21]. Greenway et al. [27] reported a case in which a 30-year-old man newly diagnosed with T2DM was treated with a cobiotic supplement containing inulin, beta-glucan, and blueberry pomace extract for 8 weeks. This patient exhibited balanced glycemic control and alleviated GI side effects of metformin. In addition, Burton et al. [28] found that the combination of metformin with GI microbiome modulator (GIMM) in T2DM patients who experienced GI intolerance to metformin resulted in better glucose tolerance compared to placebo and significantly improved fasting glucose levels. These results demonstrate that a safe dietary supplement may improve the efficacy and tolerability of metformin, possibly through the alteration of gut microbiota. Thus, gut microbiota may serve as a novel approach to alleviate metformin adverse effects and consequently improve patient compliance.

3. The Effect of Acarbose on Gut Microbiota in T2DM

Accumulating evidence suggests that postprandial blood glucose level is a powerful predictor of diabetic cardiovascular events [47, 48]. As a classical α-glucosidase inhibitor, acarbose lowers postprandial blood glucose levels by delaying glucose absorption, as it inhibits the enzyme that cleaves oligosaccharides into mono- and disaccharides in the intestinal lumen [29]. The control of postprandial hyperglycemia is especially important in Asia due to the traditional carbohydrate-rich dietary pattern [49]. In a randomized, open-label, noninferiority clinical trial recruiting Chinese patients newly diagnosed with T2DM, treatment with acarbose as initial therapy showed similar glucose-lowering efficacy to that of metformin [50]. Therefore, acarbose is an effective and safe antidiabetic agent, especially for the control of postprandial hyperglycemia. The major cause of acarbose side effects (e.g., diarrhea, flatulence, and abdominal distention) is the increased delivery of oligosaccharides to the large intestine. However, these side effects can be ameliorated by gradual upward dose titration [29]. Previous studies indicated that acarbose treatment could reduce the risk of cardiovascular events in diabetic patients [51–54]. The detailed underlying mechanisms for this cardiovascular protective function are only partially understood [55], but they can be attributed to the ability of acarbose to neutralize oxidative stress by increasing H_2 production in the GI tract (GIT) [56]. However, the results of Chang et al. did not support a cardiovascular protective effect of acarbose compared to metformin in Taiwan populations [57].

A series of recent clinical trials clarified the relationship between acarbose and gut microbiota. For example, in a clinical study, 95 Chinese T2DM patients were distributed into 2 groups; one group was treated with acarbose while the other was not. At baseline, diabetic patients showed lower levels of *Bifidobacterium longum* and higher levels of *Enterococcus faecalis* than healthy volunteers [55]. After 4 weeks of treatment, acarbose-treated patients showed increased *Bifidobacterium longum* and decreased lipopolysaccharide and prothrombin activator inhibitor-1 levels [55]. These results suggest that acarbose treatment could alter gut microbiota and reduce the levels of inflammatory cytokines in diabetic patients. Another randomized, double-blind, controlled crossover trial recruiting prediabetic Chinese individuals demonstrated that acarbose treatment significantly altered the diversity and composition of gut microbiota [58]. In addition, Gu et al. [23] revealed that acarbose could regulate the gut microbiota of T2DM patients, thereby modulating bile acid metabolism and contributing to beneficial effects on host metabolism.

Although α-glucosidase inhibitors have been widely used clinically, there is an ongoing interest in probiotics or gut microbiota as biotherapeutic agents for some metabolic diseases. Panwar et al. [59] found that *Lactobacillus* strains exhibit glucosidase-inhibitory effects and regulate blood glucose responses to carbohydrates *in vivo*. As mentioned previously, SCFAs play an important role in diabetes mellitus. Acarbose was found to increase serum butyrate levels in individuals with impaired glucose tolerance. The underlying mechanism for this effect might be that acarbose increases the fermentation of insoluble fibers in the colon [25]. Similarly, a clinical study showed that butyrate production is significantly increased during acarbose treatment, whereas the production of acetate and propionate is significantly decreased [26].

The beneficial effects of acarbose on diabetes mellitus, such as reduction of inflammatory cytokines and regulation of SCFA levels, can be related to the alteration of intestinal microbiota. However, whether there is an association between the cardiovascular protective action of acarbose and gut microbiota is not yet clear.

4. Glucagon-Like Peptide-1 (GLP-1) and Gut Microbiota

Endocrine peptides play an important role in the crosstalk between gut microbiota and host metabolism. Everard and Cani [60] reviewed the effects of certain dietary fibers on the gut microbiota and host homeostasis and on the secretion of enteroendocrine peptides. As discussed earlier in this review, gut microbiota ferments nondigestible polysaccharides in the colon producing SCFAs and thus influences host glucose and energy homeostasis. It has been elucidated that SCFAs activate GPR41 and GPR43 and thus regulate the secretion of enteroendocrine peptides [61–63]. Known as a gut hormone, GLP-1 is involved in glucose metabolism, appetite regulation, and gastric emptying. The mechanism by which gut microbiota could accelerate the GI motility was mainly attributed to the suppression of GLP-1 receptor expression in the GIT [64]. Recently, several studies have proven the significant glucose-lowering effect of GLP-1-based therapies; GLP-1 receptor agonists like exenatide and liraglutide could promote insulin secretion, suppress glucagon levels, slow gastric emptying, accelerate satiety, induce weight loss, and lower the risk of hypoglycemia [29]. Grasset et al. [65] demonstrated that GLP-1 sensitivity was modulated by gut microbiota through nitric oxide-dependent mechanism in the enteric nervous system. Their results indicated that new hypoglycemic agents based on GLP-1 should focus on the research of patients' intestinal microbiota.

Currently, the association between gut microbiota and intestinal peptides involved in energy and glucose homeostasis has been well reported. However, the relationship between GLP-1 receptor agonists and gut microbiota is not yet clear; further clinical trials are needed to understand this relationship.

5. Other Glucose-Lowering Agents and Gut Microbiota

Pioglitazone is a thiazolidinedione that can reduce insulin resistance by binding to peroxisome proliferator-activated receptor γ (PPAR-γ) nuclear receptor [29]. Previous experimental studies identified the difference in gut microbial structure between KKAy mice and C57BL/6J mice by showing a higher abundance of *Bacteroides* spp. in the intestine of KKAy mice [66]. Pioglitazone was shown to improve gut microbial structure of KKAy mice, but it decreased microbial diversity [66]. The traditional Chinese medicine *Danshensu Bingpian Zhi* (DBZ), a PPAR-γ partial agonist, not only improved the phenotypes of metabolic syndrome but also increased the Bacteroidetes/Firmicutes ratio, resulting in an increase in *Akkermansia muciniphila* and a decrease in *Helicobacter marmotae* in HFD-fed mice [67]. Sitagliptin, a dipeptidyl peptidase-4 (DPP-4) inhibitor, was also found to improve gut microbial structure. The underlying mechanism is not clear; however, it can be mediated by relieving intestinal wall edema, alleviating intestinal inflammation, and maintaining the intestinal mucosal barrier integrity [13]. Vildagliptin, another DPP-4 inhibitor, was found to significantly reduce microbiota diversity in diabetic rats and to normalize the Bacteroidetes/Firmicutes ratio [68]. Sodium/glucose cotransporter (SGLT) is a novel therapeutic target in T2DM. LX4211, a dual inhibitor of SGLT1 and SGLT2, could reduce glucose absorption by inhibiting SGLT1 and stimulate the release of GLP-1 and peptide YY. These effects may be mediated by SCFAs produced by cecal fermentation of unabsorbed glucose [69]. Although no definite evidence indicates that SGLT inhibitor has direct effects on gut microbiota to improve glycemic control, it should be noted that SGLT inhibition exerts positive effects on metabolic diseases [70].

Other glucose-lowering agents such as cathelicidin antimicrobial peptide [71], phlorizin [72], and transglucosidase [73] were also proven to have beneficial modulatory effects on gut microbiota composition, glucose homeostasis, insulin resistance, and β cell function.

Taken together, these studies are of great significance for understanding the role of gut microbiota as novel therapeutic targets in diabetes mellitus. However, further studies are still needed to confirm the hypothesis.

6. Conclusion

In conclusion, the alteration of gut microbiota is a pivotal process in the pathogenesis and progression of metabolic diseases. The association between glucose-lowering agents and gut microbiota is not yet fully understood. Understanding the effects of glucose-lowering agents on gut microbiota is of great importance to further understand the etiopathogenesis, diagnosis, treatment, adverse effects, and prognosis of metabolic diseases.

Conflicts of Interest

The authors declare that there are no conflicts of interest.

Acknowledgments

The research was supported by the Fund for Science and Technology Development Plan of Jilin Province (20170623092TC-04) to You Lv.

References

[1] K. Forslund, F. Hildebrand, T. Nielsen et al., "Disentangling type 2 diabetes and metformin treatment signatures in the human gut microbiota," *Nature*, vol. 528, no. 7581, pp. 262–266, 2015.

[2] R. Sender, S. Fuchs, and R. Milo, "Revised estimates for the number of human and bacteria cells in the body," *PLoS Biology*, vol. 14, no. 8, article e1002533, 2016.

[3] K.-A. Lê, Y. Li, X. Xu et al., "Alterations in fecal *Lactobacillus* and *Bifidobacterium* species in type 2 diabetic patients in Southern China population," *Frontiers in Physiology*, vol. 3, p. 496, 2013.

[4] A. J. Cox, N. P. West, and A. W. Cripps, "Obesity, inflammation, and the gut microbiota," *The Lancet Diabetes & Endocrinology*, vol. 3, no. 3, pp. 207–215, 2015.

[5] A. V. Hartstra, K. E. C. Bouter, F. Bäckhed, and M. Nieuwdorp, "Insights into the role of the microbiome in obesity and type 2 diabetes," *Diabetes Care*, vol. 38, no. 1, pp. 159–165, 2015.

[6] G. Blandino, R. Inturri, F. Lazzara, M. Di Rosa, and L. Malaguarnera, "Impact of gut microbiota on diabetes mellitus," *Diabetes & Metabolism*, vol. 42, no. 5, pp. 303–315, 2016.

[7] C. L. Boulange, A. L. Neves, J. Chilloux, J. K. Nicholson, and M. E. Dumas, "Impact of the gut microbiota on inflammation, obesity, and metabolic disease," *Genome Medicine*, vol. 8, no. 1, p. 42, 2016.

[8] R. J. Perry, L. Peng, N. A. Barry et al., "Acetate mediates a microbiome-brain-β-cell axis to promote metabolic syndrome," *Nature*, vol. 534, no. 7606, pp. 213–217, 2016.

[9] H. Plovier, A. Everard, C. Druart et al., "A purified membrane protein from *Akkermansia muciniphila* or the pasteurized bacterium improves metabolism in obese and diabetic mice," *Nature Medicine*, vol. 23, no. 1, pp. 107–113, 2017.

[10] J. Sato, A. Kanazawa, F. Ikeda et al., "Gut dysbiosis and detection of "live gut bacteria" in blood of Japanese patients with type 2 diabetes," *Diabetes Care*, vol. 37, no. 8, pp. 2343–2350, 2014.

[11] J. Qin, Y. Li, Z. Cai et al., "A metagenome-wide association study of gut microbiota in type 2 diabetes," *Nature*, vol. 490, no. 7418, pp. 55–60, 2012.

[12] F. H. Karlsson, V. Tremaroli, I. Nookaew et al., "Gut metagenome in European women with normal, impaired and diabetic glucose control," *Nature*, vol. 498, no. 7452, pp. 99–103, 2013.

[13] X. Yan, B. Feng, P. Li, Z. Tang, and L. Wang, "Microflora disturbance during progression of glucose intolerance and effect of sitagliptin: an animal study," *Journal of Diabetes Research*, vol. 2016, Article ID 2093171, 10 pages, 2016.

[14] A. P. Liou, M. Paziuk, J. M. Luevano, S. Machineni, P. J. Turnbaugh Jr., and L. M. Kaplan, "Conserved shifts in the gut microbiota due to gastric bypass reduce host weight and adiposity," *Science Translational Medicine*, vol. 5, no. 178, article 178ra141, 2013.

[15] P. D. Cani, A. M. Neyrinck, F. Fava et al., "Selective increases of bifidobacteria in gut microflora improve high-fat-diet-induced diabetes in mice through a mechanism associated with endotoxaemia," *Diabetologia*, vol. 50, no. 11, pp. 2374–2383, 2007.

[16] P. Tian, B. Li, C. He et al., "Antidiabetic (type 2) effects of *Lactobacillus* G15 and Q14 in rats through regulation of intestinal permeability and microbiota," *Food & Function*, vol. 7, no. 9, pp. 3789–3797, 2016.

[17] K. L. Wickens, C. A. Barthow, R. Murphy et al., "Early pregnancy probiotic supplementation with *Lactobacillus rhamnosus* HN001 may reduce the prevalence of gestational diabetes mellitus: a randomised controlled trial," *British Journal of Nutrition*, vol. 117, no. 6, pp. 804–813, 2017.

[18] A. Salonen, L. Lahti, J. Salojarvi et al., "Impact of diet and individual variation on intestinal microbiota composition and fermentation products in obese men," *The ISME Journal*, vol. 8, no. 11, pp. 2218–2230, 2014.

[19] G. den Besten, K. van Eunen, A. K. Groen, K. Venema, D. J. Reijngoud, and B. M. Bakker, "The role of short-chain fatty acids in the interplay between diet, gut microbiota, and host energy metabolism," *Journal of Lipid Research*, vol. 54, no. 9, pp. 2325–2340, 2013.

[20] J. Tan, C. McKenzie, M. Potamitis, A. N. Thorburn, C. R. Mackay, and L. Macia, "Chapter Three - the role of short-chain fatty acids in health and disease," *Advances in Immunology*, vol. 121, pp. 91–119, 2014.

[21] L. J. McCreight, C. J. Bailey, and E. R. Pearson, "Metformin and the gastrointestinal tract," *Diabetologia*, vol. 59, no. 3, pp. 426–435, 2016.

[22] S. Khan and G. Jena, "Sodium butyrate reduces insulin-resistance, fat accumulation and dyslipidemia in type-2 diabetic rat: a comparative study with metformin," *Chemico-Biological Interactions*, vol. 254, pp. 124–134, 2016.

[23] Y. Gu, X. Wang, J. Li et al., "Analyses of gut microbiota and plasma bile acids enable stratification of patients for antidiabetic treatment," *Nature Communications*, vol. 8, no. 1, p. 1785, 2017.

[24] H. Wu, E. Esteve, V. Tremaroli et al., "Metformin alters the gut microbiome of individuals with treatment-naive type 2 diabetes, contributing to the therapeutic effects of the drug," *Nature Medicine*, vol. 23, no. 7, pp. 850–858, 2017.

[25] T. M. Wolever and J. L. Chiasson, "Acarbose raises serum butyrate in human subjects with impaired glucose tolerance," *British Journal of Nutrition*, vol. 84, no. 1, pp. 57–61, 2000.

[26] G. A. Weaver, C. T. Tangel, J. A. Krause et al., "Acarbose enhances human colonic butyrate production," *The Journal of Nutrition*, vol. 127, no. 5, pp. 717–723, 1997.

[27] F. Greenway, S. Wang, and M. Heiman, "A novel cobiotic containing a prebiotic and an antioxidant augments the glucose control and gastrointestinal tolerability of metformin: a case report," *Beneficial Microbes*, vol. 5, no. 1, pp. 29–32, 2014.

[28] J. H. Burton, M. Johnson, J. Johnson, D. S. Hsia, F. L. Greenway, and M. L. Heiman, "Addition of a gastrointestinal microbiome modulator to metformin improves metformin tolerance and fasting glucose levels," *Journal of Diabetes Science and Technology*, vol. 9, no. 4, pp. 808–814, 2015.

[29] D. L. Longo, *Harrison's Principles of Internal Medicine*, McGraw-Hill, New York, 18th edition, 2012.

[30] A. Napolitano, S. Miller, A. W. Nicholls et al., "Novel gut-based pharmacology of metformin in patients with type 2 diabetes mellitus," *PLoS One*, vol. 9, no. 7, article e100778, 2014.

[31] M. D. Fullerton, S. Galic, K. Marcinko et al., "Single phosphorylation sites in Acc1 and Acc2 regulate lipid homeostasis and the insulin-sensitizing effects of metformin," *Nature Medicine*, vol. 19, no. 12, pp. 1649–1654, 2013.

[32] F. A. Duca, C. D. Côté, B. A. Rasmussen et al., "Metformin activates a duodenal Ampk-dependent pathway to lower hepatic glucose production in rats," *Nature Medicine*, vol. 21, no. 5, pp. 506–511, 2015.

[33] R. A. Miller, Q. Chu, J. Xie, M. Foretz, B. Viollet, and M. J. Birnbaum, "Biguanides suppress hepatic glucagon signalling by decreasing production of cyclic AMP," *Nature*, vol. 494, no. 7436, pp. 256–260, 2013.

[34] K. Y. Hur and M. S. Lee, "New mechanisms of metformin action: focusing on mitochondria and the gut," *Journal of Diabetes Investigation*, vol. 6, no. 6, pp. 600–609, 2015.

[35] S. E. Inzucchi, R. M. Bergenstal, J. B. Buse et al., "Management of hyperglycemia in type 2 diabetes: a patient-centered approach: position statement of the American Diabetes Association (ADA) and the European Association for the Study of Diabetes (EASD)," *Diabetes Care*, vol. 35, no. 6, pp. 1364–1379, 2012.

[36] H. Florez, J. Luo, S. Castillo-Florez et al., "Impact of metformin-induced gastrointestinal symptoms on quality of life and adherence in patients with type 2 diabetes," *Postgraduate Medicine*, vol. 122, no. 2, pp. 112–120, 2010.

[37] T. Dujic, K. Zhou, L. A. Donnelly, R. Tavendale, C. N. A. Palmer, and E. R. Pearson, "Association of organic cation transporter 1 with intolerance to metformin in type 2 diabetes: a GoDARTS study," *Diabetes*, vol. 64, no. 5, pp. 1786–1793, 2015.

[38] J. B. Buse, R. A. DeFronzo, J. Rosenstock et al., "The primary glucose-lowering effect of metformin resides in the gut, not the circulation: results from short-term pharmacokinetic and 12-week dose-ranging studies," *Diabetes Care*, vol. 39, no. 2, pp. 198–205, 2016.

[39] C. J. Bailey, C. Wilcock, and J. H. B. Scarpello, "Metformin and the intestine," *Diabetologia*, vol. 51, no. 8, pp. 1552-1553, 2008.

[40] E. Bonora, M. Cigolini, O. Bosello et al., "Lack of effect of intravenous metformin on plasma concentrations of glucose, insulin, C-peptide, glucagon and growth hormone in non-diabetic subjects," *Current Medical Research and Opinion*, vol. 9, no. 1, pp. 47–51, 1984.

[41] F. Cabreiro, C. Au, K. Y. Leung et al., "Metformin retards aging in *C. elegans* by altering microbial folate and methionine metabolism," *Cell*, vol. 153, no. 1, pp. 228–239, 2013.

[42] E. Le Chatelier, T. Nielsen, J. Qin et al., "Richness of human gut microbiome correlates with metabolic markers," *Nature*, vol. 500, no. 7464, pp. 541–546, 2013.

[43] H. Lee and G. Ko, "Effect of metformin on metabolic improvement and gut microbiota," *Applied and Environmental Microbiology*, vol. 80, no. 19, pp. 5935–5943, 2014.

[44] N. R. Shin, J. C. Lee, H. Y. Lee et al., "An increase in the *Akkermansia* spp. population induced by metformin treatment improves glucose homeostasis in diet-induced obese mice," *Gut*, vol. 63, no. 5, pp. 727–735, 2014.

[45] J. de la Cuesta-Zuluaga, N. T. Mueller, V. Corrales-Agudelo et al., "Metformin is associated with higher relative abundance of mucin-degrading *Akkermansia muciniphila* and several short-chain fatty acid–producing microbiota in the gut," *Diabetes Care*, vol. 40, no. 1, pp. 54–62, 2017.

[46] X. Zhang, Y. Zhao, J. Xu et al., "Modulation of gut microbiota by berberine and metformin during the treatment of high-fat diet-induced obesity in rats," *Scientific Reports*, vol. 5, no. 1, article 14405, 2015.

[47] The DECODE study group, European Diabetes Epidemiology Group, and Diabetes Epidemiology: Collaborative analysis Of Diagnostic criteria in Europe, "Glucose tolerance and mortality: comparison of WHO and American Diabetes Association diagnostic criteria," *The Lancet*, vol. 354, no. 9179, pp. 617–621, 1999.

[48] T. Nakagami and the DECODA Study Group, "Hyperglycaemia and mortality from all causes and from cardiovascular disease in five populations of Asian origin," *Diabetologia*, vol. 47, no. 3, pp. 385–394, 2004.

[49] S. R. Joshi, E. Standl, N. Tong, P. Shah, S. Kalra, and R. Rathod, "Therapeutic potential of α-glucosidase inhibitors in type 2 diabetes mellitus: an evidence-based review," *Expert Opinion on Pharmacotherapy*, vol. 16, no. 13, pp. 1959–1981, 2015.

[50] W. Yang, J. Liu, Z. Shan et al., "Acarbose compared with metformin as initial therapy in patients with newly diagnosed type 2 diabetes: an open-label, non-inferiority randomised trial," *The Lancet Diabetes & Endocrinology*, vol. 2, no. 1, pp. 46–55, 2014.

[51] J. L. Chiasson, R. G. Josse, R. Gomis et al., "Acarbose treatment and the risk of cardiovascular disease and hypertension in patients with impaired glucose tolerance: the STOP-NIDDM trial," *JAMA*, vol. 290, no. 4, pp. 486–494, 2003.

[52] M. Hanefeld, M. Cagatay, T. Petrowitsch, D. Neuser, D. Petzinna, and M. Rupp, "Acarbose reduces the risk for myocardial infarction in type 2 diabetic patients: meta-analysis of seven long-term studies," *European Heart Journal*, vol. 25, no. 1, pp. 10–16, 2004.

[53] J. M. Chen, C. W. Chang, Y. C. Lin, J. T. Horng, and W. H. H. Sheu, "Acarbose treatment and the risk of cardiovascular disease in type 2 diabetic patients: a nationwide seven-year follow-up study," *Journal of Diabetes Research*, vol. 2014, Article ID 812628, 6 pages, 2014.

[54] E. Standl, M. J. Theodorakis, M. Erbach, O. Schnell, and J. Tuomilehto, "On the potential of acarbose to reduce cardiovascular disease," *Cardiovascular Diabetology*, vol. 13, no. 1, p. 81, 2014.

[55] B. Su, H. Liu, J. Li et al., "Acarbose treatment affects the serum levels of inflammatory cytokines and the gut content of bifidobacteria in Chinese patients with type 2 diabetes mellitus," *Journal of Diabetes*, vol. 7, no. 5, pp. 729–739, 2015.

[56] Y. Suzuki, M. Sano, K. Hayashida, I. Ohsawa, S. Ohta, and K. Fukuda, "Are the effects of α-glucosidase inhibitors on cardiovascular events related to elevated levels of hydrogen gas in the gastrointestinal tract?," *FEBS Letters*, vol. 583, no. 13, pp. 2157–2159, 2009.

[57] C. H. Chang, Y. C. Chang, J. W. Lin, S. T. Chen, L. M. Chuang, and M. S. Lai, "Cardiovascular risk associated with acarbose versus metformin as the first-line treatment in patients with type 2 diabetes: a nationwide cohort study," *The Journal of Clinical Endocrinology & Metabolism*, vol. 100, no. 3, pp. 1121–1129, 2015.

[58] X. Zhang, Z. Fang, C. Zhang et al., "Effects of acarbose on the gut microbiota of prediabetic patients: a randomized, double-blind, controlled crossover trial," *Diabetes Therapy*, vol. 8, no. 2, pp. 293–307, 2017.

[59] H. Panwar, D. Calderwood, I. R. Grant, S. Grover, and B. D. Green, "*Lactobacillus* strains isolated from infant faeces possess potent inhibitory activity against intestinal alpha- and beta-glucosidases suggesting anti-diabetic potential," *European Journal of Nutrition*, vol. 53, no. 7, pp. 1465–1474, 2014.

[60] A. Everard and P. D. Cani, "Gut microbiota and GLP-1," *Reviews in Endocrine and Metabolic Disorders*, vol. 15, no. 3, pp. 189–196, 2014.

[61] B. S. Samuel, A. Shaito, T. Motoike et al., "Effects of the gut microbiota on host adiposity are modulated by the short-chain fatty-acid binding G protein-coupled receptor, Gpr41," *Proceedings of the National Academy of Sciences of the United States of America*, vol. 105, no. 43, pp. 16767–16772, 2008.

[62] M. K. Nøhr, M. H. Pedersen, A. Gille et al., "GPR41/FFAR3 and GPR43/FFAR2 as cosensors for short-chain fatty acids in enteroendocrine cells vs FFAR3 in enteric neurons and FFAR2 in enteric leukocytes," *Endocrinology*, vol. 154, no. 10, pp. 3552–3564, 2013.

[63] G. Tolhurst, H. Heffron, Y. S. Lam et al., "Short-chain fatty acids stimulate glucagon-like peptide-1 secretion via the G-protein-coupled receptor FFAR2," *Diabetes*, vol. 61, no. 2, pp. 364–371, 2012.

[64] M. Yang, H. Fukui, H. Eda et al., "Involvement of gut microbiota in association between GLP-1/GLP-1 receptor expression and gastrointestinal motility," *American Journal of Physiology. Gastrointestinal and Liver Physiology*, vol. 312, no. 4, pp. G367–G373, 2017.

[65] E. Grasset, A. Puel, J. Charpentier et al., "A specific gut microbiota dysbiosis of type 2 diabetic mice induces GLP-1 resistance through an enteric NO-dependent and gut-brain axis mechanism," *Cell Metabolism*, vol. 26, no. 1, p. 278, 2017.

[66] Y. Li, L. Han, M. Xu, J. Guo, M. Feng, and X. Wang, "The primary research on the gut microbes in KKAy mice," *Indian Journal of Microbiology*, vol. 54, no. 1, pp. 12–19, 2014.

[67] P. Xu, F. Hong, J. Wang et al., "DBZ is a putative PPARγ agonist that prevents high fat diet-induced obesity, insulin resistance and gut dysbiosis," *Biochimica et Biophysica Acta (BBA) - General Subjects*, vol. 1861, no. 11, Part A, pp. 2690–2701, 2017.

[68] Q. Zhang, X. Xiao, M. Li et al., "Vildagliptin increases butyrate-producing bacteria in the gut of diabetic rats," *PLoS One*, vol. 12, no. 10, article e0184735, 2017.

[69] D. R. Powell, M. Smith, J. Greer et al., "LX4211 increases serum glucagon-like peptide 1 and peptide YY levels by reducing sodium/glucose cotransporter 1 (SGLT1)–mediated absorption of intestinal glucose," *The Journal of Pharmacology and Experimental Therapeutics*, vol. 345, no. 2, pp. 250–259, 2013.

[70] A. Lehmann and P. J. Hornby, "Intestinal SGLT1 in metabolic health and disease," *American Journal of Physiology Gastrointestinal and Liver Physiology*, vol. 310, no. 11, pp. G887–G898, 2016.

[71] L. D. Pound, C. Patrick, C. E. Eberhard et al., "Cathelicidin antimicrobial peptide: a novel regulator of islet function, islet regeneration, and selected gut bacteria," *Diabetes*, vol. 64, no. 12, pp. 4135–4147, 2015.

[72] X. Mei, X. Zhang, Z. Wang et al., "Insulin sensitivity-enhancing activity of phlorizin is associated with lipopolysaccharide decrease and gut microbiota changes in obese and type 2 diabetes (*db/db*) mice," *Journal of Agricultural and Food Chemistry*, vol. 64, no. 40, pp. 7502–7511, 2016.

[73] M. Sasaki, N. Ogasawara, Y. Funaki et al., "Transglucosidase improves the gut microbiota profile of type 2 diabetes mellitus patients: a randomized double-blind, placebo-controlled study," *BMC Gastroenterology*, vol. 13, no. 1, p. 81, 2013.

14

Effect of a Nurse-Led Diabetes Self-Management Education Program on Glycosylated Hemoglobin among Adults with Type 2 Diabetes

Golnaz Azami,[1,2] Kim Lam Soh,[1] Shariff Ghazali Sazlina,[3] Md. Said Salmiah,[4] Sanaz Aazami,[2] Mosayeb Mozafari,[2] and Hamid Taghinejad[2]

[1]*Department of Nursing and Rehabilitations, Faculty of Medicine and Health Sciences, University Putra Malaysia (UPM), 43400 Serdang, Selangor, Malaysia*
[2]*Department of Nursing, Faculty of Nursing and Midwifery, Ilam University of Medical Sciences, Ilam 693917714, Iran*
[3]*Department of Family Medicine, Faculty of Medicine and Health Sciences, University Putra Malaysia (UPM), 43400 Serdang, Selangor, Malaysia*
[4]*Department of Community Health, Faculty of Medicine and Health Sciences, University Putra Malaysia (UPM), 43400 Serdang, Selangor, Malaysia*

Correspondence should be addressed to Kim Lam Soh; sklam@upm.edu.my

Academic Editor: Jordi Lluis Reverter

In recent years, great emphasis has been placed on the role of nonpharmacological self-management in the care of patients with diabetes. Studies have reported that nurses, compared to other healthcare professionals, are more likely to promote preventive healthcare seeking behaviors. The aim of this study was to investigate the effectiveness of a nurse-led diabetes self-management education on glycosylated hemoglobin. A two-arm parallel-group randomized controlled trial with the blinded outcome assessors was designed. One hundred forty-two adults with type 2 diabetes were randomized to receive either usual diabetes care (control group) or usual care plus a nurse-led diabetes self-management education (intervention group). Duration of the intervention was 12 weeks. The primary outcome was glycosylated hemoglobin (HbA1c values). Secondary outcomes were changes in blood pressure, body weight, lipid profiles, self-efficacy (efficacy expectation and outcome expectation), self-management behaviors, quality of life, social support, and depression. Outcome measures were assessed at baseline and at 12-week and 24-week postrandomizations. Patients in the intervention group showed significant improvement in HbA1c, blood pressure, body weight, efficacy expectation, outcome expectation, and diabetes self-management behaviors. The beneficial effect of a nurse-led intervention continued to accrue beyond the end of the trial resulting in sustained improvements in clinical, lifestyle, and psychosocial outcomes. This trial is registered with IRCT2016062528627N1.

1. Introduction

Iran is located in western Asia covering a total land area of 1,648,195 km^2. By 2014, with a population of 82,801,633, Iran became the 16th most populous country in the world [1]. Healthcare in Iran is the responsibilities of the Ministry of Health (MOH) [2]. The national health priorities include developing a new policy to improve health system and better health outcomes for both communicable and noncommunicable diseases [3]. One of the great challenges that healthcare continues to face is the epidemiological transition of diseases from communicable to noncommunicable [4, 5]. Diabetes is a prominent public health concern in Iran that is associated with increased premature mortality, as well as increased risk for micro- and macrovascular complications. The International Diabetes Federation estimated that there were more than 4.6 million cases of diabetes in Iran in 2015, which is 8.5% of the population (20–79 years)

[6]. The prevalence of diabetes in Iran is projected to be 9.2 million by the year 2040 [7]. Type 2 diabetes mellitus (T2DM) is the most common form of diabetes, accounting for 90–95% of all diabetes cases [8]. In Iran, T2DM occurs predominantly in middle-aged and older population, with an average age of 40–50 years. In contrast, the average age of the T2DM population in developed countries is over 65 years [9]. With the prolongation of the average life expectancy, the occurrence of T2DM in the younger age groups will lead to the escalation of the disease-related disability-adjusted life years in Iran [10]. In order to prevent or delay the development of diabetes complications, intensive efforts are required to achieve optimal glycemic control. Evidence suggested that diabetes self-management education can reduce diabetes complications and improve short-term glycemic control [11].

Different members of the healthcare team can provide diabetes self-management education. Much of research comparing the effectiveness of discipline-based education has not determined clear differences in the quality of services delivered by different healthcare professions [12]. However, published evidence favors the registered nurses, pharmacist, and registered nutritionist serving both as the members of the multidisciplinary team responsible for designing the curriculum and assisting in the delivery of education and the key primary instructors for diabetes education [12]. Nurses comprise the largest and most trusted health professional group. Nurses are uniquely positioned to inspire positive changes and transform healthcare delivery by serving as the bridge between theory and practice [13]. In diabetes self-management education (DSME), the close involvement of patients and caregivers is encouraged. Practice nurses are ideally positioned to provide monitoring, tailored feedback, and education on key aspects of self-management [14]. Despite growing interest, there is limited evidence to support the clinical effectiveness of nurse-led diabetes self-management interventions on glycemic control, particularly in Iran. The current study seeks to address these limitations by designing a randomized controlled trial with outcomes measured at baseline and postintervention at 3 and 6 months. Our primary hypothesis was that a nurse-led DSME intervention, compared with the usual care, would result in improvement in HbA1c. The secondary hypothesis was that the nurse-led DSME intervention would improve lipid profiles, blood pressure, body weight, self-management behavior, self-efficacy, quality of life, depression, and social support.

2. Method

2.1. Research Setting. This study took place in an urban primary and secondary outpatient endocrine clinic located within a teaching hospital in Ilam city, Iran. The hospital has a daily outpatient diabetes clinic with a daily turnover of approximately 20–30 patients except on Friday [15]. A multidisciplinary team is involved in the management of the patients. The clinic is currently the only leading medical service available to Ilamian residents with T2DM.

2.2. Research Design and Participants. The trial was conducted as a single-center, observer-blinded, parallel group (2 groups) randomized controlled trial.

Eligible participants were randomized into two groups:

(1) The control group receives usual diabetes care routines.

(2) The intervention group receives usual diabetes care plus 24 weeks of the nurse-led DSME intervention.

Participants were eligible if they were Iranian adults aged ≥18 years, who were clinically diagnosed with T2DM for at least 6 months, and had the medical record showing HbA1c ≥ 8%. To make sure that the lack of access to healthcare does not pose significant barriers to diabetes self-management, all patients were recommended to participate in follow-up at regular intervals. We required patients to participate in follow-up care (at least two visits per year) and have no evidence of a serious medical illness.

Exclusion criteria include cognitive dysfunction, pregnancy, uncontrolled high blood pressure (≥180/110 mmHg), hearing impairment, vision impairment, hemolytic anemias, and hemoglobinopathies. Patients were excluded if they were illiterate, had acute or chronic diabetes complications, and had major difficulties in activities of daily living.

The recruitment process was conducted in two stages. The first stage involved strategies to ensure adequate participant enrolment via placing an advertisement on the message boards of the clinic.

The second stage involved screening and assessment process by evaluating previous medical histories, measurement of HbA1c values, blood pressure, and visual acuity, and completion of three validated questionnaires regarding cognitive function (modified Mini-Mental State Examination (3MS)) [16], activity of daily living (Instrumental Activity of Daily Living (IADL)) [17], and hearing problem status (validated Single Global Screening Question) [18]. After successfully completing all screening processes and baseline assessment, eligible participants were randomized to either intervention or control groups. Randomization consisted of permuted block randomization with fixed block sizes of 4 or 6. No stratification was used. A statistician blinded to the allocation of participants to groups generates the random allocation sequence, using computer-generated random numbers. The allocation was concealed from the other researchers until randomization occurred.

In this study, we had multiple outcome variables, and the mean values were used for further analysis. Estimated sample sizes for each outcome variable were calculated independently, and the largest of the sample sizes was chosen as the target sample size. The following formula was used to calculate the sample size (Lemeshow et al., 1990: cited in [19]):

$$\mathbf{N} = \frac{2\sigma^2\left(\mathbf{Z}_{1-\alpha/2} + \mathbf{Z}_{1-\beta}\right)^2}{\left(\mu_1 - \mu_2\right)^2}. \quad (1)$$

To detect the difference in means of outcomes, a minimum of 71 patients were needed for each arm (accounting for 20% loss to follow-up) [20].

2.3. Usual Care. The usual diabetes care is based on the Iranian Ministry of Health Guideline on the management of the T2DM, which involves self-care management, lifestyle modification, and medication adherence. Individual-based education was provided at three monthly intervals with the duration of 20–30 minutes per appointment. Face to face consultations and pamphlets are used to provide the usual diabetes care education. Physical examination and laboratory tests are performed at each visit in accordance with national guidelines. Based on the physical examination and laboratory findings, prescription refills or renewal are obtained during the check-ups.

2.4. Research Intervention. In addition to usual diabetes care, participants in the intervention group received a 12-week nurse-led DSME founded in the theoretical framework from Albert Bandura's self-efficacy theory [21] and Motivational Interviewing (MI) spirit. Self-efficacy was defined as "people's judgment of their capabilities to organize and execute the course of action which require designated types of performances" [22]. MI was used as a teaching approach toward the goal of behavior change [23, 24]. The American Association of Diabetes Educators (AADE) defined the seven essential self-care behaviors for successful and effective diabetes self-management. Self-care behaviors, including healthy eating, being active, monitoring, taking medication, problem-solving, reducing risk, and healthy coping, are the core components of our intervention.

Participants in the intervention group received (1) a detailed information booklet, which includes information on conducting self-management, (2) viewed four 10-minute movie clips, (3) attended four weekly group-based educational sessions, and (4) received follow-up telephone calls weekly.

A multidisciplinary team including endocrinologists, nutritionists, nurses, and pharmacists, with the actual intervention to be carried out by a nurse, designed the intervention program. The pilot version of the intervention was then produced and validated by fourteen patients with T2DM.

2.4.1. Receiving the Booklet. The booklet consisted of six sections: (1) diet, (2) physical activity, (3) medication, (4) monitoring of blood glucose, (5) foot care, and (6) healthy living with diabetes. The booklet was developed based on the two sources of self-efficacy, that is, verbal persuasion and performance accomplishment. Participants in the intervention group received the booklet at the start of the program. The content of the booklet was used throughout the entire length of the intervention to direct further learning, elaboration, and discussion or to create resources for self-directed learning.

2.4.2. Watching Movie Clips. For the first 4 weeks of the intervention, participants were invited to watch four 10-minute weekly movies. The movie is based on the content of the booklet. The language used in the movies was Persian. They were designed and developed by the research team to provide coaching and encouragement (verbal persuasion). Based on the educational contents, four movies were produced in different field of diabetes self-management including general information about T2DM, preventing short- and long-term complications (session 1), physical activity, daily foot care (session 2), healthy eating (session 3), and healthy living with diabetes (session 4).

2.4.3. Group Discussion Session. Four group discussion sessions were carried out at weekly intervals, but the scheduling was flexible and the seating was limited to 10 participants for each session. These sessions were carried out weekly during the first 4 weeks of the intervention. Each session lasted for 120 minutes. The focus of these sessions was on building knowledge, self-efficacy, and skills regarding self-goal setting, action plan, problem-solving, sharing, and peer support. The group discussion sessions were facilitated by the first author (GA), who is a diabetes specialist nurse with 4 years of clinical experience. Participants' family members were encouraged to attend sessions that can provide multibeneficial support for the patient and their families. All group members were heartened to actively participate in each session. Group members who miss a session received a follow-up from the facilitator before the next session. Standard guidelines were developed for the group discussions and used in all the sessions held. At the last meeting of the group session, all group members received a list of residential phone numbers and were encouraged to ask for help if needed.

2.4.4. Receiving Telephone Follow-Up Calls. Two months after the end of the group discussion sessions, intervention participants received a phone call once per week. Each follow-up call lasted approximately 15–20 minutes. The purpose of the telephone calls was to foster continued performance accomplishment via positive verbal persuasion. Telephone calls were based on principles of motivational interviewing (MI) that successfully help patients to engage and support them in making better health choices [25]. The first step in MI is to set the agenda for the consultation together with the patients [23]. "Agenda setting" is an issue to keep in the back of patient's mind from the opening scene of the interview. The basic question was "what are we going to talk about today?" Patients were encouraged to choose one or more key items (agenda settings) as their main area of concern. Then, the researcher assessed the participant's current self-care behavior and motivation for behavior change by rating and exploring importance and confidence with respect to the chosen key items. Techniques that were applied in the telephone calls to invoke the spirit of MI were asking open-ended questions, affirmations, reflective listening, summarizing during a conversation, expressing empathy, developing discrepancy, rolling with resistance, supporting self-efficacy, and reinforcing positive change-talk and new behavior. It led to an action plan being drawn up to implement strategies to improve the patient's performance [26]. At the end of the intervention, educational booklet and movies were given to the participants of the control group.

2.5. Measurements

2.5.1. Laboratory Measures. A single laboratory analyzed all blood samples. For the blood tests, 10 cc of fasting venous blood was taken after fasting for at least 8–10 hours.

Whole blood levels of HbA1c, total triglyceride, total cholesterol, high-density lipoprotein (HDL), and low-density lipoprotein (LDL) were measured. NycoCard HbA1c analyzer (made in the US) was used for quantitative determination of HbA1c value. Lipid profile tests were conducted using an Auto Analyzer BT-3000 (made in Spain).

2.5.2. Clinical Measures. Blood pressure was measured as the mean of two measurements performed after 5 min of rest while patients were seated with a cuff placed on their dominant arm at the same vertical height as the heart, using an automated blood pressure monitor (UA-779, A&D Instruments Ltd., Abingdon, UK). Weight and height were measured using a weighing and height scale (BT-ETS002, Medical Hospital Electronic height scale with weight measure, China). The participant's weight and height were measured without shoes or heavy clothing according to a standardized procedure. Patients were asked to stand up as straight as possible and look straight ahead. Body mass index (BMI) was calculated with the formula weight(kg)/height(m)^2. According to the World Health Organization (WHO) criteria, there are three types of metabolic phenotypes as determined by BMI range (kg/m^2) including underweight (severe thinness (<16), moderate thinness (16-17), and mild thinness (1–18.5)), normal BMI (18.5–25), and obesity (overweight (25–30), obese class I (30–35), obese class II (35–40), and obese class III (>40)) [27].

2.5.3. Questionnaires. Efficacy expectation (self-efficacy) was measured using the Diabetes Management Self-Efficacy Scale (DMSES) [28]. The DMSES is a 20-item self-administered scale that assesses the extent to which respondents are confident that they can manage their blood glucose level, diet, level of physical activity, medications, and food care. The total score ranged from 0 to 200 points, with the higher scores indicating a greater self-efficacy [28]. This instrument has been validated for Iranian population [29] and showed to have satisfactory validity and reliability ($\alpha = 0.96$).

Outcome expectation was measured using the Perceived Therapeutic Efficacy Scale (PTES) [30] translated into a Persian version in accordance with recommendations [31]. The PTES contains ten questions designed to measure the confidence that the individuals have in performing self-management which activates for achieving desired outcomes. The total score ranged from 0 to 100 points, with the higher scores indicating a greater confidence. The reliability of the Persian version of the instrument was 0.95. To date, this questionnaire had not been validated in Iran. Thus, a pilot study was conducted where the instrument was tested and validated at a hospital outpatient clinic in Ilam city before the questionnaire was taken into use. The pilot study was conducted in September 2016 among 160 individuals with T2DM who registered at the clinic. Pilot testing demonstrated that the instrument is valid and reliable to assess outcome expectation ($\alpha = 0.95$).

Diabetes self-management behavior was measured using the validated Diabetes Self-Management Questionnaire (DSMQ). The instrument was translated from English into Persian in accordance with a recommended translation procedure [31]. The DSMQ is a 16-item self-administered questionnaire, with the higher scores indicating a more effective self-care [32]. To date, the DSMQ had not been validated for local use. Prior to the distribution of the instrument, a pilot study was conducted on 160 patients with T2DM to check the validity and reliability of the instrument. The pilot study indicated that the DSMQ is a valid and reliable instrument for assessing outcome expectations in Iran ($\alpha = 0.87$).

The quality of life was measured using the World Health Organization Quality of Life Scale (WHOQOL-BREF). The WHOQOL-BREF is a self-administered, abbreviated version of the WHOQOL-100 containing 26 items divided into four domains and two general items. The WHOQOL-BREF scores were transformed on a scale from 0 to 100 with the higher scores indicating better quality of life [33]. This instrument has previously been validated for use in Iranian population ($\alpha = 0.94$) [34].

Social support was measured with the Medical Outcome Study (MOS) Social Support Survey (SSS) tool. The MOS is a 19-item self-report instrument, measuring a multidimensional of the functional aspects of perceived social support, developed for patients with chronic conditions [35]. The total score ranged from 0 to 100 points, with the higher scores indicating more available social support. This instrument has previously been validated for use in Iranian population ($\alpha = 0.97$) [36].

Depression was assessed using the Centre for Epidemiology Studies Short Depression Scale (CES-D) [37]. The CES-D is a 10-item self-administered instrument designed to measure the presence of depressive symptoms over the previous week. The total score ranged from 0 to 30 points, with a higher score indicating a more severe depression. This instrument has previously been validated for use in Iranian population ($\alpha = 0.93$) [38].

2.6. Statistical Analysis. All data were analyzed using SPSS software (version 22, IBM Company, Chicago, IL, USA). Statistical significance was reported at the 0.05 alpha level, with two-tailed P values. Values are expressed as mean ± SD or n (%). Data analysis was carried out in two steps. Firstly, comparisons of baseline data between two experimental groups were made using Student's t-test or Mann–Whitney U test for continuous variables based on their normality, and the Chi-square or Fisher exact test for categorical variables, as appropriate. Next, main analyses were made on an intention to treat basis using repeated measures ANOVA. We investigated the impact of missing data with an expected-maximization algorithm, to compute estimates to replace missing data. Time points were used as the within-subject factor and group as the between-subject factor. Effect size is reported as partial Eta square. Our findings only concern the interaction of time × group.

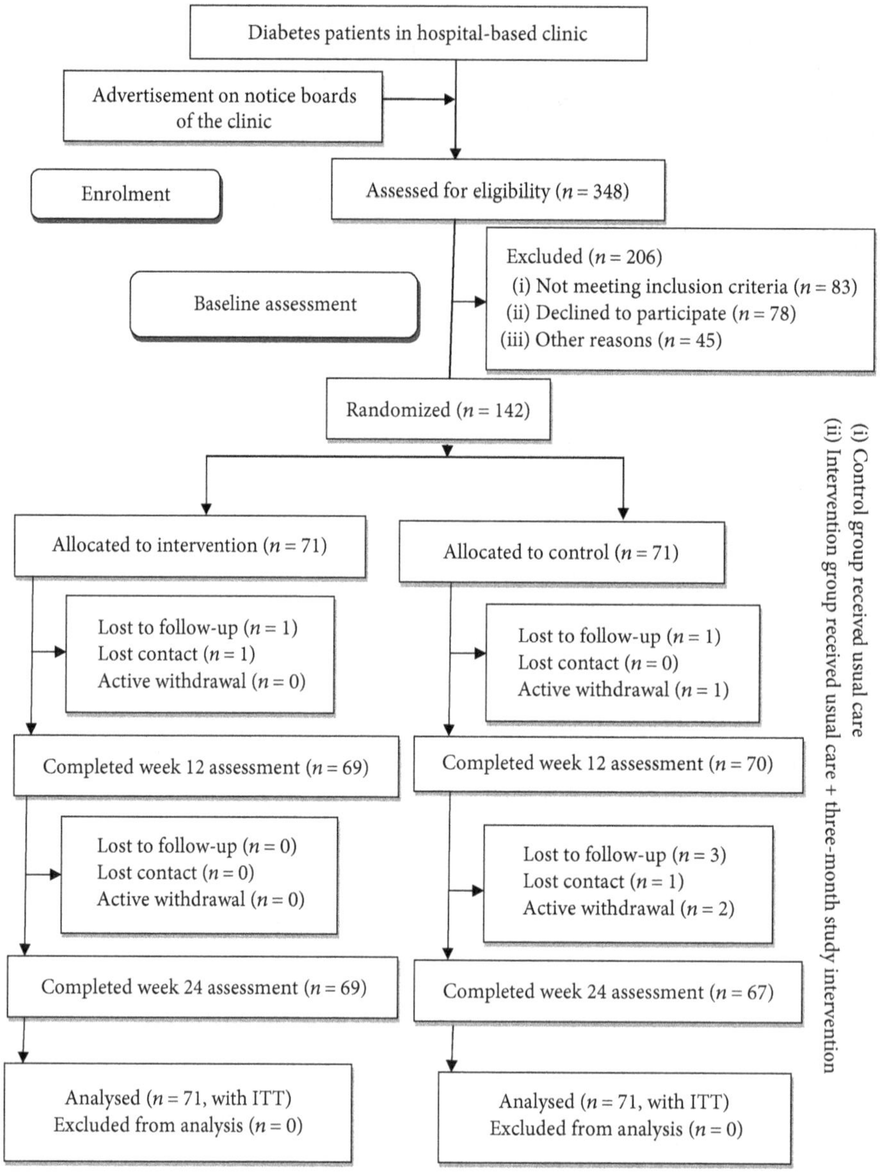

FIGURE 1: Consort flow diagram of study participation.

2.7. Research Ethics. Ethical approval was granted from the University Putra Malaysia Ethics Committee for Research Involving Human Subjects and Medical University of Ilam Ethics Committee. Patients were informed about the purpose of the study and gave their consent prior to participation.

3. Results

3.1. Baseline Data. Between October 2016 and Jun 2017, 348 patients were approached and invited to participate in this study. Eighty-three patients did not meet the study inclusion criteria, and 78 declined to participate. The main reasons for declining participation were time constraints and family obligation. Of the 187 eligible patients, 13 did not respond (either telephone contact was not achieved after 6 repeated attempts or wrong phone number), 12 agreed to attend but did not, 11 not interested after reading the information, 7 responded after the deadline, and 2 not willing to be randomized. In total, 142 eligible patients were randomized; 72 were allocated to the intervention group and 72 were allocated to the control group.

During the 24-week follow-up period, 6 patients dropped out (4.2%), of whom 5 had been allocated to the control group and 1 to the intervention group (Figure 1). The baseline characteristics of both groups were similar, indicating that randomization was effective. The differences between participants who completed and those who did not complete the study were not significant except for income. Income is a well-known factor that influences health outcomes. The analysis found that lower income individuals were more likely to withdraw from the study ($P < 0.001$).

Mean age at baseline was 54.2 ± 11.8 years (range 22–69 years), and two-thirds of the participants were female (65.5%). Majority of the participants had primary education

Table 1: Sociodemographic characteristics of study participants.

Characteristics	Total sample $N = 142$	Intervention group $N = 71$	Control group $N = 71$
Age, years[a]	56 ± 11.1	55.09 ± 10.16	53.49 ± 10.98
Gender[b]			
(i) Male	49 (34%)	23 (32.4%)	26 (36.6%)
(ii) Female	93 (65.5%)	48 (67.6%)	45 (63.4%)
Marital status[b]			
(i) Married	117 (82.4%)	58 (81.7%)	59 (83.1%)
(ii) Single (divorced/widow)	25 (17.6%)	13 (18.3%)	12 (16.9%)
Educational status[b]			
(i) Primary education	64 (45.1%)	33 (46.5%)	31 (43.7%)
(ii) Secondary education	23 (16.2%)	12 (16.9%)	11 (15.5%)
(iii) Tertiary education	55 (38.7%)	26 (36.6%)	29 (40.8%)
Occupation status[b]			
(i) Working	83 (58.5%)	28 (39.4%)	31 (43.7%)
(ii) Not working	59 (41.5%)	43 (60.6%)	40 (56.3%)
Difficulty paying for basics[b]			
(i) Very hard	7 (4.9%)	5 (7%)	2 (2.8%)
(ii) Somewhat hard	96 (67.6%)	47 (66.2%)	49 (69%)
(iii) Not hard at all	39 (27.5%)	19 (26.8%)	20 (28.2%)
Smoking status[b]			
(i) Current smoker	18 (12.7%)	9 (12.7%)	9 (12.7%)
(ii) Never	108 (76.1%)	55 (77.5%)	53 (74.6%)
(iii) Ex-smoker	16 (11.3%)	7 (9.9%)	9 (12.7%)
Duration of diabetes, years[a]	8.9 ± 7.4	8.8 ± 7.5	9.04 ± 7.31
Presence of at least one comorbidity[b]	113 (79.5%)	57 (80.3%)	56 (78.9%)
Use of SBGM[a]	71 (50%)	32 (45.1%)	39 (54.9%)
BMI (kg/m^2)[a]	28.78 ± 3.34	28.69 ± 3.25	28.87 ± 3.46
Systolic blood pressure (mmHg)[a]	132.3 ± 11.2	130.6 ± 9.6	133.9 ± 12.4
Diastolic blood pressure (mmHg)[a]	86.6 ± 5.9	85.8 ± 5.2	87.3 ± 6.4
HbA1c[a]	9.32 ± 1.11	9.32 ± 1.06	9.31 ± 1.15
(i) 8–8.9%[b]	59 (41.5%)	29 (40.8%)	30 (42.3%)
(ii) ≥9%[b]	83 (58.5%)	42 (59.2%)	41 (57.7%)
Triglyceride[a]	142.4 ± 34.9	142.83 ± 34.4	142.09 ± 35.7
Total cholesterol[a]	172.5 ± 46.8	173.14 ± 45.4	171.91 ± 48.4
HDL[a]	53.44 ± 12.62	53.68 ± 12.8	53.21 ± 12.4
LDL[a]	94.28 ± 27.86	95.89 ± 30	92.68 ± 25.6

Note: [a]Mean ± standard deviation; [b]frequency (%); HDL = high-density lipoprotein; LDL = low-density lipoprotein; BMI = body mass index; SBMG = self-blood glucose monitoring.

(45.1%), and nearly three-fifths of them (58.5%) were currently working. A vast majority of participants had middle socioeconomic status; only 4.9% reported having difficulties meeting basic needs. Approximately three-quarters of the participants (76.1%) never smoked. The mean duration of diabetes was 8.9 ± 7.4 years. Participants were characterized by poor glycemic and blood pressure control. 58.5% had HbA1c ≥ 9%, and 9.1% had blood pressure at the recommended target < 130/80 mmHg. The proportion of self-blood glucose monitoring was similar for those who conducted it and those who did not, at 50% (see Table 1).

3.2. Laboratory Measures. The intention-to-treat analysis evaluated the primary and secondary outcomes. The primary outcome of the present study was HbA1c levels as presented in Table 2. Analysis of variance with repeated measure on time revealed a significant group-by-time interaction for HbA1c levels ($P < 0.001$). At week 12, participants in the intervention group had significantly lower HbA1c values (47.9%) than those in the control group. At week 24, the differences increased to 62% ($P < 0.001$). More than a fifth (21.1%) of the patients in the intervention group achieved an HbA1c < 7% compared to none in the control group ($P < 0.001$). No significant group × time interaction effects

Table 2: Two-way ANOVA with repeated measures for primary and secondary outcomes.

Model	Intervention mean (SD)			Control mean (SD)				Significance	
	T_1	T_2	T_3	T_1	T_2	T_3	F value	P value	Effect size (Eta square)
HbA1c	9.3 (1.06)	8.6 (1.01)	7.9 (0.93)	9.3 (1.1)	9.3 (1.1)	9.3 (1.1)			
Group							14.5	$P < 0.001$	0.09
Time							277.6	$P < 0.001$	0.66
Group × time							289.5	$P < 0.001$	0.67
Systolic blood pressure	130.7 (9.4)	129.3 (9.1)	127.8 (9)	133.9 (12.3)	133.7 (12.1)	133.3 (12)			
Group							5.9	0.01	0.04
Time							59.1	$P < 0.001$	0.29
Group × time							25.7	$P < 0.001$	0.15
Diastolic blood pressure	85.8 (0.69)	84.7 (0.67)	83.4 (0.65)	87.3 (0.69)	87.3 (0.67)	87.1 (0.65)			
Group							7.4	$P < 0.001$	0.05
Time							61.3	$P < 0.001$	0.30
Group × time							39.3	$P < 0.001$	0.21
Weight	82.58 (11.08)	82.21 (11.09)	82 (10.89)	83.75 (10.93)	83.77 (10.91)	83.82 (10.89)			
Group							0.68	0.41	0.01
Time							4.69	0.01	0.03
Group × time							7.17	0.01	0.04
BMI	28.69 (3.2)	28.54 (3.2)	28.55 (3.2)	28.87 (3.4)	28.87 (3.4)	29.89 (3.4)			
Group							0.24	0.62	0.01
Time							2.59	0.07	0.01
Group × time							3.18	0.04	0.02
Triglyceride	142.83 (34.4)	141.66 (33.9)	140.90 (33.7)	142.09 (35.7)	142.04 (35.6)	142.01 (35.6)			
Group							0.00	0.96	0.01
Time							40.41	$P < 0.001$	0.22
Group × time							33.82	$P < 0.001$	0.19
Cholesterol	173.1 (45.4)	171.3 (43.8)	169.09 (43.1)	171.9 (48.4)	170.7 (47.02)	171.88 (46.8)			
Group							0.006	0.93	0.01
Time							3.15	0.06	0.02
Group × time							0.10	0.82	0.01
LDL	95.89 (30.04)	95.59 (28.4)	93.95 (27.9)	92.68 (25.6)	93.06 (25.4)	94.15 (25)			
Group							0.16	0.68	0.01
Time							0.15	0.85	0.01
Group × time							5.62	0.22	0.39
HDL	53.68 (12.8)	54.72 (11.6)	55.38 (11.8)	53.21 (12.4)	53.21 (12.5)	52.76 (12.6)			

Table 2: Continued.

Model	Intervention mean (SD)			Control mean (SD)				Significance	
	T_1	T_2	T_3	T_1	T_2	T_3	F value	P value	Effect size (Eta square)
Group							0.55	0.45	0.01
Time							2.66	0.28	0.01
Group × time							6.94	0.94	0.04
Efficacy expectation	98.35 (13.95)	113.47 (11.07)	123.47 (11.31)	98.06 (17.47)	99.77 (14.48)	98.44 (15.69)			
Group							34.3	$P < 0.001$	0.19
Time							152.2	$P < 0.001$	0.52
Group × time							138.7	$P < 0.001$	0.49
Outcome expectation	57.80 (7.11)	62.85 (5.50)	66.79 (5.35)	58.11 (7.50)	58.04 (7.33)	58.16 (7.23)			
Group							16.15	$P < 0.001$	0.10
Time							150.81	$P < 0.001$	0.51
Group × time							147.61	$P < 0.001$	0.51
DSMB	3.56 (1.22)	4.67 (1)	5.41 (1.15)	3.71 (1.40)	3.67 (1.37)	3.73 (1.40)			
Group							16.7	$P < 0.001$	0.10
Time							228.5	$P < 0.001$	0.62
Group × time							221.6	$P < 0.001$	0.61
QOL	50.42 (9.17)	50.76 (9.06)	50.67 (9.04)	50.69 (8.90)	50.34 (8.83)	50.39 (8.71)			
Group							0.00	0.92	0.01
Time							0.07	0.86	0.01
Group × time							10.5	$P < 0.001$	0.07
Social support	52.63 (9.31)	54.33 (9.42)	55.37 (9.61)	55.83 (12.11)	55.82 (12.63)	55.91 (12.75)			
Group							0.88	0.34	0.01
Time							43.6	$P < 0.001$	0.23
Group × time							39.3	$P < 0.001$	0.21
Depression	12.15 (4.99)	11.98 (4.97)	11.95 (5.03)	12.76 (4.66)	12.84 (4.61)	12.91 (4.50)			
Group							1	0.31	0.01
Time							0.51	0.55	0.01
Group × time							9.33	0.10	0.06

Note: Group: test of between-subject effects; Time: test of within-subject effect; Group × time: interaction between group by time; SD: standard deviation; T_1: baseline measurement; T_2: 3-month measurement; T_3: 6-month measurement; DSMB: diabetes self-management behavior; LDL: low-density lipoprotein; HDL: high-density lipoprotein; BMI: body mass index; QOL: quality of life; Primary outcome: HbA1c. To interpret effect sizes, 0.02 be considered a "small magnitude," 0.15 be considered a "medium magnitude," and 0.35 be considered a "large magnitude" [52].

were observed for any of the lipid profile parameters except for the triglyceride.

3.3. Clinical Measures. Two-way ANOVA with repeated measures over time revealed statistically significant differences in the changes in systolic blood pressure and diastolic blood pressure from baseline at time points (12 and 24 weeks) between the two groups ($P < 0.001$). A significant interaction effect of time and group exists with respect to the body weight of participants ($P < 0.001$).

3.4. Questionnaires. Analysis indicated a significant group-by-time interaction for efficacy expectation, outcome expectation, and diabetes self-management behavior ($P < 0.001$). Mean scores for efficacy expectation, outcome expectation, and self-management behavior differ significantly between groups at postintervention, with the intervention group showing greater improvement compared with the control group.

Interestingly, our findings showed a significant interaction effect of time × group for quality of life ($P < 0.001$), but no significant group ($P = 0.92$) or time main effects ($P = 0.86$). There was a significant difference in social support scores at all time points in both the control and intervention groups ($P < 0.001$).

No statistically significant interaction effect of time × group in depression was found in our study ($P = 0.10$), although a small reduction in depressive symptoms was more likely in the intervention participants (mean differences at 6 months = −0.2, $P > 0.05$) than in the control group (mean differences at 6 months = −0.04, $P > 0.05$). No serious adverse events or withdrawals as a result of adverse events occurred in our study.

4. Discussion

We tested the hypothesis that nurse-led DSME program is effective in improving lifestyle, clinical, and psychosocial outcomes. Participants in the intervention group showed significant improvements in glycemic control, blood pressure, body weight, efficacy expectation, outcome expectation, self-management behaviors, and social support compared with patients in the control group. These improvements were sustained over a 24-week follow-up period.

No adverse effects of our intervention were reported by our subjects. In addition, none of the patients were hospitalized or died for hypoglycemia events. These findings indicate the patient's acceptance of the intervention as well as the success of the logistics. Further multicenter studies with larger sample sizes are needed to strengthen our results.

We had a dropout rate of 5% in this 24-week follow-up study which is statistically considered to an acceptable figure. This result suggested that the intervention procedures were well tolerated and there were no complications. However, dropouts were more likely to occur in low or lower-middle income individuals. Financial problems are known to significantly affect diabetes self-management in varying ways [39]. Individuals with low income face more environmental risk factors associated with poor diabetes control, such as lack of access to healthy foods, difficulties in accessing and paying for healthcare, the high costs of medical equipment, lack of access to tailored physical activity programs, and the stress and isolation. Growing evidence suggests that tracking broader issues of poverty is the key to better diabetes management [40].

The compliance and satisfaction of patients with the program were generally high, so the feasibility of implementing this intervention in a future trial on a broader scale is promising. The total cost of implementing the study intervention was $5000.

Unlike many previous studies that examined drug treatment effect on glycemic control, we employed a nurse-led DSME to improve self-management behaviors. Most of the antidiabetes drugs have serious adverse effects that led researchers to the selection of alternative strategies aiming at achieving a better control of diabetes. A recent controlled study suggests that a nurse-led DSME can achieve a greater decrease in HbA1c at 6 months [41]. In line with the above findings, our intervention found to be effective in decreasing glycated hemoglobin levels over 24 weeks, comparable to those of drug trials. Overweight individuals with type 2 diabetes are two to four times more likely to develop cardiovascular complications. In fact, a small amount of weight loss (≥2%) in diabetic patients seems to mediate significant improvements in cardiovascular risk factors [42]. The extent of body weight loss was significantly larger in the intervention group compared to the control group (-0.58 ± 0.09 versus 0.07 ± 0.08, $P < 0.05$). Although the mean reduction in body weight was modest (0.58 kg decrease), one should not underestimate the potential benefits of weight loss and improvement in cardiovascular risk factors. The intervention group showed statistically significant improvements in blood pressure levels compared to the control group. Overall, our intervention resulted in a modest but significant reduction in weight, which, in turn, leads to significant decrease in HbA1c and blood pressure. There are numerous factors that can lead to changes in these variables, but lifestyle modifications is the key factor in the management of diabetes. Changes in lifestyle and dietary habits may have led to weight reduction over time. Losing weight can help control blood glucose levels and reduce blood pressure [43, 44]. The current study is in agreement with previous studies, demonstrating that modest weight loss can mitigate cardiovascular risk factors [11].

There were no significant differences between groups in their lipid profiles. However, there was a nonsignificant tendency towards a greater improvement in lipid profiles that might be confirmed if we had the bigger sample size and longer follow-up period. Recent studies suggest that lipid profile values varied by season, tend to be worse in cold season than in the warm season [45]. This study was conducted from October to May when the average air temperature decreased over the study period. We hypothesize that seasonal variation may be related to the changes in this parameter rather than the outcome of our intervention.

This study was based on a theoretical construct of self-efficacy by Bandura, the perception of one's ability to perform a task successfully [46]. This study has taken an initial step in involving nurses to work and collaborate beyond the traditional boundaries in order to build on the self-efficacy. This might be the key attributes for increasing patients' skills and confidence in managing health problems—so-called "self-management program" instead of just "self-monitoring" which has been proven to be not very useful. Our results were generally in accordance with the theoretical construction of the self-efficacy. Participants in the intervention group had significantly greater improvements in efficacy expectation, outcome expectation, and self-management behaviors compared with the control group. These results provide further support to drive a paradigm shift in healthcare delivery system form doctor-centered to patient-centered approaches. This potentially puts more emphasis on supporting nursing education, patients' self-management, and confidence to accomplish activities rather than mainly hospital-based management.

Our findings showed a significant interaction effect of time × group for quality of life ($P < 0.001$), but no significant group ($P = 0.92$) or time main effects ($P = 0.86$). One possible explanation for this finding is that there is a crossover interaction [47]. The existence of crossover interaction suggests that at 3-month intervention group showed better quality of life than the control group, but that this pattern reversed for the 6-month measurement. Although nonsignificant, our intervention had a positive impact on how patients perceived their quality of life.

Social support is known as one of the emotional coping mechanisms that can positively influence the quality of life [48]. There is a direct positive relationship between social support and health, so higher levels of social support are linked to better overall health [49, 50].

We found a significant improvement in social support throughout the study period. In contrast, no significant differences between groups were observed for quality of life and depression, which likely reflect the short follow-up period and lack of power to detect such changes. However, there was a nonsignificant trend towards greater improvements in quality of life and depression symptoms in the intervention group than in the control group that might be confirmed if we had the larger sample size and longer follow-up period. To substantiate the robustness of the findings, further detailed interventions with larger sample size and longer follow-up period are still required to confirm our results.

4.1. Strength and Limitation. To the best of our knowledge, this is the first study of its kind conducted in Ilam province, in the western part of Iran.

This trial has many strengths. By using a randomized clinical trial, we ensured a robust study design, with reasonably well-matched pairs in groups. Eventually, we were successful in minimizing contamination between the two groups. The program was delivered by a facilitator trained to give a high-quality education program. We aimed to ensure that necessary education materials were available to all in a local language. This approach greatly increases the generalizability of our findings and therefore the possibilities to implement this program for use in other resource-limited settings.

Data were analyzed by the intention-to-treat approach to preserve the merit of randomization. At the end of the study, the response rate was higher than expected (more than 90%), minimizing the amount of missing data. We acknowledge that there are some limitations in our study. Participants were followed-up for a short period of time. A follow-up period of 6 months may be too short to evaluate the long-term effect of the self-management intervention. Further studies are needed to evaluate the long-term effects of the intervention. Our trial may have been underpowered to detect significant changes in some variables and as a result, some of our findings may be prone to type 2 error (i.e., discarding real associations). There was a substantially and statistically significantly greater improvement in the intervention group, which might be due to the Hawthorne effect. The Hawthorne effect can influence the behavior of the participant, potentially improve or modify their behavior in response to the fact that they knew they are being observed. However, a rigorous design was used to minimize and adjust the common bias and limitations associated with research.

5. Conclusion

In a cohort of 142 adults with T2DM, a single-center nurse-led DSME offered sustained benefits in clinical and lifestyle outcomes at 24 weeks. Facilitating self-efficacy has been found to improve longer-term health outcomes in patients with chronic health conditions [51]. Our findings indicated that it is possible to achieve behavior changes by enhancing intrinsic motivation and self-efficacy. Thus, the novelty here is the application of theory into the clinical practice. Our findings support the implementation of a program that emphasizes collaborative learning, although the optimum interval and contact time require further evaluation. We recognize that there might be room for further improvement of clinical outcomes by increasing contact time and frequency. Further research, with extended contact time and longer follow-up, is needed to show if our intervention has long-term effects.

Conflicts of Interest

The authors declare that they have no competing interests.

Acknowledgments

The authors gratefully acknowledge all participants of the study. This study was supported by University Putra Malaysia (UPM) in cooperation with the Ilam University of Medical Sciences, Ilam, Iran.

References

[1] United Nations, *Most Populous Cities of the World*, 2014, http://www.infoplease.com/ipa/A0762524.html.

[2] R. Mehrdad, "Health system in Iran," *JMAJ*, vol. 52, pp. 69–73, 2009.

[3] P. Owlia, M. B. Eftekhari, A. S. Forouzan, F. Bahreini, M. Farahani, and M. Ghanei, "Health research priority setting in Iran: introduction to a bottom up approach," *Journal of Research in Medical Sciences: the Official Journal of Isfahan*

University of Medical Sciences, vol. 16, no. 5, pp. 691–698, 2011.

[4] A. Boutayeb, "The double burden of communicable and non-communicable diseases in developing countries," *Transactions of the Royal Society of Tropical Medicine and Hygiene*, vol. 100, no. 3, pp. 191–199, 2006.

[5] A. D. Lopez and C. D. Mathers, "Measuring the global burden of disease and epidemiological transitions: 2002–2030," *Annals of Tropical Medicine & Parasitology*, vol. 100, no. 5-6, pp. 481–499, 2006.

[6] International Diabetes Federation, *Diabetes in Iran*, 2015, http://www.idf.org/membership/mena/iran.

[7] International Diabetes Federation, *The IDF Diabetes Atlas*, Axford Academic, Brussels, Belgium, 7-th edition edition, 2015.

[8] Iran Diabetes Leadership Forum, *The Diabetes Challenge in Islamic Republic of Iran Tehran*, Iranian Diabetes Society, 2015.

[9] A. Esteghamati, M. M. Gouya, M. Abbasi et al., "Prevalence of diabetes and impaired fasting glucose in the adult population of Iran: national survey of risk factors for non-communicable diseases of Iran," *Diabetes Care*, vol. 31, no. 1, pp. 96–98, 2007.

[10] A. Shaghaghi, A. Ahmadi, and H. Matlabi, "Iranian patients require more pertinent care to prevent type 2 diabetes complications," *Advances in Preventive Medicine*, vol. 2014, Article ID 409391, 6 pages, 2014.

[11] S. L. Norris, J. Lau, S. J. Smith, C. H. Schmid, and M. M. Engelgau, "Self-management education for adults with type 2 diabetes a meta-analysis of the effect on glycemic control," *Diabetes Care*, vol. 25, no. 7, pp. 1159–1171, 2002.

[12] L. Haas, M. Maryniuk, J. Beck et al., "National standards for diabetes self-management education and support," *The Diabetes Educator*, vol. 38, no. 5, pp. 619–629, 2012.

[13] P. A. Grady and L. L. Gough, "Self-management: a comprehensive approach to management of chronic conditions," *Revista Panamericana de Salud Pública*, vol. 37, no. 3, pp. 187–194, 2015.

[14] M. Hollis, K. Glaister, and J. Anne Lapsley, "Do practice nurses have the knowledge to provide diabetes self-management education?," *Contemporary Nurse*, vol. 46, no. 2, pp. 234–241, 2014.

[15] Shahid Mostafa Khomeini hospital, *Endocrine clinic in Shahid Mostafa Khomeini hospital (in persian)*, 2014.

[16] E. Teng and H. Chui, "The modified mini-mental state examination (3MS)," *Canadian Journal of Psychiatry*, vol. 41, pp. 114–121, 1987.

[17] M. Lawton and E. Brody, "Instrumental Activities of Daily Living Scale (IADL)," *Psychopharmacology Bulletin*, vol. 24, no. 4, pp. 785–787, 1988.

[18] G. A. Gates, M. Murphy, T. S. Rees, and A. Fraher, "Screening for handicapping hearing loss in the elderly," *Journal of Family Practice*, vol. 52, no. 1, pp. 56–62, 2003.

[19] L. A. Aday and L. J. Cornelius, *Designing and Conducting Health Surveys: A Comprehensive Guide*, John Wiley & Sons, 2006.

[20] K. R. Amico, "Percent total attrition: a poor metric for study rigor in hosted intervention designs," *American Journal of Public Health*, vol. 99, no. 9, pp. 1567–1575, 2009.

[21] A. Bandura, "Self-efficacy: toward a unifying theory of behavioral change," *Psychological Review*, vol. 84, no. 2, pp. 191–215, 1977.

[22] A. Bandura, *Social Foundations of Thought and Action*, Prentice Hall, Englewood Cliffs, NJ, 1986.

[23] W. Miller and S. Rollnick, "Motivational interviewing: preparing people for change, 2nd ed," *Journal for Healthcare Quality*, vol. 25, no. 3, p. 46, 2003.

[24] W. R. Miller and S. Rollnick, "Ten things that motivational interviewing is not," *Behavioural and Cognitive Psychotherapy*, vol. 37, no. 2, pp. 129–140, 2009.

[25] C. Bundy, "Changing behaviour: using motivational interviewing techniques," *Journal of the Royal Society of Medicine*, vol. 97, Supplement 44, p. 43, 2004.

[26] R. Jansink, J. Braspenning, T. van der Weijden, L. Niessen, G. Elwyn, and R. Grol, "Nurse-led motivational interviewing to change the lifestyle of patients with type 2 diabetes (MILD-project): protocol for a cluster, randomized, controlled trial on implementing lifestyle recommendations," *BMC Health Services Research*, vol. 9, no. 1, p. 19, 2009.

[27] World Health Organisation, *BMI classification*, 2015, http://apps.who.int/bmi/index.jsp? intro Page=intro_3.html.

[28] J. McDowell, M. Courtney, H. Edwards, and L. Shortridge-Baggett, "Validation of the Australian/English version of the diabetes management self-efficacy scale," *International Journal of Nursing Practice*, vol. 11, no. 4, pp. 177–184, 2005.

[29] A. Noroozi and R. Tahmasebi, "The diabetes management self-efficacy scale: translation and psychometric evaluation of the Iranian version," *Nursing Practice Today*, vol. 1, pp. 9–16, 2015.

[30] J. Dunbar-Jacob, L. Burke, E. A. Schlenk, and S. Sereika, "The perceived therapeutic efficacy scale," in *The 17th international nursing research congress focusing on evidence-based Practice*, 2006.

[31] World Health Organization, *Process of translation and adaptation of instruments*, 2016, http://www.who.int/substance_abuse/research_tools/translation/en/.

[32] A. Schmitt, A. Gahr, N. Hermanns, B. Kulzer, J. Huber, and T. Haak, "The Diabetes Self-Management Questionnaire (DSMQ): development and evaluation of an instrument to assess diabetes self-care activities associated with glycaemic control," *Health and Quality of Life Outcomes*, vol. 11, no. 1, p. 138, 2013.

[33] C. Hasanah, L. Naing, and A. Rahman, "World Health Organization quality of life assessment: brief version in Bahasa Malaysia," *The Medical Journal of Malaysia*, vol. 58, no. 1, pp. 79–88, 2003.

[34] A. R. Usefy, G. R. Ghassemi, N. Sarrafzadegan, S. Mallik, A. M. Baghaei, and K. Rabiei, "Psychometric properties of the WHOQOL-BREF in an Iranian adult sample," *Community Mental Health Journal*, vol. 46, no. 2, pp. 139–147, 2010.

[35] C. D. Sherbourne and A. L. Stewart, "The MOS social support survey," *Social Science & Medicine*, vol. 32, no. 6, pp. 705–714, 1991.

[36] J. Mohammadzadeh, K. Sayehmiri, and B. Mahmoudi, "Standardization of social support scale (MOS) of adults who have chronic diseases in Ilam, 2015," *Scientific Journal of Ilam University of Medical Sciences*, vol. 23, no. 7, pp. 69–77, 2016.

[37] E. M. Andresen, J. A. Malmgren, W. B. Carter, and D. L. Patrick, "Screening for depression in well older adults: evaluation of a short form of the CES-D," *American Journal of Preventive Medicine*, vol. 10, no. 2, pp. 77–84, 1994.

[38] S. K. Malakouti, N. A. Pachana, B. Naji, S. Kahani, and M. Saeedkhani, "Reliability, validity and factor structure of

the CES-D in Iranian elderly," *Asian Journal of Psychiatry*, vol. 18, pp. 86–90, 2015.

[39] D. M. Rabi, A. L. Edwards, D. A. Southern et al., "Association of socio-economic status with diabetes prevalence and utilization of diabetes care services," *BMC Health Services Research*, vol. 6, no. 1, p. 124, 2006.

[40] Diabetes in Control, *Poverty a Leading Cause of Type 2 Diabetes, Studies Say*, 2010, http://www.diabetesincontrol.com/poverty-a-leading-cause-of-type-2-diabetes-studies-say/.

[41] P. C. Tang, J. M. Overhage, A. S. Chan et al., "Online disease management of diabetes: engaging and motivating patients online with enhanced resources-diabetes (EMPOWER-D), a randomized controlled trial," *Journal of the American Medical Informatics Association*, vol. 20, no. 3, pp. 526–534, 2013.

[42] R. R. Wing, W. Lang, T. A. Wadden et al., "Benefits of modest weight loss in improving cardiovascular risk factors in overweight and obese individuals with type 2 diabetes," *Diabetes Care*, vol. 34, no. 7, pp. 1481–1486, 2011.

[43] J. Staessen, R. Fagard, P. Lijnen, and A. Amery, "Body weight, sodium intake and blood pressure," *Journal of Hypertension*, vol. 7, Supplement 1, pp. S19–S23, 1989.

[44] L. A. Savory, S. J. Griffin, K. M. Williams et al., "Changes in diet, cardiovascular risk factors and modelled cardiovascular risk following diagnosis of diabetes: 1-year results from the ADDITION-Cambridge trial cohort," *Diabetic Medicine*, vol. 31, no. 2, pp. 148–155, 2014.

[45] I. S. Ockene, D. E. Chiriboga, E. J. Stanek III et al., "Seasonal variation in serum cholesterol levels: treatment implications and possible mechanisms," *Archives of Internal Medicine*, vol. 164, no. 8, pp. 863–870, 2004.

[46] A. Bandura, "Self-efficacy mechanism in human agency," *American Psychologist*, vol. 37, no. 2, pp. 122–147, 1982.

[47] T. J. VanderWeele and M. J. Knol, "A tutorial on interaction," *Epidemiologic Methods*, vol. 3, no. 1, pp. 33–72, 2014.

[48] M. Ersoy-Kart and Ö. Güldü, "Vulnerability to stress, perceived social support, and coping styles among chronic hemodialysis patients," *Dialysis & Transplantation*, vol. 34, no. 10, pp. 662–671, 2005.

[49] L. F. Berkman, "The role of social relations in health promotion," *Psychosomatic Medicine*, vol. 57, no. 3, pp. 245–254, 1995.

[50] P. A. Bovier, E. Chamot, and T. V. Perneger, "Perceived stress, internal resources, and social support as determinants of mental health among young adults," *Quality of Life Research*, vol. 13, no. 1, pp. 161–170, 2004.

[51] K. R. Lorig, P. L. Ritter, D. D. Laurent, and K. Plant, "Internet-based chronic disease self-management: a randomized trial," *Medical Care*, vol. 44, no. 11, pp. 964–971, 2006.

[52] J. Cohen, *Statistical Power Analysis for the Behavioral Sciences Lawrence Earlbaum Associates*, Lawrence Erlbaum Associates, Publishers, Hillsdale, NJ, 1988.

15

The Constellation of Macrovascular Risk Factors in Early Onset T2DM

Mingchen Zhang,[1,2] Jiangfeng Mao,[3] Ablikm Tuerdi,[1] Xiaoyun Zeng,[1] Li Quan,[1] Shan Xiao,[1] Jun Zhu,[1] and Hua Yao[2,4]

[1]*Department of Endocrinology, First Affiliated Hospital of Xinjiang Medical University, Urumqi, China*
[2]*Postdoctoral Research Station of Public Health, School of Public Health, Xinjiang Medical University, Urumqi, China*
[3]*Department of Endocrinology, Peking Union Medical College Hospital, Key Laboratory of Endocrinology, Ministry of Health, Beijing, China*
[4]*The Key Laboratory of Xinjiang Metabolic Disease, Clinical Medical Research Institute, First Affiliated Hospital of Xinjiang Medical University, Urumqi, China*

Correspondence should be addressed to Hua Yao; yaohua01@sina.com

Academic Editor: Secundino Cigarran

Background. Despite a rapid popular of early onset type 2 diabetes (defined as diagnosis at <40 years old) recently, there is a lack of studies on this population in economically undeveloped area. We aimed to investigate the risk factors of macrovascular complications in the early onset T2DM patients in Xinjiang, China. *Methods.* A cross-sectional survey of 1736 consecutive patients with T2DM was conducted. Macrovascular complications and risk factors were documented. Another nondiabetic population matched with age and sex was as a control group. Logistic regression analysis was performed to obtain odds ratios (OR) for macrovascular complications in early and late onset T2DM, respectively. *Results.* The final analysis consisted of 1036 late onset and 219 early onset T2DM patients. The mean HbA_{1c} in the early onset group was higher than that in the late onset group ($9.1 \pm 2.4\%$ versus $8.3 \pm 2.2\%$, P=0.039) despite a higher proportion of patients in the early onset group receiving insulin treatment (73.1% versus 58.7%, $P < 0.001$). Compared to the control, early onset patients had higher blood pressure and worse lipid profiles (all $P < 0.01$). More than half of the early onset T2DM patients already had macro- and microvascular complications, despite of their young age (39.5 ± 10.8) and short DM duration (6.6 ± 8.0). In the early onset group, women had a ~3-fold hazard of atherosclerotic plaques compared with men (OR 3.22, 95% CI 1.53–6.78). *Conclusions.* Patients with early onset T2DM have worse glycemic control and higher burden of atherogenic risk factors. The prevalence of macro- and microvascular complications is astonishingly high in these young adults with T2DM. Moreover, young women with T2DM are more susceptible to cardiovascular complications than their male counterpart.

1. Introduction

Diabetes is one of the leading causes of death and disability. The number of patients with diabetes worldwide is projected to double over the next 30 years, mainly in a developing country; 85% of patients are categorized as having type 2 diabetes (T2DM), with associated mortality predominantly from cardiovascular diseases (CVDs) [1]. The phenotypic landscape of T2DM has evolved, with increasing numbers of people younger than 40 years being affected. Many Western countries have witnessed an increase in the prevalence of early onset T2DM [2, 3]. The impact of early onset T2DM is extensive. Recent evidence suggests that early onset T2DM is a more aggressive disease phenotype than the late onset cohort, and a premature development of micro- and macrovascular complications is the main concern for these young patients [4, 5]. Because early onset T2DM is a relatively new phenomenon, having only been recognized in the past few decades, the data of clinical outcomes are limited.

During the past three decades, the prevalence of diabetes in China increased from 1.3% in 1986 to 11.6% in 2010; 5.7% of these people were younger than 40 years at diagnosis in 2010 [6, 7]. Xinjiang Province is located in the northwest of China and composed of more than 13 ethnic groups. The prevalence of T2DM in Xinjiang Province has increased considerably over recent decades to an estimated 8.2% in urban areas and 6.1% in rural areas (approximately 2 million DM patients) [8]. There are few studies on the prevalence and risk factors of diabetes-related complications in early onset T2DM Han nationality population residing in economically developed areas of China [6, 9]. However, no study focused on early onset diabetes in economically underdeveloped and multiethnic areas such as Xinjiang. To address this gap in knowledge, we conducted a cross-sectional study which aimed to estimate the phenomenon of early onset T2DM patients residing in Xinjiang, China.

2. Materials and Methods

2.1. Study Population. This cross-sectional and noninterventional study was conducted from May 2014 to September 2015. A total of 1736 consecutive T2DM patients, who underwent diabetic complication evaluation in the outpatient clinic, the First Affiliated Hospital of Xinjiang Medical University, were screened. 349 individuals were excluded for incomplete diabetic complication tests, 87 individuals for incomplete laboratory tests, and 45 individuals for incomplete physical exam. The final analysis consisted of 1255 patients who had met the inclusion and exclusion criteria. The inclusion criteria included all the following points: (1) T2DM diagnosed based on the 1999 World Health Organization's definition [10]; (2) age 18 years or older; (3) and fulfilled comprehensive physical examination, laboratory tests, and complication evaluation tests. Exclusion criteria were as follows: (1) patients with type 1 diabetes mellitus, other specific types of diabetes mellitus, and unclear types of diabetes; (2) pregnancy or breast feeding; (3) being unable to complete the survey owing to mental illness or other reasons; (4) recent history of acute illness; and (5) drug or alcohol abuse. The patient's gender, age, weight, height, smoking status, date of diabetes diagnosis, and family history of DM were recorded. Past medical history and medications for T2DM were documented. Evaluations comprised detailed medical history, physical examination, laboratory measurements, and diabetic complication studies. The control group, including 478 subjects after matching for age and gender with early onset DM, is derived from another epidemiological study, which is aiming to investigate the prevalence of metabolic syndrome in Urumqi community, Xinjiang Province. Each of them had normal plasma glucose level after OGTT.

2.2. Anthropometric and Laboratory Measurements. Height and weight were measured to the nearest 0.1 cm and 0.1 kg, respectively. Body mass index (BMI) was defined as weight (kg) divided by height (m) squared. Blood pressure was measured after the subject had rested for at least 10 min in a sitting position. Blood samples were collected in the morning at fasting state. Laboratory data on fasting glucose, HbA_{1c}, lipid profiles, and diabetic complication evaluation were recorded. Biochemical parameters such as plasma glucose and lipids (triglycerides, total cholesterol, HDL cholesterol, and LDL cholesterol) were measured by an autoanalyzer (ADVIA1650; Siemens, NY, USA) with commercially available kits. HbA_{1c} was measured by high-performance liquid chromatography using the VARIANT II Hemoglobin Testing System (Bio-Rad Laboratories). Urinary albumin was analyzed with an enzyme-linked immunosorbent assay.

2.3. Definition. In consistent with the previous studies, early onset T2DM in this study was defined as T2DM diagnosed younger than 40 years [3, 6, 9]. Type 1 diabetes mellitus was defined as patients with a history of ketoacidosis or GAD antibody positive when they were diagnosed with diabetes mellitus, with a large amount of ketonuria, and required persistent insulin therapy within the 1st year after the diagnosis. Hypertension was defined as systolic blood pressure (SBP) $\geq$ 140 mmHg or diastolic blood pressure (DBP) $\geq$ 90 mmHg or treatment with antihypertensive medications. Microalbuminuria was defined as urinary albumin $\geq$ 30 mg/24 h after excluding other causes of kidney damage, urinary tract infection, and hematuria [11]. The diagnosis of diabetic retinopathy was made by ophthalmologist(s) based on typical funduscopic findings of diabetes, including background, preproliferative, proliferative, and maculopathy. The diagnosis of diabetic neuropathy was made based on electromyography (EMG). EMG was considered to be positive when it demonstrated distal symmetric polyneuropathy and other causes of neuropathy were excluded. Carotid atherosclerosis was determined by B-mode ultrasound (ATL HDI 3000-CV; Phillips Medical Systems). This procedure was performed by an experienced ultrasonographer while the patient was supine with the neck extended in a slightly lateral rotation. Average carotid intima media thickness was calculated, and a *B*-score was formed as follows: 0 = no alteration, 1 = wall thickness < 1 mm, 2 = plaque 1 to 2 mm, 3 = plaque 2 to 3 mm, 4 = plaque > 3 mm, and 5 = total occlusion of the lumen. A single *B*-score > 2 on any measurement was defined as carotid atherosclerotic plaque. All the evaluators were blinded to the other test results.

2.4. Statistical Analysis. We conducted all statistical analyses using the IBM SPSS version 21.0 (IBM Corp., Armonk, NY). Data were given as means ± SD for continuous variables or percentages (%) for categorical variables. The distribution of continuous variables was checked by a normality test. If normal distributions were not rejected, continuous variables were compared by Student's *t*-test. Otherwise, the comparison was done by Kruskal-Wallis test. Categorical variables were compared using chi-square test. Logistic regression analysis was used to obtain odds ratios (OR) and their 95% confidence intervals (CI) for macrovascular complications in the early and late onset T2DM groups, respectively. All the statistical tests are two-sided, and a P value < 0.05 was considered statistically significant.

2.5. Ethical Consideration. The study was designed to comply with the Declaration of Helsinki. Written informed consent was obtained from all participants, and the study was approved by the ethics committee of the First Affiliated Hospital of Xinjiang Medical University, China.

3. Results

3.1. Population Characteristics. Among the 1736 enrolled patients, 481 with key variables missing were excluded, and the remaining 1255 (219 early onset and 1036 late onset) were used in the analysis. These patients had a mean age of 55.5 years (SD 10.2), with 7.7 years (SD 6.7) history of diabetes. Their mean HbA_{1c}, fasting plasma glucose, and 2-h postprandial glucose were 8.5% (SD 2.3), 9.9 mmol/L (SD 4.5), and 14.4 mmol/L (SD 5.4), respectively.

Clinical and biochemical data on patients with early and late onset diabetes are summarized in Table 1. A total of 219 (17.5%) were diagnosed with diabetes before 40 years of age, and the mean age of diagnosis was 34.3 years (SD 7.6).

The mean HbA_{1c} of adults with early onset was higher than that with late onset ($9.1 \pm 2.4\%$ versus $8.3 \pm 2.2\%$, $P = 0.039$), despite a higher proportion of patients in the early onset group receiving insulin treatment (73.1% versus 58.7%, $P < 0.001$). Compared to the late onset group, patients in the early onset group were more likely to be younger, to have a higher prevalence of diabetic family history, to be a smoker, to have a shorter duration of T2DM, and to have a lower BMI. Although patients in the early onset group were markedly younger than patients in the late onset group, the prevalence of hypertension and dyslipidemia was similar between the two groups, reflecting metabolic abnormalities occurred earlier in this group.

Since many metabolic parameters are highly correlated with age and gender, a total of 478 subjects with normal plasma glucose levels were selected as the control group after matching for age and gender with the early onset group. Compared to the control subjects, patients with early onset T2DM had a much higher incidence of hypertension (56.2% versus 33.9%, $P < 0.001$). Systolic and diastolic blood pressure, triglyceride concentrations, total cholesterol, and LDL cholesterol levels in the early onset group were increased, while HDL cholesterol level was decreased compared with the control group (Table 1).

3.2. The Prevalence of Diabetic Complications. Early onset diabetes may be associated with the development of complications at an early stage of life; therefore, we compared the prevalence of diabetic complications between the early and late onset groups. Patients in the late onset group had a much higher incidence of atherosclerotic plaques, diabetic retinopathy (DR), diabetic neuropathy, and microalbuminuria compared with the early onset group (late onset versus early onset: 80.3% versus 50.7% for atherosclerotic plaques; 61.3% versus 52.5% for DR; 82.0% versus 53.4% for diabetic neuropathy; 65.0% versus 53.0% for microalbuminuria; all $P < 0.01$) (Figure 1). (The detailed information about macrovascular complications is shown in Supplementary Table 1.)

3.3. The Management of Traditional Cardiovascular Risk Factors. Both groups had poor management on traditional cardiovascular risk factors (Figure 2): in either group, less than half achieved blood pressure targets and less than 10% achieved lipid targets. In the early onset T2DM group, smaller portion of patients achieved the target of glucose control (14.2% versus 23.1% for $HbA_{1c} < 7\%$; 19.6% versus 29.2% for 2-h postprandial glucose < 11.1 mmol/L; all $P < 0.01$). They were more likely to be smokers (45.2% versus 36.8%, $P < 0.05$). (The detailed information about antihypertensive and statin therapies is shown in Supplementary Table 2.)

3.4. The Independent Risk Factors on Atherosclerotic Plaques. Multiple logistic regression analysis was done to assess the independent risk factors on atherosclerotic plaques in early and late onset T2DM, respectively. The variables in the multivariate model included age, gender, age of diabetes diagnosis, duration of diabetes, BMI, systolic and diastolic blood pressure, hypertension, smoking, fasting glucose, 2-h postprandial glucose, HbA_{1c}, total cholesterol, LDL cholesterol, HDL cholesterol, and triglyceride. In the early onset group, females had a ~3-fold hazard of atherosclerotic plaques compared with male adults (OR 3.22, 95% CI 1.53–6.78). Other risk factors included age (OR 1.05, 95% CI 1.02–1.08), SBP (OR 1.04, 95% CI 1.02–1.07), and 2-h postprandial glucose (OR 1.01, 95% CI 1.00–1.03). The results are presented in Table 2. By contrast, in the late onset group, females had a much lower risk of atherosclerotic plaques relative to male adults (OR 0.25, 95% CI 0.17–0.37). Other risk factors associated with atherosclerotic plaques in the late onset group included age (OR 1.05, 95% CI 1.03–1.07), DBP (OR 1.01, 95% CI 1.00–1.03), 2-h postprandial glucose (OR 1.04, 95% CI 1.01–1.07), and LDL cholesterol (OR 1.18, 95% CI 1.01–1.38). The results are presented in Table 3.

4. Discussion

There is a marked increase in the prevalence of diabetes in China with more and more young people affected by the disease [12]. Our study found that (1) early onset T2DM accounted for 17.5% of the diabetes outpatient population in our tertiary care center in Xinjiang, China. Poorer glycemic control (compared to the late onset group) and higher burden of atherogenic risk factors (compared to the control group) were documented in the early onset cohort; (2) the incidence of micro- and macrovascular complications was astonishingly high (up to ~50%) in these young adults with T2DM; (3) risk factors for macrovascular complications were different in the early and late onset groups, and women were more susceptible to cardiovascular complications in the early onset group.

Although T2DM is traditionally considered as a disease mainly affecting the elderly, the age at diagnosis has gradually reduced in recent years. A rapid increase in the incidence of early onset T2DM has become a new trend all over the world. From 1990 to 2000, the number of patients with early onset T2DM increased 9 times in New York [13]. Recent large survey in China showed that 5.7% and 44% of adults aged below 40 years have diabetes or prediabetes, respectively [14]. Consistent with the previous studies, our data found early onset

TABLE 1: Clinical and biochemical characteristics of patients with early versus late onset of T2DM and control subjects matched for age and sex.

Variable	Early onset $n = 219$	Late onset $n = 1036$	P value	Control subjects $n = 478$	P value[#]
Age (years)	39.5 ± 10.8	60.2 ± 8.3	<0.001	39.4 ± 7.1	0.103
Female gender	78 (35.6)	476 (45.)	0.005	182 (38.1)	0.556
Age of diabetes diagnosis (years)	34.3 ± 7.6	51.4 ± 7.2	<0.001	—	—
Duration of diabetes (years)	6.6 ± 8.0	8.8 ± 6.1	<0.001	—	—
Diabetic family history	138 (63.0)	499 (39.8)	<0.001	102 (21.3)	<0.001
BMI (kg/m^2)	25.2 ± 4.9	26.1 ± 3.6	0.002	24.2 ± 2.8	0.009
Current cigarette smoking*	99 (45.2)	381 (36.8)	0.012	213 (47.2)	0.680
Hypertension	112 (51.1)	582 (56.2)	0.330	153 (33.9)	<0.001
SBP (mmHg)	141.9 ± 25.1	137.4 ± 22.8	0.015	120.6 ± 18.0	<0.001
DBP (mmHg)	79.8 ± 14.7	77.1 ± 14.5	0.023	72.3 ± 12.7	<0.001
Fasting blood glucose (mmol/L)	10.3 ± 4.4	9.9 ± 4.6	0.680	4.9 ± 0.5	<0.001
2-h postprandial glucose (mmol/L)	15.7 ± 5.4	14.1 ± 5.2	0.535	5.7 ± 1.3	<0.001
HbA$_{1c}$,% (mmol/mol)	9.1 ± 2.4 (76 ± 26)	8.3 ± 2.2 (67 ± 23)	0.039	5.2 ± 1.1 (33 ± 11)	<0.001
Required insulin therapy	160 (73.1)	608 (58.7)	<0.001	—	—
Triglyceride (mmol/L)	2.4 ± 1.6	2.2 ± 1.4	0.405	1.6 ± 0.9	<0.001
Total cholesterol (mmol/L)	4.1 ± 1.3	4.6 ± 1.5	0.952	3.7 ± 1.2	<0.001
HDL cholesterol (mmol/L)	1.1 ± 0.4	1.2 ± 0.4	0.397	1.2 ± 0.2	<0.001
LDL cholesterol (mmol/L)	2.6 ± 1.1	2.5 ± 1.0	0.500	2.1 ± 0.6	<0.001

Data are means ± SD or n (%). P values were derived from chi-square test or Student's t-test. BMI: body mass index; SBP/DBP: systolic/diastolic blood pressure; HbA$_{1c}$: hemoglobin A1c; HDL cholesterol: high-density lipoprotein cholesterol; LDL cholesterol: low-density lipoprotein cholesterol. *Current cigarette smoking, 1 or more cigarettes per day. #P value, early onset DM versus control subjects matched with age and sex.

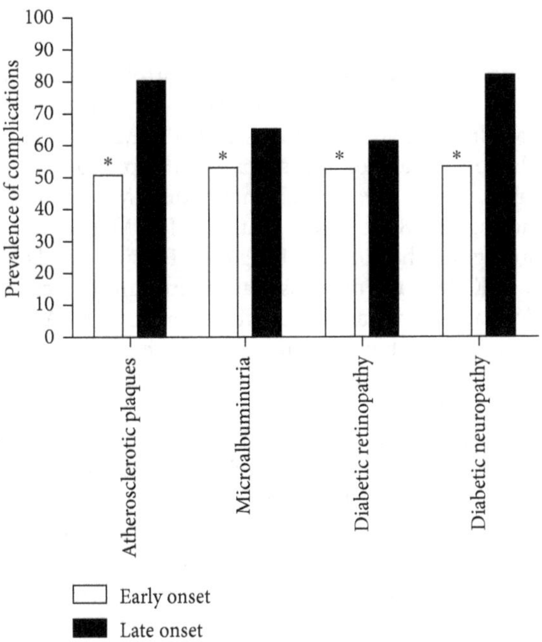

FIGURE 1: The prevalence of diabetic complications in early versus late onset T2DM. *All P values for chi-square test < 0.01.

T2DM accounted for 17.5% of the diabetes outpatient population in Xinjiang, China. These data suggest that adults with early onset T2DM represent a substantial proportion of patients consuming medical resource even in economically underdeveloped areas of China. Of note, patients with early onset T2DM, despite of younger ages and shorter durations of diabetes, had poorer plasma glucose control than those patients with late onset [8, 15, 16]. Thus, prevention of diabetes, especially among individuals aged below 40 years, should be regarded as a public health emergency in such area.

Diabetic nephropathy (DN) and diabetic retinopathy (DR) are major microvascular complications of T2DM [17]. Previous reports showed that microalbuminuria was present in ~25% of T2DM patients when diagnosis was made. The incidence would increase to 28–42% and 60% at 5 and 10 years after the diagnosis was made [18]. Beyond our expectation, the incidence of microalbuminuria was 53.0% in our early onset patients, despite of their short disease duration and young age. The reported rates of DR in early onset T2DM population were 4–40%, varied considerably depending on the different study methods [18–20]. The incidence of DR in our early onset population was 53.4%, higher than previous reported [18–20]. In a UK study, 40% patients aged 13–35 years had evidence of neuropathy, and among them, 20% had evidence of skin ulceration [21]. In consistent, our study found that 53.4% of early onset T2DM patients had neuropathy. Our findings revealed that microvascular complications may occur early in the natural history of T2DM in young adults. Therefore, screening for microvascular complications is indispensable and should be initiated when young adult is diagnosed. Since it is conclusively established that the microvascular complications are directly related to

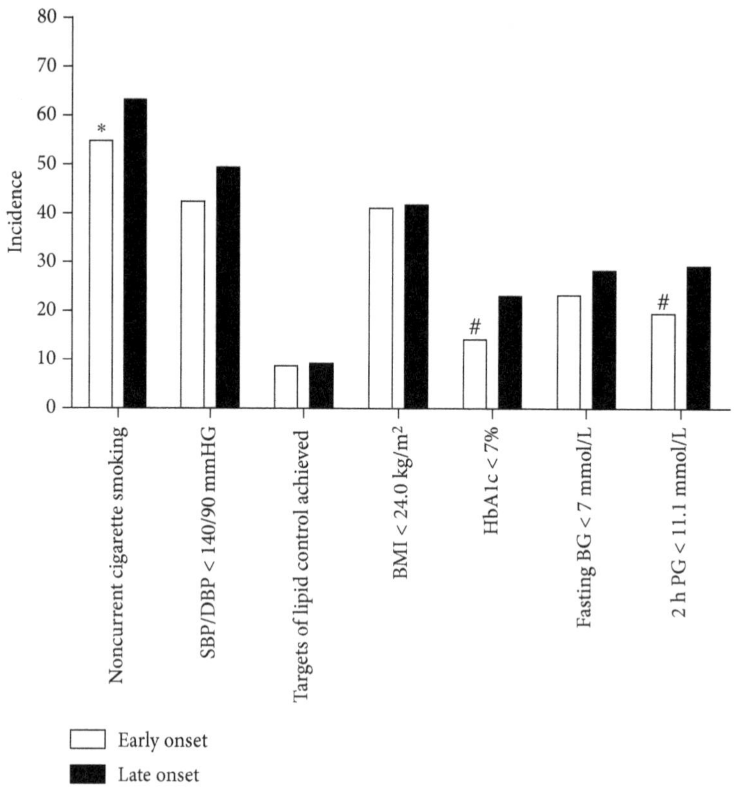

Figure 2: Control of traditional cardiovascular risk factors in patients with early and late onset T2DM. *y*-axis: incidence of achieved control targets of traditional cardiovascular risk factors. Targets of lipid control were defined as LDL cholesterol less than 2.6 mmol/L, HDL cholesterol greater than 1.0 mmol/L in men and 1.3 mmol/L in women, and triglyceride less than 1.7 mmol/L whether patients were on lipid-lowering drugs or not. BG, blood glucose; PG, postprandial glucose. $^{*}P < 0.05$, $^{\#}P < 0.01$; all P values for chi-square test.

Table 2: Multivariate logistic regression analysis in patients with early onset T2DM ($n = 219$) in order to obtain odds ratios (OR) for macrovascular complications.

Variables	OR	95% CI	*P* value
Sex (male = 1)	3.22	1.53–6.78	0.002
Age (years)	1.05	1.02–1.08	0.001
SBP (mmHg)	1.04	1.02–1.07	0.036
2-h postprandial glucose (mmol/L)	1.01	1.00–1.03	<0.001

CI: confidence interval; SBP: systolic blood pressure.

Table 3: Multivariate logistic regression analysis in patients with late onset T2DM ($n = 1039$) in order to obtain odds ratios (OR) for macrovascular complications.

Variables	OR	95% CI	*P* value
Sex (male = 1)	0.25	0.17–0.37	<0.001
Age (years)	1.05	1.03–1.07	<0.001
DBP (mmHg)	1.01	1.00–1.03	0.043
2-h postprandial glucose (mmol/L)	1.04	1.01–1.07	0.002
LDL-CHO (mmol/L)	1.18	1.01–1.38	0.035

CI: confidence interval; DBP: diastolic blood pressure; LDL-CHO: low density lipoprotein cholesterol.

glycemic [22] and blood pressure control [23, 24], more intensive control on hyperglycemia and hypertension is required in these young patients with T2DM.

Macrovascular complications are the primary cause of mortality, with myocardial infarction (MI) and stroke accounting for 80% of all death in T2DM patients [25]. According to the United Kingdom Prospective Diabetes Study (UKPDS), the main risk factors for cardiovascular disease in diabetes are raised LDL cholesterol and HbA_{1c}, lower HDL cholesterol, higher systolic blood pressure, and current smoking [26]. Our data documented that early onset T2DM patients had a more adverse cardiovascular risk profile compared with age- and sex-matched controls. Hillier and Pedula demonstrated that the hazard of MI in early onset T2DM patients was 14-fold higher than in control subjects (HR 14.0, 95% CI 6.2–31.4) [4]. These data suggested that young patients with T2DM may lose the protection of youth. Previous studies demonstrated that early onset cohorts have similar or more adverse risk factors for cardiovascular diseases compared to late onset population [27]. Consistently, we observed that a high proportion had hypertension (51.1%), morbid obesity (58.9%), and dyslipidemia (91.3%) in early onset T2DM cohort. Furthermore, 53.0% early onset T2DM subjects developed microalbuminuria, a known risk factor for CVD. Although the macrovascular outcomes in our early onset population have not been obtained, the constellation of risk factors commonly encountered in this group suggests an extremely high tendency for cardiovascular disease. In consistent with previous studies, our data demonstrated that 50.7% early onset T2DM patients had developed atherosclerotic plaques in carotid artery at the mean age of 39.5 years. The evidence for increased cardiovascular morbidity in younger patients was confirmed by a large prospective cohort study of 4857 American Indian children who were followed up for 24 years [28]. In this study, obesity, glucose intolerance, and hypertension increased the risk of premature death by 130%, 73%, and 57%, respectively.

What makes things worse is that the patients with early onset T2DM had poor control of cardiovascular risk factors [8, 15]. Similar findings were observed in our study: 57.6% and 91.3% of patients with early onset T2DM did not achieve the recommended targets for blood pressure and lipids, respectively. Meanwhile, 45.2% of them were current smokers. Recent studies demonstrated that early onset T2DM subjects had poor compliance to cardioprotective medications [29]. Only 31% and 37% of this population insisted on statins and antihypertensive medications, respectively [30]. Consistently, our findings showed that only 6.3%, 8.0%, and 66.4% patients of the early onset DM group insisted on statins, aspirin, and antihypertensive medications, respectively (Supplementary Table 2). Therefore, increasing the awareness of controlling the risk factors and improving the compliance to medications on hypertension and dyslipidemia are crucial to modify these risk factors.

Our data demonstrated that young females with T2DM had a ~3-fold hazard of atherosclerotic plaques compared with male counterparts, in agreement with studies in non-Chinese populations [4]. A previous study showed that young women with T2DM had an increasing risk of developing MI than men (10.8-fold versus 3.9-fold) [4]. Diabetes may increase the detrimental effects of the other risk factors and alleviate the protective effect of estrogens. However, there is no evidence to date that normalization of glucose level in young women with T2DM may reduce the risk of CVD. For this reason, guidelines for such patients are aimed at keeping the other risk factors under strict control in order to significantly reduce their detrimental effects on CVD. However, studies demonstrated that women with early onset T2DM were less likely to be treated. Only 11.1% and 22.2% of female subjects received statins and antihypertensive medications, respectively, compared with 38.7% and 35.5% of male subjects with a similar age [31]. This gender disparity in cardioprotective treatment is of concern since it may compound the burden of excess risk for cardiovascular disease in women with diabetes. The elevated cardiovascular risk in women with early onset T2DM should be kept in the mind of health care professionals. And cardiovascular risk factors should be actively identified and tightly controlled in this population.

4.1. Limitations. Our study has several limitations. First, the study patients were not representative of the general patients with T2DM in Xinjiang, China. Patients with severe diabetes were more likely to seek care in tertiary medical center; therefore, the reported prevalence of diabetic complications in this study would be higher than in the general population with T2DM. Second, we fully recognize that distinguishing type 1 from type 2 diabetes is increasingly more challenging for clinicians since the incidence of T2DM is dramatically rising in young adults. Some of these young patients with T2DM present with diabetic ketoacidosis. As the body weight of the general increases, many people with type 1 diabetes are also obese. In order to reduce misclassification bias, we excluded 132 cases (7.6% of entire cases). By excluding these more severe cases, we may underestimate the full impact of T2DM in young adults. Third, though, we found early and late onset T2DM patients had different risk factors for macrovascular disease, but the sample number was limited, especially for early onset T2DM. As a cross-sectional designed study, it does not lead to any causative conclusions and more large prospective designed investigations are needed.

5. Conclusions

In summary, our data delineate that early onset T2DM patients in Xinjiang, China, had a poor glycemic control and a high burden of atherogenic risk factors. The prevalence of micro- and macrovascular complications was astonishingly high in this population. Moreover, young women with T2DM were more susceptible to cardiovascular complications. This population requires more aggressive management on all cardiovascular risk factors.

Abbreviations

T2DM: Type 2 diabetes mellitus
CVD: Cardiovascular disease
PG: Plasma glucose
2-h PG: 2-hour postprandial glucose
HbA_{1c}: Hemoglobin A1c
BP: Blood pressure
MI: Myocardial infarction.

Conflicts of Interest

The authors declare that they have no competing interests.

Authors' Contributions

Hua Yao, Mingchen Zhang, and Jiangfeng Mao conceptualized this study. Mingchen Zhang and Jiangfeng Mao are assigned in the data curation. Mingchen Zhang and Jiangfeng Mao worked on the formal analysis. Mingchen Zhang acquired the funding of the study. Mingchen Zhang, Ablikm Tuerdi, Xiaoyun Zeng, Li Quan, Jun Zhu, and Shan Xiao are assigned in the investigation of the study. Mingchen Zhang worked on the methodology. Hua Yao and Jun Zhu administered the project. Hua Yao supervised the study. Mingchen Zhang and Jiangfeng Mao validated the data. Hua Yao and Mingchen Zhang visualized the study. Mingchen Zhang wrote the original draft. Mingchen Zhang and Jiangfeng Mao wrote the reviewed and edited version of the draft.

Acknowledgments

The study was supported by grants from the Natural Science Foundation of China (no. 81760161) to Mingchen Zhang.

The authors are grateful to Dr. Nai-Wen Chi in the Department of Medicine, University of California, San Diego, for his valuable comments. And the authors would also like to thank all the health professionals who participated in this cross-sectional survey for their efforts.

References

[1] L. S. Geiss, J. Wang, Y. J. Cheng et al., "Prevalence and incidence trends for diagnosed diabetes among adults aged 20 to 79 years, United States, 1980-2012," *JAMA*, vol. 312, no. 12, pp. 1218–1226, 2014.

[2] R. G. Feltbower, P. A. McKinney, F. M. Campbell, C. R. Stephenson, and H. J. Bodansky, "Type 2 and other forms of diabetes in 0-30 year olds: a hospital based study in Leeds, UK," *Archives of Disease in Childhood*, vol. 88, no. 8, pp. 676–679, 2003.

[3] S. H. Song and C. A. Hardisty, "Early onset type 2 diabetes mellitus: a harbinger for complications in later years–clinical observation from a secondary care cohort," *QJM*, vol. 102, no. 11, pp. 799–806, 2009.

[4] T. A. Hillier and K. L. Pedula, "Complications in young adults with early-onset type 2 diabetes: losing the relative protection of youth," *Diabetes Care*, vol. 26, no. 11, pp. 2999–3005, 2003.

[5] M. E. Pavkov, P. H. Bennett, W. C. Knowler, J. Krakoff, M. L. Sievers, and R. G. Nelson, "Effect of youth-onset type 2 diabetes mellitus on incidence of end-stage renal disease and mortality in young and middle-aged Pima Indians," *JAMA*, vol. 296, no. 4, pp. 421–426, 2006.

[6] A. O. Y. Luk, E. S. H. Lau, W. Y. So et al., "Prospective study on the incidences of cardiovascular-renal complications in Chinese patients with young-onset type 1 and type 2 diabetes," *Diabetes Care*, vol. 37, no. 1, pp. 149–157, 2013.

[7] X. R. Pan, G. W. Li, Y. H. Hu et al., "Effects of diet and exercise in preventing NIDDM in people with impaired glucose tolerance. The Da Qing IGT and Diabetes Study," *Diabetes Care*, vol. 20, no. 4, pp. 537–544, 1997.

[8] H. Gong, L. Pa, K. Wang et al., "Prevalence of diabetes and associated factors in the Uyghur and Han population in Xinjiang, China," *International Journal of Environmental Research and Public Health*, vol. 12, no. 10, pp. 12792–12802, 2015.

[9] X. Huo, L. Gao, L. Guo et al., "Risk of non-fatal cardiovascular diseases in early-onset versus late-onset type 2 diabetes in China: a cross-sectional study," *The Lancet Diabetes and Endocrinology*, vol. 4, no. 2, pp. 115–124, 2016.

[10] K. G. M. M. Alberti and P. Z. Zimmet, "Definition, diagnosis and classification of diabetes mellitus and its complications. Part 1: diagnosis and classification of diabetes mellitus provisional report of a WHO consultation," *Diabetic Medicine*, vol. 15, no. 7, pp. 539–553, 1998.

[11] R. J. Hogg, S. Furth, K. V. Lemley et al., "National Kidney Foundation's kidney disease outcomes quality initiative clinical practice guidelines for chronic kidney disease in children and adolescents: evaluation, classification, and stratification," *Pediatrics*, vol. 111, no. 6, pp. 1416–1421, 2003.

[12] M. Z. Li, L. Su, B. Y. Liang et al., "Trends in prevalence, awareness, treatment, and control of diabetes mellitus in mainland China from 1979 to 2012," *International Journal of Endocrinology*, vol. 2013, Article ID 753150, 14 pages, 2013.

[13] G. Grinstein, R. Muzumdar, L. Aponte, P. Vuguin, P. Saenger, and J. DiMartino-Nardi, "Presentation and 5-year follow-up of type 2 diabetes mellitus in African-American and Caribbean-Hispanic adolescents," *Hormone Research in Paediatrics*, vol. 60, no. 3, pp. 121–126, 2003.

[14] Y. Xu, L. Wang, J. He et al., "Prevalence and control of diabetes in Chinese adults," *JAMA*, vol. 310, no. 9, pp. 948–959, 2013.

[15] L. Li, L. Ji, X. Guo et al., "Prevalence of microvascular diseases among tertiary care Chinese with early versus late onset of type 2 diabetes," *Journal of Diabetes and its Complications*, vol. 29, no. 1, pp. 32–37, 2015.

[16] H. Yu, L. F. Xie, K. Chen et al., "Initiating characteristics of early-onset type 2 diabetes mellitus in Chinese patients," *Chinese Medical Journal*, vol. 129, no. 7, pp. 778–784, 2016.

[17] S. van Dieren, J. W. J. Beulens, Y. T. van der Schouw, D. E. Grobbee, and B. Neal, "The global burden of diabetes and its complications: an emerging pandemic," *European Journal of Preventive Cardiology*, vol. 17, Supplement 1, pp. S3–S8, 2010.

[18] M. C. Eppens, M. E. Craig, J. Cusumano et al., "Prevalence of diabetes complications in adolescents with type 2 compared with type 1 diabetes," *Diabetes Care*, vol. 29, no. 6, pp. 1300–1306, 2006.

[19] TODAY Study Group, "Rapid rise in hypertension and nephropathy in youth with type 2 diabetes: the TODAY clinical trial," *Diabetes Care*, vol. 36, no. 6, pp. 1735–1741, 2013.

[20] M. E. Pavkov, W. C. Knowler, P. H. Bennett, H. C. Looker, J. Krakoff, and R. G. Nelson, "Increasing incidence of proteinuria and declining incidence of end-stage renal disease in diabetic Pima Indians," *Kidney International*, vol. 70, no. 10, pp. 1840–1846, 2006.

[21] R. B. Paisey, R. M. Paisey, M. P. Thomson et al., "Protection from clinical peripheral sensory neuropathy in Alström syndrome in contrast to early-onset type 2 diabetes," *Diabetes Care*, vol. 32, no. 3, pp. 462–464, 2009.

[22] I. M. Stratton, A. I. Adler, H. A. Neil et al., "Association of glycaemia with macrovascular and microvascular complications of type 2 diabetes (UKPDS 35): prospective observational study," *BMJ*, vol. 321, no. 7258, pp. 405–412, 2000.

[23] UK Prospective Diabetes study group, "Tight blood pressure control and risk of macrovascular and microvascular complications in type 2 diabetes: UKPDS 38," *BMJ*, vol. 317, no. 7160, pp. 703–713, 1998.

[24] ADVANCE Collaborative Group, A. Patel, S. MacMahon et al., "Intensive blood glucose control and vascular outcomes in patients with type 2 diabetes," *The New England Journal of Medicine*, vol. 358, no. 24, pp. 2560–2572, 2008.

[25] N. J. Morrish, S. L. Wang, L. K. Stevens, J. H. Fuller, H. Keen, and WHO Multinational Study Group, "Mortality and causes of death in the WHO Multinational Study of Vascular Disease in Diabetes," *Diabetologia*, vol. 44, Supplement 2, pp. S14–S21, 2001.

[26] R. C. Turner, H. Millns, and R. R. Holman, "Coronary heart disease and risk factors in NIDDM–experience from the United Kingdom Prospective Diabetes Study," *Diabetologia*, vol. 40, Supplement 2, pp. S121–S122, 1997.

[27] B. L. Rodriguez, W. Y. Fujimoto, E. J. Mayer-Davis et al., "Prevalence of cardiovascular disease risk factors in U.S. children and adolescents with diabetes: the SEARCH for diabetes in youth study," *Diabetes Care*, vol. 29, no. 8, pp. 1891–1896, 2006.

[28] P. W. Franks, R. L. Hanson, W. C. Knowler, M. L. Sievers, P. H. Bennett, and H. C. Looker, "Childhood obesity, other cardiovascular risk factors, and premature death," *The New England Journal of Medicine*, vol. 362, no. 6, pp. 485–493, 2010.

[29] M. Hatunic, N. Burns, F. Finucane, C. Mannion, and J. J. Nolan, "Contrasting clinical and cardiovascular risk status between early and later onset type 2 diabetes," *Diabetes and Vascular Disease Research*, vol. 2, no. 2, pp. 73–75, 2016.

[30] R. O. Yeung, Y. Zhang, A. Luk et al., "Metabolic profiles and treatment gaps in young-onset type 2 diabetes in Asia (the JADE programme): a cross-sectional study of a prospective cohort," *The Lancet Diabetes & Endocrinology*, vol. 2, no. 12, pp. 935–943, 2014.

[31] E. G. Wilmot, M. J. Davies, T. Yates, K. Benhalima, I. G. Lawrence, and K. Khunti, "Type 2 diabetes in younger adults: the emerging UK epidemic," *Postgraduate Medical Journal*, vol. 86, no. 1022, pp. 711–718, 2010.

16

Relationship of Hyperglycaemia, Hypoglycaemia, and Glucose Variability to Atherosclerotic Disease in Type 2 Diabetes

Caroline Jane Magri,[1,2] Dillon Mintoff,[3] Liberato Camilleri,[4] Robert G. Xuereb,[2] Joseph Galea,[5] and Stephen Fava[5]

[1]Department of Cardiology, Mater Dei Hospital and University of Malta, Msida, Malta
[2]Department of Cardiology, Mater Dei Hospital, Msida, Malta
[3]Mater Dei Hospital, Msida, Malta
[4]Statistics & Operations Research, Faculty of Science, University of Malta, Msida, Malta
[5]Mater Dei Hospital and University of Malta, Msida, Malta

Correspondence should be addressed to Stephen Fava; stephen.fava@um.edu.mt

Academic Editor: Andrea Flex

Objective. Type 2 diabetes mellitus (T2DM) is known to be associated with increased cardiovascular risk. The aim of this study was therefore to investigate the independent effects of hyperglycaemia, hypoglycaemia, and glucose variability on microvascular and macrovascular disease in T2DM. *Methods.* Subjects with T2DM of <10 years duration and on stable antiglycaemic treatment underwent carotid intima-media thickness (CIMT), ankle-brachial index (ABI), albumin-creatinine ratio (ACR), and HbA_{1c} measurement, as well as 72-hour continuous glucose monitoring. Macrovascular disease was defined as one or more of the following: history of ischaemic heart disease (IHD), cerebrovascular accident (CVA), ABI < 0.9, or abnormal CIMT. *Results.* The study population comprised 121 subjects with T2DM (89 males : 32 females). The mean age was 62.6 years, and the mean DM duration was 3.7 years. Macrovascular disease was present in 71 patients (58.7%). In multivariate logistic regression analysis, body surface area (BSA) (OR 18.88 (95% CI 2.20–156.69), $p = 0.006$) and duration of blood glucose (BG) < 3.9 mmol/L (OR 1.12 (95% CI 1.014–1.228), $p = 0.024$) were independent predictors of macrovascular disease. BSA (OR 12.6 (95% CI 1.70–93.54), $p = 0.013$) and duration of BG < 3.9 mmol/L (OR 1.09 (95% CI 1.003–1.187), $p = 0.041$) were independent predictors of abnormal CIMT. Area under the curve for BG > 7.8 mmol/L ($\beta = 15.83$, $p = 0.005$) was the sole independent predictor of albuminuria in generalised linear regression. *Conclusions.* This study demonstrates that hypoglycaemia is associated with the occurrence of atherosclerotic disease while hyperglycaemia is associated with microvascular disease in a Caucasian population with T2DM of recent duration.

1. Introduction

Diabetes is known to be associated with both microvascular and macrovascular disease [1]. Whilst good glycaemic control has been consistently shown to reduce microvascular disease, most intervention studies have failed to document a reduction in macrovascular disease outcomes [2, 3].

One possible explanation for this discrepancy is the detrimental effect of hypoglycaemia. Östgren and colleagues have recently reported a U-shaped relationship of HbA_{1c} with cardiovascular events, including mortality [4]. A recent meta-analysis has also confirmed that hypoglycaemia is associated with a twofold increased risk of cardiovascular disease in type 2 diabetes [5]. Furthermore, both hyperglycaemia and hypoglycaemia following acute coronary syndrome have been associated with increased mortality [6, 7] The traditional explanations of these observations are the proarrhythmogenic effect of hypoglycaemia as a consequence of catecholamine release and QTc prolongation [8, 9] and the unavailability of an energy substrate to the myocardium during hypoglycaemia leading to an ischaemia equivalent [10]. However, the increased mortality extends beyond the hypoglycaemic episode itself. Although a hypoglycaemic episode is known to predict future ones [11], this is unlikely to be the sole mechanism. Another possible contributory mechanism that has not been well investigated is the possibility that hypoglycaemia may accelerate atherosclerosis, as suggested by some animal studies. For example, Yasunari and colleagues reported that repeated hypoglycaemia worsens injury-provoked intimal thickening in a male Goto-Kakizaki rat carotid artery [12], whilst Jin and colleagues reported that hypoglycaemia induced monocyte adhesion to rat aortic endothelium [13]. Furthermore, a small study found higher carotid and femoral intima-media thickness in 25 subjects with type 1 diabetes and with repeated hypoglycaemic episodes when compared to 20 subjects with type 1 diabetes but without hypoglycaemia [14]. However, continuous glucose monitoring was not performed, and therefore, hyperglycaemic episodes were not captured. Since the two groups had similar HbA_{1c}, it is likely that the hypoglycaemic group also had more hyperglycaemia, which might conceivably have contributed to increased intima-media thickness.

Another possible explanation of the failure of clinical trials to demonstrate a beneficial effect of glycaemic control is that none of them targeted reducing fluctuations in blood glucose. Indeed, many forms of treatment may increase blood glucose fluctuations. Acute fluctuations in blood glucose have been shown to be associated with increased mortality [15]. This may be mediated by endothelial dysfunction, oxidative stress, and endothelial cell apoptosis [16]. Such effects of glucose fluctuations could predispose to both microvascular and macrovascular disease.

The aim of this study was therefore to investigate the independent effects of hyperglycaemia, hypoglycaemia, and glucose variability on microvascular and macrovascular disease in type 2 diabetes. Urinary albumin-creatinine served as a marker of microvascular disease. Ankle-brachial index, carotid intima-media thickness, and documented cardiovascular disease served as markers of macrovascular disease. 72-hour continuous glucose monitoring was used to assess hypoglycaemia, hyperglycaemia, and glucose variability. HBA_{1c} and fructosamine served as additional glycaemic indexes.

2. Methods

The study was cross-sectional in nature; data collection was performed over a one-year period, from April 2015 to April 2016. Patients were randomly selected from the list of outpatients attending the Diabetes Centre, Mater Dei Hospital, Malta, during the year 2014. The inclusion criteria were subjects who were diagnosed with type 2 DM according to World Health Organization criteria within the last ten years and were on stable antiglycaemic treatment. Patients suffering from dementia or mental illnesses with the consequent inability to give an informed consent with regard to participation in the study were excluded from the study. Other exclusion criteria included recent admission to hospital with a diabetes-related complication such as hyperglycaemic hyperosmolar ketoacidosis, liver failure, or kidney failure, as well as any other factors that result in glycaemic fluctuations. The study protocol was approved by the University of Malta Research Ethics Committee. All participants gave written informed consent.

2.1. Clinical and Laboratory Measurements. The presence of history of ischaemic heart disease and of cerebrovascular disease was ascertained by use of a questionnaire and by review of medical notes. Height and weight were measured using a calibrated balance and a stadiometer, with the subjects wearing light clothing and without shoes. Body mass index (BMI) was calculated as weight divided by height squared. Waist circumference was measured to the nearest 0.5 cm in the horizontal plane at the midpoint between the lowest rib and the iliac crest [17]. The waist index was calculated as waist circumference (cm) divided by 94 for men and 80 for women [18] Office blood pressure was measured in the supine position after 5 min of rest.

All subjects underwent routine blood investigations in the fasting state on the day of the clinical examination. No medication was taken on the morning of the examination. Patients who were treated with insulin discontinued injections after 22:00 on the day preceding the examination. Estimated glomerular filtration rate (eGFR) was calculated using the Modified Diet in Renal Disease (MDRD) formula (National Kidney Foundation Calculator for Healthcare Professionals). Haemoglobin A_{1c} (measured using high-performance liquid chromatography) and fructosamine were taken as markers of glycaemic control. Urine albumin was measured by an immunoturbidometric technique (Roche Diagnostics, Mannheim, Germany). Creatinine was measured by a kinetic colorimetric test using the Jaffe reaction (Roche Diagnostics). Albumin-creatinine ratio (ACR) was assessed in all patients as a marker of microvascular disease. Body surface area was provided by the Esaote machine used to perform CIMT by inputting weight and height.

2.2. Continuous Glucose Monitoring. Seventy-two-hour subcutaneous continuous glucose monitoring (CGM) was performed in all study participants on an ambulatory basis using the iPro2 continuous glucose-monitoring system (Medtronic MiniMed, Northridge, CA, USA). Participants were advised to pursue their normal daily living without alterations in their usual diet, exercise, and medications taken. Data from the iPro2 were uploaded online via the CareLink iPro software. The following parameters were extracted for each patient: mean blood glucose (MBG), standard deviation of blood glucose (SD), the highest and lowest blood glucose values, the number of high and low excursions, the area under the curve when the blood glucose was higher than 7.8 mmol/L (AUC > 7.8), the area under the curve when the blood glucose was lower than 3.9 mmol/L (AUC < 3.9), the duration (%) when the blood glucose was higher than 7.8 mmol/L, the duration (%) when the blood glucose was lower than 3.9 mmol/L, and the duration (%) when the blood glucose was between 3.9 mmol/L and 7.8 mmol/L.

2.3. Carotid Intima-Media Thickness Measurement. Carotid intima-media thickness (CIMT) was assessed in both common carotid arteries in each participant using the Esaote

Quality intima media thickness (QIMT®). The common carotid artery was utilised since, according to the Mannheim consensus, it increases the accuracy and reproducibility of the measurements obtained. The Esaote QIMT utilises a radio frequency signal to enable measurement of the CIMT with high spatial resolution. The QIMT tool automatically provides accurate measurements of all the parameters which are independent from both the investigator and device settings. Results were categorised as normal or abnormal using age-specific cut-offs, which have been validated in large worldwide databases [19]. Furthermore, all study participants were screened for the presence of carotid plaques in view that the combination of plaque area and thickness have greater value in predicting CVD compared to the thickness alone [17]. Patients with an increased CIMT as assessed by QIMT and/or presence of carotid plaque were categorised as having an abnormal CIMT.

2.4. Clinical Definitions. eGFR was defined as being low if it was <60 mL/min/1.73m^2. PAD was defined as an ABI of ≤0.9. The mean arterial pressure was the average arterial pressure during a single cardiac cycle and pulse pressure the difference between the systolic and diastolic blood pressure readings. Macrovascular disease was defined as the presence of one or more of the following: history of ischaemic heart disease (IHD) or cerebrovascular accident (CVA), ABI < 0.9, or abnormal CIMT.

2.5. Statistical Analysis. All data were analysed using SPSS version 24.0 for Windows. Results are presented as mean ± standard deviation (SD) or median (interquartile range (IQR)). Continuous variables were checked for normality of distribution using the Kolmogorov-Smirnov method. Comparisons of continuous variables between two groups were made using independent sample *t*-test for normally distributed variables. For nonparametric variables, the Mann–Whitney *U* test was used for comparison of 2 groups. Categorical variables were compared using the χ^2 test. The Pearson test was used to test correlation of normally distributed variables, and the Spearman test was used for comparison of non-normally distributed variables.

Univariate followed by multivariate analyses (logistic regression analyses) were performed to identify independent determinants of both the occurrence of macrovascular disease and abnormal CIMT in the study population. Variables were entered into the regression model if their p value was <0.1 in univariate analysis. Predictors were removed from the model if their p value exceeded 0.05.

With regard to ACR, univariate followed by multivariate analysis was again performed with variables with a p value < 0.1 in univariate analysis being included in the multivariate model; however, a generalised linear model was performed as multivariate analysis in view that ACR exhibited a gamma distribution (a right-skewed distribution). All tests were two-sided, and a p value of <0.05 was considered to be statistically significant.

Sample size was determined so as to have statistical power of 90% to detect a moderate effect size ($f^2 = 0.15$) at $\alpha = 0.05$.

2.6. Role of Funding Source. The study sponsor had no role in study design; in the collection, analysis, and interpretation of data; in the writing of the report; and in the decision to submit the paper for publication. The authors had full access to the data.

3. Results

3.1. Characteristics of Study Population. The study population comprised 121 T2DM subjects of Caucasian origin. The baseline characteristics are outlined in Table 1, whilst continuous glucose-monitoring data are shown in Table 2. Patients had reasonably well-controlled diabetes with a median HbA_{1c} of 6.8% (45 mmol/mol), a median fasting plasma glucose of 7.08 mmol/L, and a mean blood glucose (MBG) during CGM of 7.9 mmol/L. Hyperglycaemic episodes were more prevalent than hypoglycaemic episodes as shown by the number of high and low excursions, the AUC > 7.8 mmol/L and AUC< 3.9 mmol/L, as well as duration of BG > 7.8 mmol/L, between 3.9 and 7.8 mmol/L, and < 3.9 mmol/L. However, none of the study participants reported hypoglycaemic episodes, indicating that all these episodes were subclinical. There were no patients with missing data.

3.2. Predictors of Macrovascular Disease. Seventy-two subjects exhibited macrovascular disease. Univariate followed by multivariate analysis was performed to identify predictors of macrovascular disease in the study population. The results of univariate analysis are shown in Tables 3–5. In univariate analysis, the following variables had a p value < 0.1 and were thus included in the multivariate model: body surface area (BSA), smoking pack years, HDL cholesterol, triglycerides, ESR, lowest blood glucose (BG) value, AUC for BG < 3.9 mmol/L, and duration of BG < 3.9 mmol/L. In multivariate logistic regression analysis, BSA (OR 18.88 (95% CI 2.20–156.69), $p = 0.006$) and duration of BG < 3.9 mmol/L (OR 1.12 (95% CI 1.014–1.228), $p = 0.024$) were shown to be independent predictors of macrovascular disease. The relation between presence of cardiovascular disease and duration of BG < 3.9 mmol/L is shown in Figure 1.

3.3. Predictors of Abnormal Carotid Intima-Media Thickness. In the study population, 64 subjects had abnormal CIMT (composite of increased CIMT and presence of carotid plaque). In univariate analysis, the following variables had a p value < 0.1: age, DM duration, smoking pack years, BSA, white cell count, eGFR, ESR, and duration of BG < 3.9 mmol/L. These variables were consequently included in the multivariate model.

Binary logistic regression analysis revealed that BSA (OR 12.6 (95% CI 1.70–93.54), $p = 0.013$) and duration of BGM < 3.9 mmol/L (OR 1.09 (95% CI 1.003–1.187), $p = 0.041$) were independent predictors of abnormal CIMT. The relation between abnormal CIMT and duration of BG < 3.9 mmol/L is shown in Figure 1.

3.4. Predictors of Albuminuria. The following had p value < 0.1 in univariate analysis: low eGFR (<60 mL/min/1.73m^2), white cell count, HDL cholesterol, triglycerides, uric acid,

Table 1: Baseline demographic and clinical findings of study population.

Patient characteristics ($n = 121$)	Values
Age (years)†	64 (57–68)
Male : female (n (%))	89 (73.6) : 32 (26.4)
Diabetes duration (years)†	3 (2–5)
Smoking (current/ex/nonsmokers) (n (%))	22 (18.2)/41 (33.9)/58 (47.9)
Hypertension (n (%))	80 (66.1)
Hyperlipidaemia (n (%))	87 (71.9)
Ischaemic heart disease (n (%))	15 (12.4)
Peripheral arterial disease (n (%))	7 (5.8)
Cerebrovascular accident/transient ischaemic attack (n (%))	3 (2.5)
Abnormal carotid intima-media thickness (n (%))	64 (52.9)
Macrovascular disease (n (%))	72 (59.5)
Chronic kidney disease (n (%))	9 (7.4)
On metformin (n (%))	109 (90.1)
On sulphonylurea (n (%))	36 (29.8)
On gliptins (n (%))	6 (5)
On insulin (n (%))	6 (5)
On angiotensin-converting enzyme inhibitor/on angiotensin receptor blocker (n (%))	77 (63.6)
On β-blocker (n (%))	22 (18.2)
On calcium channel blocker (n (%))	23 (19)
On diuretic (n (%))	33 (23.7)
On aspirin (n (%))	38 (31.4)
On statin (n (%))	81 (66.9)
On fibrate (n (%))	7 (5.8)
On allopurinol (n (%))	5 (4.1)
Body mass index (kg/m^2)†	31.22 (27.94–34.53)
Body surface area (m^2)*	1.89 ± 0.21
Waist index*	1.19 ± 0.14
Pulse rate (bpm)†	68 (61.5–78.5)
Mean systolic pressure (mmHg)*	144.19 ± 17.82
Mean diastolic pressure (mmHg)*	84.60 ± 8.76
Pulse pressure (mmHg)*	61.53 ± 13.66
Mean arterial pressure (mmHg)†	107 (93–113)
White cell count (×10^9/L)†	7.16 (6.26–8.69)
Haemoglobin (g/dL)†	14.35 (13.33–15.18)
Platelet count (×10^9/L)†	240.5 (206–284.75)
Red blood cell distribution width (%)†	13.1 (12.53–13.7)
Mean platelet volume (fL)†	10.9 (10.2–11.6)
Estimated glomerular filtration rate (mL/min/1.73 m^2)*	91.22 ± 24.61
Total cholesterol (mmol/L)†	4.12 (3.55–5.15)
HDL cholesterol (mmol/L)†	1.24 (1.06–1.51)
LDL cholesterol (mmol/L)†	2.19 (1.67–3.19)
Non-HDL cholesterol (mmol/L)†	2.8 (2.26–3.82)
Triglycerides (mmol/L)†	1.36 (0.97–1.7)
Alkaline phosphatase (mmol/L)†	69 (55–83.5)
Alanine transaminase (mmol/L)†	23 (18–32.5)
Uric acid (μmol/L)*	313.05 ± 79.98
Erythrocyte sedimentation rate (mm 1st hr)†	10.5 (6–18)
Albumin-creatinine ratio (mg/mmol)†	7.08 (1–23.34)
Fasting plasma glucose (mmol/L)†	7.08 (6.11–8.18)
Fructosamine (μmol/L)†	278 (257–303)
Glycated haemoglobin (%)†	6.8 (6.3–7.6)

Values are expressed as number (%) of patients, *mean ± SD, or †median (IQR).

Table 2: Baseline continuous glucose-monitoring findings of study population.

Patient characteristics ($n = 121$)	Values
Highest value (mmol/L)	13.2 (11.3–15.5)
Lowest value (mmol/L)	3.95 (2.93–5.1)
Mean blood glucose (mmol/L)	7.35 (6.63–8.65)
Standard deviation (mmol/L)	1.9 (1.5–2.3)
Number of high excursions	8 (5–10)
Number of low excursions	0 (0–2)
AUC above 7.8 mmol/L	0.63 (0.23–1.43)
AUC below 3.9 mmol/L	0 (0–0.02)
Duration during 72 hr period with BG above 7.8 mmol/L (%)	37 (19.25–60.75)
Duration during 72 hr period with BG within 3.9–7.8 mmol/L (%)	60 (37.5–77)
Duration during 72 hr period with BG below 3.9 mmol/L (%)	0 (0–4)

Values are expressed as median (IQR). AUC: area under curve.

BMI, WI, MBG, SD, AUC for BG > 7.8 mmol/L, duration of BG > 7.8 mmol/L, duration of BG between 3.9 and 7.8 mmol/L, and highest BG value recorded. Generalised linear regression model revealed AUC for BG > 7.8 mmol/L ($\beta = 15.83$, $p = 0.005$) to be the sole independent predictor of albuminuria.

4. Discussion

The present study found that the duration of blood glucose < 3.9 mmol/L was significantly and independently associated with abnormal CIMT and with the composite of abnormal CIMT, ABI, coronary artery disease, and cerebrovascular disease in subjects with type 2 diabetes. This suggests that hypoglycaemia may predispose to atherosclerosis.

Table 3: Demographic and clinical findings of subjects with and without macrovascular disease.

Variable	No macrovascular disease ($n = 49$)	Macrovascular disease ($n = 72$)	p value
Age (years)†	66 (62–69)	61 (54.25–67)	0.001
Male : female (n (%))	34 (**69.4**) : 15 (30.6)	55 (**76.4**) : 17 (**23.6**)	0.41
Diabetes duration (years)†	3.5 (2–5)	3 (2–4)	0.23
Smoking (current/ex/nonsmokers) (n (%))	4 (8.1)/19 (38.8)/26 (53.1)	18 (25.0)/22 (30.6)/32 (44.4)	0.06
Hypertension (n (%))	29 (59.18)	51 (70.83)	0.24
Hyperlipidaemia (n (%))	36 (73.47)	51 (70.83)	0.84
CKD (n (%))	2 (4.08)	7 (9.72)	0.31
Metformin (n (%))	44 (89.80)	65 (90.28)	1.00
Sulphonylurea (n (%))	14 (28.57)	50 (69.44)	0.84
Gliptins (n (%))	4 (8.16)	2 (2.77)	0.22
Insulin (n (%))	1 (2.04)	5 (6.94)	0.40
ACEI/ARB (n (%))	29 (59.18)	48 (66.67)	0.44
β-blocker (n (%))	7 (14.29)	15 (20.83)	0.47
CCB (n (%))	11 (22.45)	12 (16.67)	0.48
Diuretic (n (%))	14 (28.57)	19 (26.39)	0.84
Aspirin (n (%))	9 (18.36)	29 (40.28)	0.02
Statin (n (%))	29 (59.18)	52 (72.22)	0.17
Fibrate (n (%))	6 (12.24)	1 (1.39)	0.02
Allopurinol (n (%))	2 (4.08)	3 (4.17)	1.00
BMI (kg/m^2)†	31.22 (27.67–33.97)	31.31 (27.9–35.19)	0.35
BSA (m^2)*	1.83 ± 0.20	1.93 ± 0.21	0.007
Waist index*	1.17 ± 0.15	1.20 ± 0.13	0.22
Pulse rate (bpm)†	65 (61–80.25)	71 (62–78)	0.84
Mean SBP (mmHg)*	146 ± 18.28	142.96 ± 17.54	0.36
Mean DBP (mmHg)*	85.66 ± 7.34	83.88 ± 9.58	0.25
Pulse pressure (mmHg)*	62.18 ± 15.6	61.07 ± 12.22	0.68
MAP (mmHg)†	106 (97.5–112.5)	90.75 (107.5–113)	0.77

Values are expressed as number (%) of patients, *mean ± SD, or †median (IQR). ACEI: angiotensin-converting enzyme inhibitor; ARB: angiotensin receptor blocker; BMI: body mass index; BSA: body surface area; CCB: calcium channel blocker; CKD: chronic kidney disease; CVD: cardiovascular disease; DM: diabetes mellitus; DBP: diastolic blood pressure; MAP: mean arterial pressure; SBP: systolic blood pressure.

These findings are consistent with those of the Diabetes Control and Complications Trial (DCCT), which reported that the rate of severe hypoglycaemic episodes in subjects with type 1 diabetes was associated with increased coronary calcium score in those with a HbA_{1c} below 7.5% (58 mmol/L) [18]. It is, however, possible that severe hypoglycaemia was acting as a marker for increased glucose fluctuations. Since we performed CGM, we can exclude this possibility in our study. Furthermore, whilst the DCCT data showed an association of severe hypoglycaemia with increased coronary calcium score in type 1 diabetes, the present study shows a relationship of mild asymptomatic hypoglycaemia, as detected by CGM, to atherosclerosis in type 2 diabetes.

We did not find significant associations of any of the hyperglycaemic indexes (including HbA_{1c}, fructosamine, AUC > 7.8 mmol/L, and duration > 7.8 mmol/L) or of glucose fluctuations (as assessed by standard deviation of blood glucose during CGM) with macrovascular disease. However, duration of blood glucose > 7.8 mmol/L was independently associated with ACR. These observations may be related to the short median duration of diabetes in our patients. Our findings are consistent with clinical trial data which have shown that lowering blood glucose for a few years is effective in reducing microvascular but not macrovascular disease [2, 3]. In the UKPDS, it took 10 years of intensive control and a further 10 years of follow-up to demonstrate a beneficial effect of lowering blood glucose on macrovascular outcomes [20]. Another reason could be the relatively good glycaemic control in our cohort.

Our data suggest that hypoglycaemia may have a more rapid effect in promoting atherosclerosis than mild hyperglycaemia or glucose fluctuations. They may help explain the relationship between hypoglycaemia and adverse cardiovascular outcomes even in the short term and why these deleterious effects extend well beyond the period of hypoglycaemia itself. They may also explain why too aggressive lowering of blood glucose in the Action to Control Cardiovascular Risk in Diabetes (ACCORD) trial was associated with increased mortality [21] and why agents such

TABLE 4: Laboratory findings of subjects with and without macrovascular disease.

Variable	No macrovascular disease ($n = 49$)	Macrovascular disease ($n = 72$)	p value
White cell count ($\times 10^9$/L)†	7.09 (5.88–7.87)	7.29 (6.42–9.24)	0.13
Haemoglobin (g/dL)†	14.2 (13.3–15.1)	14.4 (13.6–15.2)	0.48
Platelet count ($\times 10^9$/L)†	242 (204.5–283.5)	239 (206–287)	0.78
RDW (%)†	13 (12.5–13.45)	13.1 (12.6–13.8)	0.13
MPV (fL)†	10.95 (10.23–11.5)	10.9 (10.1–11.6)	0.53
eGFR (mL/min/1.72 m^2)*	87.76 ± 22.21	93.58 ± 26.0	0.19
Total cholesterol (mmol/L)†	4.14 (3.65–5.25)	4.1 (3.53–5.11)	0.80
HDL cholesterol (mmol/L)†	1.32 (1.1–1.58)	1.24 (1.04–1.46)	**0.07**
LDL cholesterol (mmol/L)†	2.3 (1.65–3.36)	2.18 (1.7–3.13)	0.81
Non-HDL cholesterol (mmol/L)†	2.74 (2.18–3.86)	2.83 (2.29–3.78)	0.67
Triglycerides (mmol/L)†	1.13 (0.91–1.64)	1.47 (1.14–1.85)	**0.03**
ALP (mmol/L)†	66 (52–93)	69 (59.25–80)	0.89
ALT (mmol/L)†	22 (17.5–32)	24 (18–32.75)	0.6
Uric acid (μmol/L)*	319.56 ± 83.19	308.65 ± 78.03	0.47
ESR (mm 1st hr)†	13 (7–23)	9 (5–17)	**0.08**
FPG (mmol/L)†	7.14 (6.02–8.53)	7.08 (6.23–8.05)	0.55
Fructosamine (μmol/L)†	281 (259.25–305)	277 (256–303.5)	0.77
HbA_{1c} (%)†	7.0 (6.3–8.1)	6.7 (6.3–7.4)	0.23
HbA_{1c} (mmol/L)†	53 (45–65)	50 (45–57)	0.23

Values are expressed as *mean ± SD or †median (IQR). Abbreviations: ALP: alkaline phosphatase; ALT: alanine transaminase; eGFR: estimated glomerular filtration rate; ESR: erythrocyte sedimentation rate; FPG: fasting plasma glucose; HbA_{1c}: glycated haemoglobin; MPV: mean platelet volume; RDW: red blood cell distribution width.

TABLE 5: Continuous glucose-monitoring findings of subjects with and without macrovascular disease.

Variable	No macrovascular disease ($n = 49$)	Macrovascular disease ($n = 72$)	p value
Highest value (mmol/L)†	13.4 (11.3–15.85)	13.0 (11.3–15)	0.35
Lowest value (mmol/L)†	4.4 (3.2–5.25)	3.7 (2.8–5)	**0.09**
Mean blood glucose (mmol/L)†	7.6 (6.85–9.0)	7.3 (6.6–8.4)	0.3
Standard deviation (mmol/L)†	3.0 (1.3–2.3)	1.8 (1.5–2.4)	0.9
Number of high excursions†	8 (6–10)	8 (5–10)	0.49
Number of low excursions†	0 (0–2)	1 (0–2)	0.10
AUC above 7.8 mmol/L†	0.64 (0.24–1.76)	0.57 (0.21–1.35)	0.39
AUC below 3.9 mmol/L†	0 (0–0.01)	0 (0–0.03)	**0.05**
Duration during 72 hr period with BG above 7.8 mmol/L (%)†	37 (18.5–66.5)	35 (20–58)	0.39
Duration during 72 hr period with BG within 3.9–7.8 mmol/L (%)†	58 (31.5–79)	60 (41–77)	0.63
Duration during 72 hr period with BG below 3.9 mmol/L (%)†	0 (0-1)	1 (0–5)	**0.02**

Values are expressed as number (%) of patients or †median (IQR). AUC: area under curve.

as sulphonylureas [22, 23]and insulin [24] which are prone to cause hypoglycaemia have also been associated with increased mortality and cardiovascular events by some authors.

Hypoglycaemia can promote atherogenesis in a number of ways. Acute hypoglycaemia has been shown to result in decreased nitric oxide bioavailability, increased oxidative stress [25], platelet activation [26], and release of proinflammatory [27], proatherogenic, and prothrombotic cytokines such as PAI-1, VEGF, vascular adhesion molecules, and interleukin-6 [26, 28]. Many of these effects may extend to beyond the hypoglycaemic period [26]. Furthermore, Fadini and colleagues have recently reported that hypoglycaemia may impair endothelial progenitor cell response [29]. Interestingly, Peña and colleagues have reported that hypoglycaemia, but not glucose variability, is associated with endothelial dysfunction in children with type 1 diabetes [30].

Body surface area was also found to be independently associated with atherosclerotic markers. This is probably related to insulin resistance and/or hyperinsulinaemia.

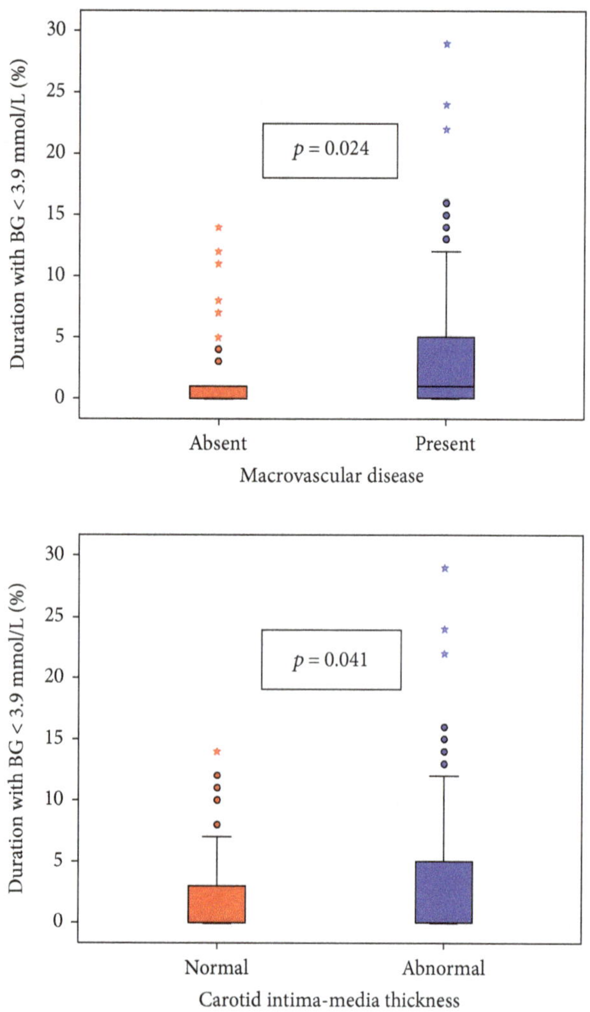

Figure 1: Box-and-whisker plot demonstrating relation of duration of glucose < 3.9 mmol/L (expressed as percentage of the entire 72 hr period) and macrovascular disease and carotid intima-media thickness. *denoting outliers.

The patients with macrovascular disease were on average younger than those without macrovascular disease. This could be due to the cross-sectional nature of our study. Macrovascular disease shortens life expectancy resulting in a lower average age of subjects with macrovascular disease compared to subjects without. Furthermore, macrovascular disease was associated with hypoglycaemia, which is also known to decrease survival [21]. Duration of diabetes was similar in both groups, meaning that those with macrovascular disease had younger onset type 2 diabetes, which might be associated with higher mortality [31].

A limitation of our study is that we have no information on antecedent glycaemic indexes. This problem is inherent to the study area as it is not practical or ethical to perform CGM over a number of years and not alter management in order to keep glycaemic parameters stable. However, we tried to reduce the impact of this limitation in a number of ways. Firstly, we only recruited patients with stable control, namely, not needing escalation of treatment. Secondly, we studied patients with short duration of diabetes because such patients are less likely to have variation in their glycaemic parameters over the course of their disease. Thirdly, we performed blind, rather than real-time, CGM so that patients did not alter their behaviour as result of the glucose readings. Additionally, patients were instructed not to change their usual routines. In this way, the CGM data are more likely to be representative of the patients' usual glycaemic profile. Furthermore, many glycaemic indices such as HbA_{1c} [32] and hypoglycaemia [11] have been shown to exhibit significant temporal tracking. Another limitation is that in view of the cross-sectional nature of our study, we cannot prove causal relationships. It is possible that those with macrovascular disease were treated more aggressively, hence causing more hypoglycaemia. However, this would not explain the observed relationship with CIMT, which is a subclinical marker of atherosclerosis.

In conclusion, the study suggests that mild asymptomatic hypoglycaemia in subjects with type 2 diabetes is associated with atherosclerotic disease. This cannot be explained by an association of hypoglycaemia with hyperglycaemia or glucose fluctuations. Hyperglycaemic load, as measured by AUC for BG > 7.8 mmol/L, was associated with microalbuminuria.

Disclosure

The study was presented in abstract form at the EuroPrevent meeting held in Ljubljana, Slovenia, April 19–21, 2017.

Conflicts of Interest

The authors have no conflict of interest to declare.

Acknowledgments

The study was sponsored by the Dean's Funds of the University of Malta Medical School.

References

[1] Emerging Risk Factors Collaboration, N. Sarwar, P. Gao et al., "Diabetes mellitus, fasting blood glucose concentration, and risk of vascular disease: a collaborative meta-analysis of 102 prospective studies," *The Lancet*, vol. 375, no. 9733, pp. 2215–2222, 2010.

[2] UK Prospective Diabetes Study (UKPDS) Group, "Intensive blood-glucose control with sulphonylureas or insulin compared with conventional treatment and risk of complications in patients with type 2 diabetes (UKPDS 33)," *The Lancet*, vol. 352, no. 9131, pp. 837–853, 1998.

[3] ADVANCE Collaborative Group, A. Patel, S. MacMahon et al., "Intensive blood glucose control and vascular outcomes in patients with type 2 diabetes," *The New England Journal of Medicine*, vol. 358, no. 24, pp. 2560–2572, 2008.

[4] C. J. Östgren, J. Sundström, B. Svennblad, L. Lohm, P. M. Nilsson, and G. Johansson, "Associations of HbA1c and educational level with risk of cardiovascular events in 32,871 drug-

treated patients with type 2 diabetes: a cohort study in primary care," *Diabetic Medicine*, vol. 30, no. 5, pp. e170–e177, 2013.

[5] A. Goto, O. A. Arah, M. Goto, Y. Terauchi, and M. Noda, "Severe hypoglycaemia and cardiovascular disease: systematic review and meta-analysis with bias analysis," *BMJ*, vol. 347, article f4533, 2013.

[6] S. Fava, O. Aquilina, J. Azzopardi, H. A. Muscat, and F. F. Fenech, "The prognostic value of blood glucose in diabetic patients with acute myocardial infarction," *Diabetic Medicine*, vol. 13, no. 1, pp. 80–83, 1996.

[7] A.-M. Svensson, D. K. McGuire, P. Abrahamsson, and M. Dellborg, "Association between hyper- and hypoglycaemia and 2 year all-cause mortality risk in diabetic patients with acute coronary events," *European Heart Journal*, vol. 26, no. 13, pp. 1255–1261, 2005.

[8] E. Tu, S. M. Twigg, and C. Semsarian, "Sudden death in type 1 diabetes: the mystery of the "dead in bed" syndrome," *International Journal of Cardiology*, vol. 138, no. 1, pp. 91–93, 2010.

[9] C. M. Reno, D. Daphna-Iken, Y. S. Chen, J. VanderWeele, K. Jethi, and S. J. Fisher, "Severe hypoglycemia-induced lethal cardiac arrhythmias are mediated by sympathoadrenal activation," *Diabetes*, vol. 62, no. 10, pp. 3570–3581, 2013.

[10] C. Desouza, H. Salazar, B. Cheong, J. Murgo, and V. Fonseca, "Association of hypoglycemia and cardiac ischemia: a study based on continuous monitoring," *Diabetes Care*, vol. 26, no. 5, pp. 1485–1489, 2003.

[11] S. Sreenan, M. Andersen, B. L. Thorsted, M. L. Wolden, and M. Evans, "Increased risk of severe hypoglycemic events with increasing frequency of non-severe hypoglycemic events in patients with type 1 and type 2 diabetes," *Diabetes Therapy*, vol. 5, no. 2, pp. 447–458, 2014.

[12] E. Yasunari, T. Mita, Y. Osonoi et al., "Repetitive hypoglycemia increases circulating adrenaline level with resultant worsening of intimal thickening after vascular injury in male Goto-Kakizaki rat carotid artery," *Endocrinology*, vol. 155, no. 6, pp. 2244–2253, 2014.

[13] W. L. Jin, K. Azuma, T. Mita et al., "Repetitive hypoglycaemia increases serum adrenaline and induces monocyte adhesion to the endothelium in rat thoracic aorta," *Diabetologia*, vol. 54, no. 7, pp. 1921–1929, 2011.

[14] M. Giménez, R. Gilabert, J. Monteagudo et al., "Repeated episodes of hypoglycemia as a potential aggravating factor for preclinical atherosclerosis in subjects with type 1 diabetes," *Diabetes Care*, vol. 34, no. 1, pp. 198–203, 2011.

[15] J. G. Timmons, S. G. Cunningham, C. A. R. Sainsbury, and G. C. Jones, "Inpatient glycemic variability and long-term mortality in hospitalized patients with type 2 diabetes," *Journal of Diabetes and its Complications*, vol. 31, no. 2, pp. 479–482, 2017.

[16] N. Wu, H. Shen, H. Liu, Y. Wang, Y. Bai, and P. Han, "Acute blood glucose fluctuation enhances rat aorta endothelial cell apoptosis, oxidative stress and pro-inflammatory cytokine expression in vivo," *Cardiovascular Diabetology*, vol. 15, no. 1, p. 109, 2016.

[17] M. F. Piepoli, A. W. Hoes, S. Agewall et al., "2016 European guidelines on cardiovascular disease prevention in clinical practice: the sixth joint task force of the European Society of Cardiology and other societies on cardiovascular disease prevention in clinical practice (constituted by representatives of 10 societies and by invited experts). Developed with the special contribution of the European Association for Cardiovascular Prevention & Rehabilitation (EACPR)," *Giornale Italiano Di Cardiologia*, vol. 18, no. 7, pp. 547–612, 2017.

[18] E. R. Fährmann, L. Adkins, C. J. Loader et al., "Severe hypoglycemia and coronary artery calcification during the diabetes control and complications trial/epidemiology of diabetes interventions and complications (DCCT/EDIC) study," *Diabetes Research and Clinical Practice*, vol. 107, no. 2, pp. 280–289, 2015.

[19] L. Engelen, I. Ferreira, C. D. Stehouwer, P. Boutouyrie, S. Laurent, and Reference Values for Arterial Measurements Collaboration, "Reference intervals for common carotid intima-media thickness measured with echotracking: relation with risk factors," *European Heart Journal*, vol. 34, no. 30, pp. 2368–2380, 2013.

[20] R. R. Holman, S. K. Paul, M. A. Bethel, D. R. Matthews, and H. A. W. Neil, "10-year follow-up of intensive glucose control in type 2 diabetes," *The New England Journal of Medicine*, vol. 359, no. 15, pp. 1577–1589, 2008.

[21] D. E. Bonds, M. E. Miller, R. M. Bergenstal et al., "The association between symptomatic, severe hypoglycaemia and mortality in type 2 diabetes: retrospective epidemiological analysis of the ACCORD study," *BMJ*, vol. 340, article b4909, 2010.

[22] O. J. Phung, E. Schwartzman, R. W. Allen, S. S. Engel, and S. N. Rajpathak, "Sulphonylureas and risk of cardiovascular disease: systematic review and meta-analysis," *Diabetic Medicine*, vol. 30, no. 10, pp. 1160–1171, 2013.

[23] C. L. Morgan, J. Mukherjee, S. Jenkins-Jones, S. E. Holden, and C. J. Currie, "Combination therapy with metformin plus sulphonylureas versus metformin plus DPP-4 inhibitors: association with major adverse cardiovascular events and all-cause mortality," *Diabetes, Obesity & Metabolism*, vol. 16, no. 10, pp. 977–983, 2014.

[24] S. E. Holden, S. Jenkins-Jones, C. L. Morgan, G. Schernthaner, and C. J. Currie, "Glucose-lowering with exogenous insulin monotherapy in type 2 diabetes: dose association with all-cause mortality, cardiovascular events and cancer," *Diabetes, Obesity and Metabolism*, vol. 17, no. 4, pp. 350–362, 2015.

[25] J. Wang, A. Alexanian, R. Ying et al., "Acute exposure to low glucose rapidly induces endothelial dysfunction and mitochondrial oxidative stress: role for AMP kinase," *Arteriosclerosis, Thrombosis, and Vascular Biology*, vol. 32, no. 3, pp. 712–720, 2012.

[26] N. G. Joy, D. B. Tate, L. M. Younk, and S. N. Davis, "Effects of acute and antecedent hypoglycemia on endothelial function and markers of atherothrombotic balance in healthy humans," *Diabetes*, vol. 64, no. 7, pp. 2571–2580, 2015.

[27] L. Razavi Nematollahi, A. E. Kitabchi, F. B. Stentz et al., "Proinflammatory cytokines in response to insulin-induced hypoglycemic stress in healthy subjects," *Metabolism*, vol. 58, no. 4, pp. 443–448, 2009.

[28] B. Kiec-Wilk, B. Matejko, U. Razny et al., "Hypoglycemic episodes are associated with inflammatory status in patients with type 1 diabetes mellitus," *Atherosclerosis*, vol. 251, pp. 334–338, 2016.

[29] G. P. Fadini, M. Albiero, S. Vigili de Kreutzenberg, and A. Avogaro, "Hypoglycemia affects the changes in endothelial progenitor cell levels during insulin therapy in type 2 diabetic patients," *Journal of Endocrinological Investigation*, vol. 38, no. 7, pp. 733–738, 2015.

[30] A. S. Peña, J. J. Couper, J. Harrington et al., "Hypoglycemia, but not glucose variability, relates to vascular function in

children with type 1 diabetes," *Diabetes Technology & Therapeutics*, vol. 14, no. 6, pp. 457–462, 2012.

[31] S. Zoungas, M. Woodward, Q. Li et al., "Impact of age, age at diagnosis and duration of diabetes on the risk of macrovascular and microvascular complications and death in type 2 diabetes," *Diabetologia*, vol. 57, no. 12, pp. 2465–2474, 2014.

[32] J. A. Edge, T. James, and B. Shine, "Persistent individual tracking within overall improvement in HbA1c in a UK paediatric diabetes clinic over 15 years," *Diabetic Medicine*, vol. 27, no. 11, pp. 1284–1288, 2010.

17

Low Birth Weight, Cumulative Obesity Dose, and the Risk of Incident Type 2 Diabetes

Cindy Feng,[1] Nathaniel D. Osgood,[2] and Roland F. Dyck[3]

[1]*School of Public Health, University of Saskatchewan, Saskatoon, SK, Canada*
[2]*Department of Computer Science, University of Saskatchewan, Saskatoon, SK, Canada*
[3]*Department of Medicine, Canadian Centre for Health and Safety in Agriculture, University of Saskatchewan, Saskatoon, SK, Canada*

Correspondence should be addressed to Roland F. Dyck; roland.dyck@usask.ca

Academic Editor: Andrea Scaramuzza

Background. Obesity history may provide a better understanding of the contribution of obesity to T2DM risk. *Methods.* 17,634 participants from the 1958 National Child Development Study were followed from birth to 50 years. Cumulative obesity dose, a measure of obesity history, was calculated by subtracting the upper cut-off of the normal BMI from the actual BMI at each follow-up and summing the areas under the obesity dose curve. Hazard ratios (HRs) for diabetes were calculated using Cox regression analysis. Three separate models compared the predictive ability of cumulative obesity dose on diabetes risk with the time-varying BMI and last BMI. *Results.* In final models, 341 of 15,043 (2.27%) participants developed diabetes; male sex and low birth weight were significant confounding variables. Adjusted HRs were 1.080 (95% CI: 1.071, 1.088) per 10-unit cumulative obesity dose, 1.098 (95% CI: 1.080, 1.117) per unit of the time-varying BMI, and 1.146 (95% CI: 1.084, 1.212) per unit of the last BMI. Cumulative obesity dose provided the best predictive ability for diabetes. *Conclusions.* Cumulative obesity dose is an improved method for evaluating the impact of obesity history on diabetes risk. The link between low birth weight and T2DM is strengthened by adjusting for cumulative obesity dose.

1. Introduction

A pandemic of type 2 diabetes (T2DM) is affecting diverse populations worldwide [1] and is strongly linked to global increases in rates of overweight and obesity which have risen dramatically over the past several decades [2]. While the immediate relationship between increased adiposity and T2DM is firmly established [1, 2], emerging evidence suggests that obesity duration and its age of onset (obesity history) may provide greater insight into the contribution of obesity to T2DM risk than into cross-sectional relationships alone [3–11]. Moreover, while there is also an established link between both low birth weight and high birth weight and the development of T2DM [12], it is not clear if and how birth weight contributes to higher diabetes risk through its possible impact on the onset, degree, and duration of excess weight.

Several approaches have been used to evaluate the relationship between obesity history and subsequent morbidity/mortality, but models incorporating a duration-of-obesity component have performed most strongly [13]. One such model type combines time interval with a measure of the degree to which an individual's body mass index (BMI) exceeds either a normal BMI or some other BMI baseline [13]. This has been described as being akin to pack years of smoking [4], and different versions of this methodology have all shown a significant correlation between an increasing area under the excess BMI curve and diabetes risk [14–17]. However, the four main studies that have used this approach [14–17] have limitations with the absence of data from the younger period of the life cycle, short study duration, the manner in which the excess BMI was calculated, or a combination of those and other drawbacks. Importantly, none of these studies have included birth weight as a potential confounder.

Using a British birth cohort from the 1958 National Child Development Study (NCDS) [18], we now report on the largest and longest study to date that has examined the relationship between the duration-of-obesity measure and T2DM risk. By following individuals from birth to age 50, our primary objective was to determine the influence of what we believe is an improved method of calculating the duration of obesity—what we refer to as cumulative obesity dose—on the incidence of diabetes, while adjusting for birth weight as well as for other known diabetes risk factors. Our secondary objective was to compare the strength of this relationship with the performance of the time-varying BMI and most recent BMI, in predicting diabetes risk. Deciphering the impact and dynamics of cumulative obesity dose on diabetes risk, while taking into account the influence of birth weight, could help us to better understand the emergence of type 2 diabetes, to guide in the timing and the nature of public health measures designed to curb the epidemics of both obesity and T2DM, and finally to provide a more informed basis on which to provide individual-level obesity counselling.

2. Methods

2.1. Study Population. The participants were from the National Child Development Study [18], an ongoing longitudinal study of a cohort of 17,634 children born in England, Wales, and Scotland during the week of March 9, 1958. To date, there have been eight follow-up sweeps that have traced the members of the cohort throughout childhood (aged 7, 11, and 16 years) and into adulthood (aged 23, 33, 42, 46, and 50 years). The main sample of the present study included 16,573 who had had at least two follow-ups. Written informed consent was obtained from the participants, and ethical approval for the study was obtained from the South East Multi-Centre Research Ethics Committee.

2.2. The Main Outcome Measure—Incidence of Diabetes. The occurrence of diabetes was determined by a self-reported response to the question, "Have you ever been diagnosed with diabetes?" at each sweep and by using information from sweep 6, when the 42-year-old participants were asked: "At what age were you diagnosed with diabetes?" No information was provided about the diabetes type, and no medical verification of diagnosis was available. While it is possible that T2DM may have been underdiagnosed among youth and young adults in the 1970s, because of the long follow-up period of this study, these individuals would likely have been diagnosed at a later age.

The self-reported age of diabetes diagnosis for those participants who remained in the study at age 42 was used as the diabetes incidence age for those individuals. For those who dropped out of the study before age 42 or who developed diabetes after sweep 6, the incidence age of diabetes diagnosis was estimated as the midpoint between the last diabetes-free follow-up and the follow-up visit when diabetes was first reported. Participants were censored at the age of their last follow-up visit if they remained diabetes-free at that time.

2.3. Key Risk Factors of Interest—Body Mass Index and Cumulative Obesity Dose. For each sweep, we calculated the BMI based on participants' weight and height (BMI = weight in kg/height in m^2). Height was not reported at sweeps 7 and 8, so height at sweep 6 was used as a proxy for later sweeps. To account for missing BMI values, we used the predicted values by fitting a generalized linear mixed-effects model on the logarithm of the BMI with age and sex as predictors. To calculate the degree of obesity dose, we first subtracted the reference BMI from the actual BMI. For the purposes of this study, the reference BMI was defined as the upper cut-off for normal BMIs which varies with age and sex. The cut-off values were 17.9 kg/m^2 for boys and 17.8 kg/m^2 for girls at age 7, 20.6 kg/m^2 for boys and 20.7 kg/m^2 for girls at age 11, 23.9 kg/m^2 for boys and 24.4 kg/m^2 for girls at age 16, and 25 kg/m^2 for both genders at age 23 and above [19]. If the difference was negative, it was treated as zero. The cumulative obesity dose takes into account the duration and degree of obesity and was calculated by summing the areas under the obesity dose curve over all previous years beginning at age 7 up to the current sweep. For ease of computation, we calculated the area numerically. Cumulative obesity dose was modeled as a time-dependent variable in the analysis, which was presented as multiple observations for a single subject, each of which applied to a time interval of observation.

The time-varying BMI [20] was determined by the repeated measurements of the BMI for a subject, which may change over the period of time that the subject is observed. The follow-up time for each patient was divided into different time windows. For each time window, a separate Cox analysis was carried out using the time-dependent variable at the beginning of that specific time window. Then, a weighted average of all the time window-specific results was calculated as the estimated relative ratio (please see Appendix A for a more detailed description).

The last BMI was the most recent BMI calculated before the diagnosis of diabetes. For those without diabetes, the last BMI was the BMI calculated at age 50 for those who remained in the study at sweep 8 or the final BMI calculated for those who dropped out of the study before age 50.

2.4. Measurement of Other Diabetes Predictors. The age of the participants was defined as the years from the date of birth to the last interview year. Ethnicity was grouped into Caucasian versus others. The participants' birth weights were grouped as low (less than 2.5 kg), normal (2.5–4.0 kg), and high (above 4.0 kg). The baseline social class of each participant's mother's husband was used as a proxy for the socioeconomic status of the participant. These were categorized as I (professional occupations), II (managerial and technical occupations), III (skilled occupations), IV (partly skilled occupations), and V (unskilled occupations).

2.5. Statistical Analysis. Potential confounding variables that may be related to the BMI and onset of diabetes and that were included in the analysis were ethnicity, sex, participants' birth weight, and social class. The univariate relationships between the potential confounding variables and incidence of diabetes were expressed as hazard ratios (HRs) and determined using Cox proportional hazard regression analysis. In multivariate analysis, the effects of cumulative obesity dose, time-varying BMI, and last BMI were examined as time-dependent covariates in separate models using Cox proportional hazard modeling, with the onset of diabetes as the dependent variable. We also included a model without measures of obesity with which to compare the others. Each of the models was adjusted for potential confounding variables that were significant at the 0.2 level of significance in the univariate analysis and were modeled as fixed (non-time-dependent) covariates. In the final multivariate models, backward model selection was carried out and the final models only included covariates that were significant at the 0.05 level of significance.

To study the specific effect of age of obesity onset on the risk of developing diabetes, while adjusting for the effect of cumulative obesity dose, a subset analysis using multivariate Cox regression analysis was carried out. This was restricted to those participants who had developed overweight/obesity during the follow-up because no age of overweight/obesity onset can be determined for those who had never experienced it. In this analysis, covariate effects were assumed to be constant over time.

Finally, to study if the effect of cumulative obesity dose on diabetes risk varies by age groups, we evaluated the interaction between cumulative obesity dose and the three age groups (7–16, 23–42, and older than 42) in the model.

The Akaike information criterion (AIC) and Bayesian information criterion (BIC) were used to select the preferred model which was the one with the lowest AIC and BIC scores. All statistical analyses were performed using SAS software version 9.4 (SAS, Cary, NC, USA). All tests of significance were two-sided.

3. Results

The total number of participants who reported their diabetes status, the number of people newly diagnosed with diabetes, the number of people with an elevated BMI, and the total number of participants who were lost to follow-up at each sweep are shown in Table 1. Overall, 373 out of 16,573 (2.25%) participants reported their onset of diabetes. Although the proportion of participants who had an elevated BMI was relatively constant among children and youths, there was a progressive increase in those with an elevated BMI from age 23 on, and this increase was greater among men. By sweep 8, 13,655 (82.4%) of the initial cohort had been lost to follow-up.

The univariate relationships between the potential confounding variables and onset of diabetes are shown in Table 2. Ethnicity was borderline significant, with Caucasians displaying a lower hazard for diabetes than other groups. Males had a significantly higher risk of developing diabetes compared with females (HR 1.389; 95% CI: 1.131, 1.704). The association between birth weight of participants and the hazard of developing diabetes was borderline significant for low birth weight but was not significant for high birth weight. Participants from the lower social classes were at a significantly increased risk of developing diabetes. HR for class III versus class I was 1.963 (95% CI: 1.007, 3.825), for class IV versus class I was 2.159 (95% CI: 1.058, 4.406), and for class V versus class I was 2.543 (95% CI: 1.227, 5.271). The cumulative obesity dose, time-varying BMI, and last BMI were all significantly associated with an increased risk of diabetes onset. The unadjusted HR was 1.076 (95% CI: 1.068–1.084) for every 10-unit increase in cumulative obesity dose, the unadjusted HR was 1.098 (95% CI: 1.081–1.115) for every one-unit increase in the time-varying BMI, and the unadjusted HR was 1.137 (95% CI: 1.078–1.198) for the last BMI.

In the multivariate analysis (Table 3), 341 out of 15,043 (2.27%) participants developed diabetes during the study period after removing the participants with missing values in any of the covariates. All four final models contained participants' sex and birth weight as confounding variables. Ethnicity and social class did not remain in the final models after backward model selection. The adjusted HR (AHR) was 1.080 (95% CI: 1.071, 1.088) for every 10-unit increase in cumulative obesity dose, the AHR was 1.098 (95% CI: 1.080, 1.117) for every one-unit increase in the time-varying BMI, and the AHR was 1.146 (95% CI: 1.084, 1.212) for every one-unit increase in the last BMI. Finally, the AIC and BIC scores were much smaller for model number 1 with cumulative obesity dose as the covariate than the AIC and BIC scores for models number 2 and number 3, indicating that cumulative obesity dose provides much better predictive ability as compared to the time-varying BMI and last BMI.

Table 3 also shows the impact of birth weight on diabetes risk with and without the inclusion of measures of obesity. Without any of the measures of obesity in model number 0, the adjusted HR for low birth weight is very similar to the unadjusted HR in Table 2 (1.444 compared to 1.408) and remains not quite significant ($P = 0.0732$). In contrast, the AHRs for low birth weight are significant when any of the three measures of obesity are added in but particularly so for COD (1.686 for COD, 1.511 for the time-varying BMI, and 1.522 for the last BMI).

Table 4 shows the AHRs of developing diabetes among the 10,172/16,753 (61.38%) participants who developed overweight/obesity during follow-up. Among those, 310 (3.05%) developed diabetes. The three models all showed that older age of obesity onset is significantly associated with a decreased risk of developing diabetes, even after adjusting for other variables. Furthermore, male and low-birth weight participants who had a history of overweight/obesity were still at significantly higher risk of developing diabetes. Model number 1 still outperformed the other two models. However, in this subset analysis, the AIC and BIC results with and without age of obesity onset as a covariate showed that age of obesity onset improved the model fit to a greater degree for the time-varying BMI and last BMI than for cumulative obesity dose.

Table 5 shows that the effect of cumulative obesity dose on diabetes risk tends to decrease with older age groups. While the effect was not significant during childhood (possibly because of small numbers—AHR 1.187; CI 0.877, 1.607), it was higher for younger adults aged 23–42 (AHR 1.097; CI

Table 1: Study participants by sweep, age, sex, diabetes status, proportion of elevated BMI, and loss to follow-up.

		Male				Female				All				
Sweep	Age	Diabetes-free	Newly diagnosed diabetes	Total	Elevated BMI (*N* (%))	Diabetes-free	Newly diagnosed diabetes	Total	Elevated BMI (*N* (%))	Diabetes-free	Newly diagnosed diabetes	Total	Elevated BMI (*N* (%))	Loss to follow-up
1	7	8537	2	8539	613 (7.18%)	8030	2	8032	770 (9.59%)	16,567	4	16,571	1383 (8.35%)	2
2	11	7683	6	7689	504 (6.55%)	7381	0	7381	688 (9.32%)	15,064	6	15,070	1192 (7.91%)	1503
3	16	7674	14	7688	449 (5.84%)	7374	9	7383	602 (8.15%)	15,048	23	15,071	1051 (6.97%)	1502
4	23	5297	5	5302	1006 (18.97%)	5495	10	5505	800 (14.53%)	10,792	15	10,807	1806 (16.71%)	5766
5	33	5571	18	5589	2753 (49.26%)	5766	27	5793	1985 (34.27%)	11,337	45	11,382	4738 (41.63%)	5191
6	42	5498	61	5559	3477 (62.55%)	5690	41	5731	2503 (43.67%)	11,188	102	11,290	5980 (52.97%)	5283
7	46	1191	76	1267	896 (70.72%)	1392	48	1440	765 (53.13%)	2583	124	2707	1661 (61.36%)	13,866
8	50	1319	29	1348	988 (73.29%)	1545	25	1570	923 (58.79%)	2864	54	2918	1911 (65.49%)	13,655
Total			211				162				373			

Elevated BMI (*N* (%)): number and proportion of subjects with BMI above normal (including overweight and obese).

TABLE 2: Unadjusted hazard ratios (HRs) of developing diabetes using univariate Cox regression analyses.

Characteristic	Levels	N (%)	Unadjusted HR (95% CI)	P value
Ethnicity ($n = 11316$)	Others	251 (2.22)	Reference	
	White	11,065 (97.78)	0.575 (0.306, 1.081)	0.0856
Sex ($n = 16573$)	Females	8034 (48.48)	Reference	
	Males	8539 (51.52)	1.389 (1.131, 1.704)	0.0017*
Birth weight ($n = 15043$)	Normal	12,761 (84.83)	Reference	
	Low birth weight	879 (5.84)	1.408 (0.942, 2.104)	0.0948
	High birth weight	1403 (9.33)	1.138 (0.801, 1.618)	0.4695
Social class ($n = 14764$)	I (professional occupations)	654 (4.43)	Reference	
	II (managerial and technical occupations)	1934 (13.10)	1.332 (0.639, 2.777)	0.4446
	III (skilled occupations)	8943 (60.57)	1.963 (1.007, 3.825)	0.0476*
	IV (partly skilled occupations)	1809 (12.25)	2.159 (1.058, 4.406)	0.0344*
	V (unskilled occupations)	1424 (9.65)	2.543 (1.227, 5.271)	0.0121*
Cumulative obesity dose ($n = 16573$)	10-unit increase		1.076 (1.068, 1.084)	<0.0001*
Time-varying BMI ($n = 16573$)	1-unit increase		1.098 (1.081, 1.115)	<0.0001*
Last BMI ($n = 16573$)	1-unit increase		1.137 (1.078, 1.198)	<0.0001*

* indicates significance at 0.05 level.

1.081, 1.113) than for adults older than 42 (AHR slightly lower at 1.074; CI 1.064, 1.084). Nonetheless, there was no difference in AIC between this model and model number 1 in Table 3 indicating that the differential effect of cumulative obesity dose on diabetes risk across different age groups is minimal.

4. Discussion

Using the data from the 1958 National Child Development Study (NCDS) [18], we have now confirmed that combining a measure of excess weight with its duration from age 7 - cumulative obesity dose - is a strong and independent predictor of diabetes risk over the life course. We have additionally shown that cumulative obesity dose provides a greater predictive ability for diabetes risk than models incorporating either the time-varying BMI or last BMI before diabetes diagnosis. Thus, the larger the cumulative obesity dose, the greater the hazard for diabetes, with each increase of 10 units in cumulative obesity dose conferring an approximately 8% increase in diabetes risk. Moreover, as a function of obesity duration in particular, we found that the older the age of overweight/obesity onset, the less likely the individual is to develop diabetes. This suggests that, for a given amount of cumulative obesity dose, a longer duration of obesity is relatively (but only slightly) more important than the degree of obesity. The most novel finding of this study is that adjusting for cumulative obesity dose greatly strengthened the relationship between low birth weight and diabetes risk. Finally, although male sex independently added to the risk of diabetes, we were unable to demonstrate that ethnicity (small numbers) [1], social class [21], and high birth weight [22] contributed to diabetes risk in this population of predominantly white British subjects, as have been shown in other jurisdictions.

Longer duration and younger onset of obesity have both been shown to increase T2DM risk [3–11], but only recently has there emerged a relatively consistent approach in using obesity history to predict diabetes occurrence. Preston and colleagues described four main approaches that have been used to evaluate the links between obesity history and subsequent morbidity/mortality [13]. These include strictly additive models, duration-of-obesity models, additive weight change models, and interactive models. Models including a duration-of-obesity component performed most strongly. At least four groups have now reported on slightly differing versions of the duration-of-obesity model, which combines time interval with the measure of the degree to which an individual's BMI exceeds either a normal BMI or some other BMI baseline to forecast T2DM risk [14–17]. This measure has been likened to pack years of smoking [4]. However, all of these studies have limitations with the absence of data from the younger portion of the life cycle, short study duration, the way in which the excess BMI was calculated, or a combination of those and other drawbacks.

Using the data from the National Longitudinal Study of Youth, the first major study (2012) [14] using a duration-of-obesity methodology calculated what was termed "excess BMI-years" by subtracting a reference BMI of 25 (or the 85th BMI percentile for adolescents) from participants' BMIs, averaging the differences between survey years, and determining the total excess BMI-years by multiplying average differences by the study duration. Lee et al. found that a greater absolute number of excess BMI-years was significantly associated with higher T2DM risk and the risk was amplified by longer duration (i.e., those who experienced excess BMIs at younger ages). The limitation to the study is that the 8446 participants were enrolled between ages 14 and 21 years, thus missing the possible impact of childhood obesity and high/low birth weight. Moreover, it only followed

TABLE 3: Adjusted hazard ratios (AHRs) of developing diabetes using multivariate Cox regression analyses.

Characteristic	Model number 0 AHR (95% CI)	Model number 0 *P* value	Model number 1 AHR (95% CI)	Model number 1 *P* value	Model number 2 AHR (95% CI)	Model number 2 *P* value	Model number 3 AHR (95% CI)	Model number 3 *P* value
Sex								
Males versus females	1.328 (1.072, 1.646)	0.0095	1.483 (1.192, 1.843)	0.0004	1.297 (1.046, 1.608)	0.0177	1.329 (1.072, 1.647)	0.0094
Birth weight								
Low birth weight versus normal	1.444 (0.966, 2.158)	0.0732	1.686 (1.125, 2.526)	0.0113	1.511 (1.010, 2.260)	0.0444	1.522 (1.017, 2.277)	0.0410
High birth weight versus normal	1.101 (0.774, 1.567)	0.5920	0.922 (0.647, 1.315)	0.6548	1.013 (0.712, 1.442)	0.9422	1.024 (0.719, 1.459)	0.8947
Cumulative obesity dose			1.080 (1.071, 1.088)	<0.0001				
Time-varying BMI					1.098 (1.080, 1.117)	<0.0001		
Last BMI							1.146 (1.084, 1.212)	<0.0001
Model evaluation								
AIC	5940.762		5716.317		5851.199		5922.872	
BIC	5952.257		5731.645		5866.526		5938.200	

Model number 1 included sex, birth weight, and cumulative obesity dose as covariates; model number 2 includes sex, birth weight, and time-varying BMI as covariates; model number 3 includes sex, birth weight, and last BMI as covariates.

TABLE 4: Adjusted hazard ratios (AHRs) of developing diabetes using multivariate Cox regression analyses: participants with the overweight/obesity onset during follow-up.

Characteristic	Model number 1 AHR (95% CI)	*P* value	Model number 2 AHR (95% CI)	*P* value	Model number 3 AHR (95% CI)	*P* value
Sex						
Males versus females	1.544 (1.211, 1.968)	0.0004	1.399 (1.101, 1.777)	0.0060	1.405 (1.106, 1.784)	0.0053
Birth weight						
Low birth weight versus normal	1.783 (1.137, 2.798)	0.0118	1.593 (1.017, 2.493)	0.0418	1.565 (1.000, 2.450)	0.0410
High birth weight versus normal	0.946 (0.651, 1.375)	0.7713	1.028 (0.708, 1.491)	0.8853	1.060 (0.731, 1.537)	0.8947
Age of obesity onset	0.988 (0.977, 1.000)	0.0434	0.976 (0.965, 0.986)	<0.0001	0.973 (0.962, 0.983)	<0.0001
Cumulative obesity dose	1.072 (1.062, 1.081)	<0.0001				
Time-varying BMI			1.080 (1.059, 1.101)	<0.0001		
Last BMI					1.044 (1.022, 1.066)	<0.0001
Model comparison						
Model with age of obesity onset						
AIC	4473.633		4605.563		4639.406	
BIC	4491.824		4623.772		4657.616	
Model without age of obesity onset						
AIC	4475.874		4625.230		4666.389	
BIC	4490.427		4639.798		4680.957	

TABLE 5: Interaction between cumulative obesity dose and age groups in risk for diabetes.

Characteristic	AHR (95% CI)	*P* value
Sex		
Males versus females	1.480 (1.190, 1.839)	0.0004
Birth weight		
Low birth weight versus normal	1.684 (1.124, 2.522)	0.0115
High birth weight versus normal	0.914 (0.641, 1.304)	0.6209
Cumulative obesity dose		
Childhood (age 7–16)	1.187 (0.877, 1.607)	0.2678
Young adult (age 23–42)	1.097 (1.081, 1.113)	<0.0001
Older adult (age above 42)	1.074 (1.064, 1.084)	<0.0001
Model evaluation		
AIC	5714.463	
BIC	5737.455	

participants for a total of 27 years when participants were aged 41–48. The second study (2013) [15] followed 1026 Framingham Offspring Study participants from their midthirties to midfifties using "cumulative excess weight" (CEW) as the outcome. CEW was calculated in a similar fashion to excess BMI-years (above) but was only associated with T2DM incidence for those with a normal BMI (<25) at baseline. Once again, the study was limited by a relatively short duration and an even larger omission of data from birth to early adulthood. Also, both of these studies in effect considered participants' BMIs below 25 as reducing diabetes risk since lower BMIs created a negative balance in their calculations.

Two more recent studies that have reported on this methodology both used different baseline BMIs in their calculations. Wei and colleagues [16] combined the data from the ARIC, CARDIA, and Framingham Heart studies to examine the relationship between "BMI-years" and incident diabetes. They followed over 17,000 participants stratified into two baseline age groups (30–44 and 45–59) for a median of 9 years and found that the younger cohort experienced a greater risk for incident diabetes than the older group for a given increase in BMI-years. However, unlike the other three studies, they used each subject's baseline BMI as the reference BMI and were once again limited by the short study duration and absence of early life data. Interestingly, another report (2015) [23] that analyzed the data from the CARDIA Study found a significant relationship between "excess BMI-years" (as well as "excess waist circumference-years") and incident cardiovascular disease. In doing so, they examined other outcomes including diabetes, which was also significantly associated with these measures. Finally, Abdullah and colleagues most recently [17] reported on the relationship between "obese-years" and T2DM risk, again using the data from the Framingham Offspring Study. They followed 5132 participants aged 5–85 (mean baseline age 37) for up to 45 years and, like the other studies, found a strong association between an increase in obese-years and T2DM risk. While study duration was longer than that of the other three studies and some children were included, the mean baseline age of 37 indicates that most participants were adults at the study onset. Moreover, a BMI of 29 was employed as the reference value to subtract from participants' BMIs. If the result was a negative value, it was considered to be 0. Thus, the main limitation to this study was the inability to consider the possible impact of overweight (BMIs 25–29) on diabetes risk.

While the studies summarized above are important in demonstrating a strong relationship between excess weight, its duration, and diabetes risk, we believe that our analysis of the data from the NCDS has methodological advantages compared to the others and is more robust in helping us to understand the contribution of increased adiposity to the pathophysiology of T2DM. With respect to methodology, we have first used a reference BMI of 25 (or corresponding values for children/youth) so we are able to take into account the impact of overweight (as well as obesity) on diabetes risk. Second, when subtracting participants' BMIs below 25 from our BMI reference, we have considered the difference to be zero. Although the studies by Lee et al. and Bouchard et al. also used a BMI reference of 25, participants' BMIs below that value created a negative balance which implies a reduced diabetes risk for which we can find no evidence. Because of these differences, we have used the new term "cumulative obesity dose" to describe our method. Third, our study is the only one to examine the relationship between cumulative obesity dose and diabetes risk in a birth cohort with data covering the time from birth to 50 years of age. It is therefore unique in its ability to include BMI values from childhood and adolescence in its analysis. Fourth, we were able to adjust for other important diabetes predictors including sex and socioeconomic status. Lower social class was a significant diabetes risk factor in univariate analysis but did not remain in final models, possibly because of the relationship between lower socioeconomic status and low birth weight. In a recent meta-analysis of the relationship between birth weight and type 2 diabetes, adjustment for social class did not appreciably influence that relationship [12]. Finally, ours is the only study to incorporate the impact of birth weight in analyzing the relationship between cumulative obesity dose and T2DM.

In the meta-analysis examining the birth weight/T2DM relationship [12], both high birth weight and low birth weight were shown to increase T2DM risk. The association of high birth weight with diabetes was initially demonstrated among indigenous peoples in North America and appears related to the impact of elevated rates of diabetic pregnancies and associated macrosomia in elevating T2DM risk in the offspring of diabetic mothers [22]. In contrast, low birth weight has been most commonly implicated as a T2DM risk factor among populations of middle-aged and older Europeans. Hales and Barker have proposed that this linkage is initiated through fetal undernutrition leading to a "thrifty phenotype" [24] wherein a maladaptive response to impaired islet cell development contributes to the later development of insulin resistance. However, it is not clear from previous studies whether the influence of low birth weight on the later development of T2DM is mediated through obesity or some other factors. The meta-analysis above found that the low birth weight/T2DM relationship was only minimally strengthened by adjustment for the current BMI. In the more recent Black Women's Health Study [25], low birth weight was also associated with increased T2DM risk but once again, adjustment for the current BMI did not materially change the incidence risk ratios.

As far as we are aware, no one has previously examined the possible interaction between birth weight and any measure of obesity history (i.e., rather than the current BMI) in strengthening the risk of T2DM. We have now shown that the relationship between low birth weight and diabetes is modestly strengthened by adjusting for the time-varying BMI and last BMI (AHR increased from 1.444 without measures of obesity to 1.511 and 1.522 for the time-varying BMI and last BMI, resp.). However, after adjusting for cumulative obesity dose, the AHR for the relationship between low birth weight and diabetes increased substantively from 1.444 to 1.686 and became significant ($P = 0.0113$). Thus, it appears that the degree and duration of excess weight do indeed play an intermediate role in the link between low birth weight and T2DM. Whether this is because the metabolic impact of the "thrifty phenotype" contributes to the predisposition to the early development of obesity and the subsequent increase in diabetes risk or the link between low birth weight and diabetes is simply enhanced by an unrelated and prolonged exposure to increased adiposity is not clear from our study. However, as far as we are aware, our findings provide the strongest evidence to date for an intermediary role of obesity in the link between low birth weight and diabetes and this has been made possible by considering obesity history rather than the current BMI.

We have summarized the strengths of our study above. Limitations include the large 82.4% loss to follow-up (although this is not unexpected in a cohort followed for 50 years) and the homogeneity of a white British population which prevented us from examining the possible impact of ethnicity on diabetes risk. We were unable to differentiate between type 1 and type 2 diabetes, but given that over 90% of incident cases of diabetes occurring during adulthood are T2DM, we believe that our findings largely relate to the impact of cumulative obesity dose on T2DM risk.

5. Conclusions

Cumulative obesity dose is an improved method for evaluating the impact of obesity degree and duration on diabetes risk and provides a better predictive ability for determining diabetes risk than either the time-varying BMI or current BMI. This supports the concept that it is the prolonged exposure to the metabolic consequences of excess weight that confers its pathophysiological link with T2DM, and this is consistent with an adverse effect on beta cell function and insulin resistance. Moreover, we have now made the unique observation that the link between low birth weight and T2DM is strengthened by an elevation in cumulative obesity dose, suggesting that this link is either mediated through or amplified by an early and sustained exposure to obesity.

Disclosure

UCL Institute of Education and the UK Data Archive and UK Data Service bear no responsibility for the analysis or interpretation of these data.

Conflicts of Interest

The authors declare that there is no conflict of interest regarding the publication of this article.

Acknowledgments

The authors are grateful to the Centre for Longitudinal Studies, UCL Institute of Education, for the use of NCDS data and to the UK Data Archive and UK Data Service for making them available.

References

[1] L. Chen, J. Magliano, and P. Z. Zimmet, "The worldwide epidemiology of type 2 diabetes mellitus—present and future perspectives," *Nature Reviews Endocrinology*, vol. 8, no. 4, pp. 228–236, 2012.

[2] M. I. McCarthy, "Genomics, type 2 diabetes and obesity," *The New England Journal of Medicine*, vol. 363, no. 24, pp. 2339–2350, 2010.

[3] J. E. Everhart, D. J. Pettitt, P. H. Bennett, and W. C. Knowler, "Duration of obesity increases the incidence of NIDDM," *Diabetes*, vol. 41, no. 2, pp. 235–240, 1992.

[4] F. L. Brancatti, N. Y. Wang, L. A. Mead, K. Y. Liang, and M. J. Klag, "Body weight patterns from 20 to 49 years of age and subsequent risk for diabetes mellitus: the Johns Hopkins Precursors Study," *Archives of Internal Medicine*, vol. 159, no. 9, pp. 957–963, 1999.

[5] J. A. Morrison, C. J. Glueck, J. G. Woo, and P. Wang, "Risk factors for cardiovascular disease and type 2 diabetes retained from childhood to adulthood predict adult outcomes: the Princeton LRC follow-up study," *International Journal of Pediatric Endocrinology*, vol. 2012, no. 1, p. 6, 2012.

[6] T. H. Inge, W. C. King, T. M. Jenkins et al., "The effect of obesity in adolescence on adult health status," *Pediatrics*, vol. 132, no. 6, pp. 1098–1104, 2013.

[7] N. S. The, A. S. Richardson, and P. Gordon-Larsen, "Timing and duration of obesity in relation to diabetes - findings from an ethnically diverse, nationally representative sample," *Diabetes Care*, vol. 36, no. 4, pp. 865–872, 2013.

[8] N. K. Mehta, S. Stenholm, I. T. Elo, A. Aromaa, M. Heliövaara, and S. Koskinen, "Weight histories and mortality among Finnish adults: the role of duration and peak body mass index," *Epidemiology*, vol. 25, no. 5, pp. 707–710, 2014.

[9] M. Charakida, T. Khan, W. Johnson et al., "Lifelong patterns of BMI and cardiovascular phenotype in individuals aged 60–64 years in the 1946 British birth cohort study: an epidemiological study," *The Lancet Diabetes & Endocrinology*, vol. 2, no. 8, pp. 648–654, 2014.

[10] C. G. Owen, V. V. Kapetanakis, A. R. Rudnicka et al., "Body mass index in early and middle adult life: prospective associations with myocardial infarction, stroke and diabetes over a 30-year period: the British Regional Heart Study," *BMJ Open*, vol. 5, no. 9, article e008105, 2015.

[11] M. Wang, Y. Yi, B. Roebothan et al., "Body mass index trajectories among middle-aged and elderly Canadians and associated health outcomes," *Journal of Environmental and Public Health*, vol. 2016, Article ID 7014857, 9 pages, 2016.

[12] P. H. Whincup, S. J. Kaye, C. G. Owen et al., "Birth weight and risk of type 2 diabetes: a systematic review," *JAMA*, vol. 300, no. 24, pp. 2886–2897, 2008.

[13] S. H. Preston, N. K. Mehta, and A. Stokes, "Modeling obesity histories in cohort analyses of health and mortality," *Epidemiology*, vol. 24, no. 1, pp. 158–166, 2013.

[14] J. M. Lee, A. Gebremariam, S. Vijan, and J. G. Gurney, "Excess body mass index-years, a measure of degree and duration of excess weight, and risk for incident diabetes," *Archives of Pediatrics & Adolescent Medicine*, vol. 166, no. 1, pp. 42–48, 2012.

[15] D. R. Bouchard, B. Porneala, I. Janssen et al., "Risk of type 2 diabetes and cumulative excess weight exposure in the Framingham Offspring Study," *Journal of Diabetes and its Complications*, vol. 27, no. 3, pp. 214–218, 2013.

[16] G. S. Wei, S. A. Coady, J. P. Reis et al., "Duration and degree of weight gain and incident diabetes in younger versus middle-aged black and white adults: ARIC, CARDIA, and the Framingham Heart Study," *Diabetes Care*, vol. 38, no. 11, pp. 2042–2049, 2015.

[17] A. Abdullah, F. A. Amin, F. Hanum et al., "Estimating the risk of type-2 diabetes using obese-years in a contemporary population of the Framingham Study," *Global Health Action*, vol. 9, no. 1, article 30421, 2016.

[18] June 2017, http://www.cls.ioe.ac.uk/page.aspx?&sitesectionid=724&sitesectiontitle=Welcome+to+the+1958+National+Child+Development+Study.

[19] T. J. Cole, M. C. Bellizzi, K. M. Flegal, and W. H. Dietz, "Establishing a standard definition for child overweight and obesity worldwide: international survey," *BMJ*, vol. 320, no. 7244, pp. 1240–1243, 2000.

[20] L. D. Fisher and D. Y. Lin, "Time-dependent covariates in the Cox proportional-hazards regression model," *Annual Review of Public Health*, vol. 20, no. 1, pp. 145–157, 1999.

[21] E. Agardh, P. Allebeck, J. Hallqvist, T. Moradi, and A. Sidorchuk, "Type 2 diabetes incidence and socio-economic position: a systematic review and meta-analysis," *International Journal of Epidemiology*, vol. 40, no. 3, pp. 804–818, 2011.

[22] R. F. Dyck, H. Klomp, and L. Tan, "From "thrifty genotype" to "hefty fetal phenotype": the relationship between high birthweight and diabetes in Saskatchewan registered Indians," *Canadian Journal of Public Health*, vol. 92, no. 5, pp. 340–344, 2001.

[23] J. P. Reis, N. Allen, E. P. Gunderson et al., "Excess body mass index- and waist circumference-years and incident cardiovascular disease: the CARDIA study," *Obesity*, vol. 23, no. 4, pp. 879–885, 2015.

[24] C. N. Hales and D. J. P. Barker, "Type 2 (non-insulin-dependent) diabetes mellitus: the thrifty phenotype hypothesis," *International Journal of Epidemiology*, vol. 42, no. 5, pp. 1215–1222, 2013.

[25] E. A. Ruiz-Narváez, J. R. Palmer, H. Gerlovin et al., "Birth weight and risk of type 2 diabetes in the Black Women's Health Study: does adult BMI play a mediating role?," *Diabetes Care*, vol. 37, no. 9, pp. 2572–2578, 2014.

18

Sex Differences in the Prevalence and Modulators of Sleep-Disordered Breathing in Outpatients with Type 2 Diabetes

T. Kroner,[1] M. Arzt,[1] M. Rheinberger,[2] M. Gorski,[3] I. M. Heid,[3] C. A. Böger,[2] and S. Stadler[1]

[1]*Department of Internal Medicine II, University Hospital Regensburg, Franz-Josef-Strauss-Allee 11, 93053 Regensburg, Germany*
[2]*Department of Nephrology, University Hospital Regensburg, Franz-Josef-Strauss-Allee 11, 93053 Regensburg, Germany*
[3]*Department of Genetic Epidemiology, University of Regensburg, Franz-Josef-Strauss-Allee 11, 93053 Regensburg, Germany*

Correspondence should be addressed to S. Stadler; stefan.stadler@ukr.de

Academic Editor: Raffaele Marfella

In patients with type 2 diabetes, sleep-disordered breathing is a widespread cause of deteriorated quality of life. However, robust prevalence estimates for sleep-disordered breathing in patients with type 2 diabetes are limited due to scarce data. We investigated sex differences in sleep-disordered breathing prevalence and its modulators in the DIACORE SDB substudy, a sample of outpatient type 2 diabetes. 721 participants were tested for sleep-disordered breathing using a two-channel sleep apnoea monitoring device. Patients were stratified according to the severity of sleep-disordered breathing, defined as an apnoea-hypopnoea index < 15, ≥ 15 to 29, and ≥ 30 events per hour as no/mild, moderate, and severe sleep-disordered breathing, respectively. In the 679 analysed patients (39% women, age 66 ± 9 years, body mass index $31.0 \pm 5.4\,\mathrm{kg/m^2}$), the prevalence of sleep-disordered breathing was 34%. The prevalence of sleep-disordered breathing was higher in men than in women (41% versus 22%, $p < 0.001$) and increased with age (15%, 21%, and 30% in women and 35%, 40%, and 47% in men in those aged 18–59, 60–69, or ≥ 70, respectively; age trend $p = 0.064$ in women and $p = 0.15$ in men). In linear regression analysis, age, BMI, and waist-hip ratio were associated with apnoea-hypopnoea index. Modulators for higher apnoea-hypopnoea index seem to be similar in men and women.

1. Introduction

The International Diabetes Federation reports a worldwide prevalence of diabetes mellitus of 8.8%, where type 2 diabetes (T2D) makes up 87–91% in high-income countries and is more common in men than in women [1]. Because of the aging population and the increasing number of obese people, the prevalence of T2D has become more than doubled during the last three decades [2]. T2D may lead to several late diabetic comorbidities like neuropathy, nephropathy, and arteriosclerosis.

Sleep-disordered breathing (SDB), which is classified into obstructive and central sleep apnoea, is characterised by repetitive apnoeas and hypopnoeas, arousals from sleep as well as alterations of heart rate, and elevated blood pressure [3, 4]. Using an apnoea-hypopnoea index (AHI) cut-off of ≥ 15/h, the prevalence of SDB ranges from 7 to 14% in men and 2 to 7% in women, with increases over the last two decades [5, 6].

It is well documented that treatment with positive airway pressure effectively suppresses obstructive sleep apnoea, reduces sleep fragmentation, and restores normal sleep structure in patients with cardiac disease [7, 8]. It leads to significant improvement of daytime sleepiness and quality of life, even in patients reporting only mild SDB-related symptoms [9]. Previous studies investigated the association between SDB and T2D. When focusing on moderate to severe forms of SDB (AHI ≥ 15/h) with an indication for treatment [4], 24 to 53% of patients with T2D suffer from SDB [10–12], compared to 16% without T2D [10].

However, previous studies provide only limited information about the prevalence and its modulators for SDB in women with diabetes. Even if there was a nearly balanced ratio in the number of men and women in most studies, they used smaller sample sizes [10–12] or included only selected patients such as obese [12] or hospitalized patients [13]. Both T2D and SDB are common in men and women, but often underdiagnosed in women [14, 15]. We analysed a sample of patients with T2D with an equal number of men and women (61%/$n = 412$ men and 39%/$n = 267$ women) and investigated sex differences in the prevalence of SDB as well as modulators that were associated with SDB.

2. Material and Methods

2.1. Study Design. The investigated patients were participants of the DIACORE (DIAbetes COhoRtE) SDB substudy [16]. DIACORE is designed as a two-center, prospectively planned study of T2D patients of European descent, with a baseline survey conducted in 2010–2014 and recruitment and ascertainment described previously [16, 17]. Briefly, written invitations were mailed to all T2D patients registered with five medical insurance companies in the respective year of the mailing and to all T2D outpatients of two diabetologists in Regensburg that had visited the offices within the last 6 months of the mailing. Further, invitations were sent to T2D patients who had received inpatient treatment at the University Hospital Regensburg's Internal Medicine Departments within two years prior to the mailing. Overall, 4226 patients contacted DIACORE, of which 1226 did not fulfil the inclusion and exclusion criteria. Diabetes status was ascertained by assessing diabetes medication or by validating self-report. Patients were subjected to a standardized online questionnaire, blood sampling, and physical examination at the two study centers.

Of 1036 individuals invited to participate in the DIACORE SDB substudy, 721 individuals with T2D from the region around Regensburg, Germany, agreed to participate and were tested with a two-channel ambulatory SDB monitoring device (ApneaLink®, ResMed). In 679 patients (94% of the 721 tested), complete SDB parameters were recorded. Apparative monitoring for SDB was not performed in the Mannheim study center. A two-year follow-up is currently ongoing [17]; for this investigation, the cross-sectional baseline dataset was used. The protocol, data protection strategy, and study procedures were approved by the ethics committees of both participating institutions and are in accordance with the Declaration of Helsinki. Patients participated in DIACORE only after providing informed written consent.

2.2. Study Population. All T2D outpatients inhabiting the city and county of Regensburg or Speyer were eligible for DIACORE. Further inclusion criteria were the ability to fully understand the study information and to provide written informed consent, age ≥ 18 years, and self-reported Caucasian ethnicity. Exclusion criteria were chronic renal replacement therapy (haemodialysis, peritoneal dialysis, or transplantation), history of active malignancy within the last five years, autoimmune-disease potentially affecting kidney function, hemochromatosis, known pancreoprivic or self-reported type 1 diabetes, acute infection, fever, pregnancy, and chronic viral hepatitis or HIV-infection. For the DIACORE SDB substudy, patients were included if they consented to perform SDB monitoring and excluded if they currently use positive airway pressure therapy.

2.3. Assessment of SDB. Nasal flow and pulse oximetry were measured using the ApneaLink device (ResMed, Sydney, Australia), which has been validated in several studies for testing of SDB as described previously [18, 19] and is easy to mount at home by the patient himself. Trained study personnel instructed participants in the use of the device in a standardized fashion. Comparing ApneaLink to the gold standard polysomnography, studies have reported a sensitivity of 73–94% and a specificity of 85–95% using an AHI cut-off value of 15/h [19, 20]. AHI, oxygen desaturation index (ODI), mean oxygen saturation (SpO_2), and minimum SpO_2 were documented. The default settings of the monitoring device were used for the definitions of apnoea, hypopnoea, and desaturation: apnoea was defined as a ≥ 80% decrease in airflow for ≥10 seconds; hypopnoea was defined as a decrease in airflow by 50–80% versus baseline for ≥10 seconds followed by a ≥ 4% decrease in oxygen saturation.

No or mild SDB was defined as AHI < 15/h, moderate SDB as AHI ≥ 15/h to 29/h, and severe SDB was defined as AHI ≥ 30/h. Periodic breathing (Cheyne-Stokes respiration) was detected by automatic pattern recognition [21]. Due to the lack of a chest band, a clear differentiation between types of SDB, such as obstructive and central apnoea, was not possible.

Additionally, subjective daytime sleepiness was assessed using the self-administered validated Epworth Sleepiness Scale (ESS). Individuals were asked to rate their likelihood of falling asleep in several common situations. Scores range from 0 (least sleepy) to 24 (sleepiest). Excessive daytime sleepiness is defined as a score of 11 or higher [22].

2.4. Statistical Analysis. Descriptive data are presented as absolute and relative numbers or as mean ± standard deviation (SD). Normally distributed values of baseline characteristics were evaluated with analysis of variance (ANOVA). Differences in AHI between age groups were tested with ANOVA and followed by pair-wise *t*-tests (Bonferroni corrected level of significance); sex differences in AHI were tested with *t*-tests.

Linear regression models were used for continuous variables and logistic regression for categorical variables, in order to investigate the association between different clinical variables. Sex, age, body mass index (BMI), waist-hip ratio, systolic blood pressure, and duration of T2D were included as covariates in these models. Variables included in the linear regression models were either normally distributed or transformed prior to incorporation in the models. Results are given as regression coefficient *B* in linear models and as odds ratio OR in logistic regression models with 95% confidence interval (CI); *p* values less than 0.05 were considered statistically significant. Data were analysed using the SPSS statistical software package (SPSS 20.0, IBM SPSS Statistics, Armonk, New York, USA).

TABLE 1: Clinical characteristics of the 679 analysed subjects of the DIACORE baseline visit.

Characteristic	Women ($n = 267$)	Men ($n = 412$)	All ($n = 679$)
Age [years]	65 ± 10	66 ± 8	66 ± 9
BMI [kg/m^2]	31.9 ± 6.0	30.3 ± 4.8	31.0 ± 5.4
Waist-hip ratio	0.9 ± 0.07	1.00 ± 0.06	0.96 ± 0.08
Waist circumference [cm]	98 ± 14	102 ± 18	101 ± 17
Triglycerides [mg/dl]	163 ± 80	177 ± 156	171 ± 131
HDL-C [mg/dl]	58 ± 16	50 ± 13	53 ± 15
T2D duration [years]	9.4 ± 7.5	10.6 ± 8.3	10.1 ± 8.0
HbA_{1c} [%]	6.8 ± 1.0	6.9 ± 1.2	6.8 ± 1.1
HbA_{1c} [mmol/mol]	50.8 ± 12.6	51.9 ± 10.4	50.8 ± 11.5
HOMA-IR†	6.3 ± 8.5	6.0 ± 6.7	6.1 ± 7.4
Systolic BP [mmHg]	136 ± 18	139 ± 18	138 ± 18
Metabolic syndrome [%]*	83.5	68.8	74.6
Coronary artery disease [%]	9.7	28.4	21.1
Acute myocardial infarction [%]	6.0	15.8	11.9
Insulin [%]	24.0	28.6	26.8
Oral antidiabetics [%]	76.4	76.5	76.4
Sulfonylureas [%]	13.5	21.8	18.6
Incretins [%]	21.3	23.5	22.7

Data are expressed as percentage (%) for categorical variables and mean ± standard deviation for continuous variables. BMI = body mass index; HDL-C = high-density lipoprotein cholesterol; T2D = type 2 diabetes; BP = blood pressure; HbA_{1c} = glycated hemoglobin; HOMA-IR = homeostasis model assessment insulin resistance (fasting, use of long-acting insulin). $^\dagger n = 413$. *Metabolic syndrome is defined according to NCEP criteria [26].

3. Results

3.1. Patient Characteristics. Of the 721 patients with T2D that were tested for SDB, 42 patients had incomplete data recordings and could not be analysed (online Supplement Figure S1). Of these, 679 participants were entered into the analysis, of which 39% ($n = 267$) were women. Patients were 66 ± 9 years old, and BMI was 31.0 ± 5.4 kg/m^2. Their glycated haemoglobin (HbA_{1c}) was 6.8 ± 1.1%, and the average duration of T2D was 10.1 ± 8.0 years (Table 1). Women were of about the same age compared to men, but had a higher BMI ($p < 0.001$) and lower diabetes duration ($p = 0.057$) than men.

Patients with severe SDB were older, predominantly male, and had a significant higher BMI as well as waist-hip ratio compared to patients with no/mild SDB ($p = 0.088$, $p = 0.002$, $p < 0.001$, and $p < 0.001$, resp.) (Table 2). Patients with severe SDB had also a significant larger waist circumference ($p < 0.001$). They showed lower high-density lipoprotein cholesterol (HDL-C) as well as higher systolic blood pressure, higher triglyceride levels, and more severe insulin resistance quantified by homeostasis model assessment (HOMA-IR [23]), but these values were not statistically significant. HbA_{1c} levels and T2D duration were comparable. Administration of incretin may have implications on prognosis for myocardial infarction in patients with T2D [24, 25]. In our study, there was no difference in incretin administration between women and men (Table 1) as well as between different severities of SDB (Table 2).

3.2. SDB Parameters. Table 2 presents the different SDB parameters and symptoms. ODI increased with higher severity of SDB. AHI was significantly higher in men than in women (mean 16 versus 11 per hour, resp., $p < 0.001$), also when patients were divided into different age groups (Figure 1). Additionally, AHI increased between the different age groups ($p = 0.102$ in men, $p = 0.045$ in women, and $p = 0.006$ overall, tested by ANOVA). Furthermore, patients with moderate or severe SDB spent more than 2 hours with $SpO_2 < 90\%$ (Table 2).

3.3. The Prevalence of SDB in Patients with T2D. The prevalence of SDB in our study sample was 22% in women, 41% in men, and 34% overall. The prevalence of SDB was significantly higher in men compared to women overall ($p < 0.001$) (Figure 2) and in each age group ($p = 0.004$, $p = 0.001$, and $p = 0.009$) (Figure 3). Using an alternative definition of clinically relevant SDB (AHI ≥ 5/h + ESS ≥ 11 or AHI ≥ 15/h) led to similar results (44% in men, 24% in women, and 36% overall; $p < 0.001$) (Figure 2). The prevalence of SDB in both men and women increased with age, but this was statistically only significant in the whole sample ($p = 0.151$ in men; $p = 0.069$ in women; and $p = 0.014$ in either sex, tested by logistic regression analysis) (Figure 3).

3.4. Modulators Associated with SDB in Patients with Type 2 Diabetes. Using logistic regression by sex, age ≥ 70 years, BMI ≥ 30 kg/m^2, waist-hip ratio ≥ 0.85 in women and ≥0.9 in men [27] as well as systolic blood pressure ≥ 130 mmHg, and T2D duration were analysed as covariates all in one

TABLE 2: Clinical and SDB parameters of the 679 analysed participants at the DIACORE baseline visit by SDB class.

	No or mild SDB (AHI < 15)	Moderate SDB (AHI ≥ 15 to 29)	Severe SDB (AHI ≥ 30)	p value[∞]	Moderate versus no/mild SDB[$]	Severe versus no/mild SDB[$]
Number of patients, n (%)	451 (66%)	163 (24%)	65 (10%)			
Age [years]	64 ± 9	66 ± 8	67 ± 7	**0.008**	**0.030**	0.088
Female, n (%)	208 (46%)	43 (26%)	16 (25%)	**<0.001**	**<0.001**	**0.002**
BMI [kg/m^2]	30.4 ± 5.1	31.3 ± 5.2	34.0 ± 6.8	**<0.001**	0.139	**<0.001**
Waist-hip ratio	0.95 ± 0.08	0.98 ± 0.07	1.00 ± 0.08	**<0.001**	**<0.001**	**<0.001**
Waist circumference [cm]	99 ± 16	102 ± 16	112 ± 15	**<0.001**	0.054	**<0.001**
Triglycerides [mg/dl]	166 ± 125	181 ± 155	187 ± 107	0.273	0.597	0.699
HDL-C [mg/dl]	54 ± 16	51 ± 14	50 ± 13	**0.016**	0.080	0.080
T2D duration [years]	10 ± 7	12 ± 10	9 ± 7	**0.001**	**0.001**	1.000
HbA_{1c} [%]	6.8 ± 1.1	6.9 ± 1.2	6.6 ± 0.7	0.111	0.867	0.340
HbA_{1c} [mmol/mol]	51 ± 7	52 ± 8	49 ± 5	0.111	0.867	0.340
HOMA-IR[†]	5.6 ± 5.9	6.7 ± 9.1	7.9 ± 10.9	0.137	0.607	0.242
Systolic BP [mmHg]	137 ± 18	140 ± 19	141 ± 17	**0.041**	0.135	0.179
Metabolic syndrome [%] *	71.8	78.4	84.6	**0.038**	0.290	0.079
Coronary artery disease [%]	16.0	23.3	20.0	0.101	0.083	0.235
Acute myocardial infarction [%]	10.9	13.5	15.4	0.448	1.000	0.882
Insulin [%]	22.6	37.4	29.2	**0.001**	**0.001**	0.771
Oral antidiabetics [%]	77.6	74.2	73.8	0.601	1.000	1.000
Sulfonylureas [%]	19.3	18.4	13.8	0.573	1.000	0.877
Incretins [%]	24.4	18.4	21.5	0.288	0.355	1.000
SDB parameters						
AHI [/h]	7 ± 4	21 ± 4	46 ± 12	**0.001**	**<0.001**	**<0.001**
ODI [/h]	7 ± 5	20 ± 5	41 ± 12	**0.001**	**<0.001**	**<0.001**
SpO_2 < 90% [min]	73 ± 106	125 ± 122	120 ± 85	**0.001**	**<0.001**	**0.004**
SpO_2 [%]	93 ± 2	92 ± 2	92 ± 2	**0.001**	**<0.001**	**<0.001**
Min SpO_2 [%]	80 ± 12	75 ± 16	74 ± 15	**0.001**	**0.001**	**0.002**
Nocturnal breathing rate [/min]	15 ± 3	14 ± 3	12 ± 3	**0.001**	0.064	**<0.001**
Nocturnal heart rate [/min]	66 ± 9	66 ± 10	67 ± 10	0.667	1.000	1.000
ESS	5.1 ± 3.3	5.4 ± 3.6	5.9 ± 3.1	0.148	1.000	0.195
ESS ≥ 11, n (%)	29 (6.5)	10 (6.4)	6 (9.5)	0.661	1.000	1.000
Nocturia (≥3x/night) [%]	64 (14%)	25 (16%)	11 (17%)	0.785	1.000	1.000

Data are expressed as percentage (%) for categorical variables and mean ± standard deviation for continuous variables. [∞]Difference of parameters between the three SDB groups assessed by chi-square tests for categorical variables and by ANOVA for continuous variables. [$]Difference of parameters between two SDB groups assessed by post hoc analysis (Bonferroni). $p < 0.05$ was considered statistically significant and marked in bold. SDB = sleep-disordered breathing; BMI = body mass index; HDL-C = high-density lipoprotein cholesterol; T2D = type 2 diabetes; BP = blood pressure; HbA_{1c} = glycated hemoglobin; HOMA-IR = homeostasis model assessment insulin resistance (fasting, use of long-acting insulin); AHI = apnoea-hypopnoea index; ODI = oxygen desaturation index; SpO_2 = peripheral oxygen saturation; ESS = Epworth Sleepiness Scale. [†]n = 413. *Metabolic syndrome is defined according to NCEP criteria [26].

model to investigate an association with SDB (AHI ≥ 15/h). In women, age ≥ 70 years (OR 1.95, 95% CI [1.04, 3.66], $p = 0.039$) and systolic blood pressure ≥ 130 mmHg (OR 2.09, 95% CI [1.09, 4.02], $p = 0.026$) were significantly and independently associated with SDB. BMI ≥ 30 kg/m^2, waist-hip ratio ≥ 0.85, and T2D duration were not significantly associated with SDB (OR 1.56 [0.82, 2.97], $p = 0.175$; OR 2.64 [0.97, 7.14], $p = 0.057$; and OR 0.99 [0.95, 1.04], $p = 0.733$, resp.).

In men, BMI ≥ 30 kg/m^2 (OR 2.27, 95% CI [1.49, 3.47], $p < 0.001$) and T2D duration (per year; OR 1.03, 95% CI [1.00, 1.05], $p = 0.033$) were significant and independent modulators were associated with SDB. Age ≥ 70 years, waist-hip ratio ≥ 0.9, and systolic blood pressure ≥ 130 mmHg were not significantly associated with SDB in men (OR 1.52 [0.97, 2.37], $p = 0.056$; OR 1.05 [0.37, 2.96], $p = 0.929$; and OR 1.10 [0.70, 1.73], $p = 0.676$, resp.).

Using a general regression model including both sexes with sex, age ≥ 70 years, BMI ≥ 30 kg/m^2, waist-hip ratio ≥ 0.85, systolic blood pressure ≥ 130 mmHg, and T2D duration as covariates, besides age ≥ 70 years (OR 1.65, 95% CI 1.2, 2.4, $p = 0.007$) and BMI ≥ 30 kg/m^2 (OR 2.08, 95% CI

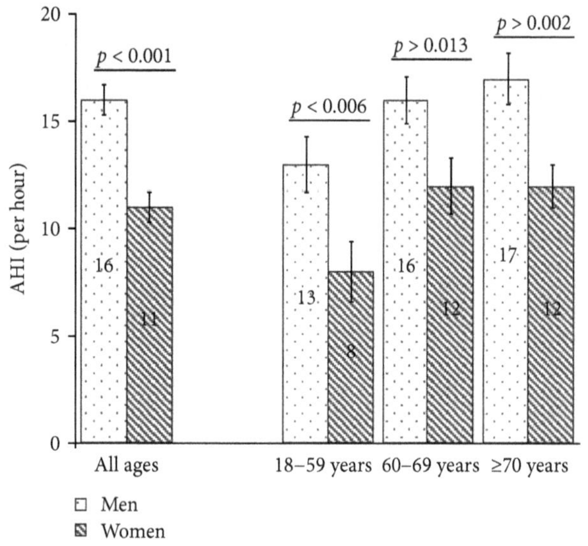

FIGURE 1: Apnoea-hypopnoea index (AHI) in men and women of the total sample ($n = 679$) and of different age groups (18–59, 60–69, and ≥70 years) ($n = 164$, $n = 286$, and $n = 229$), stating mean values in the bar and including standard errors and p values from t-tests. AHI was significantly higher in men than in women in the whole sample as well as in different age groups.

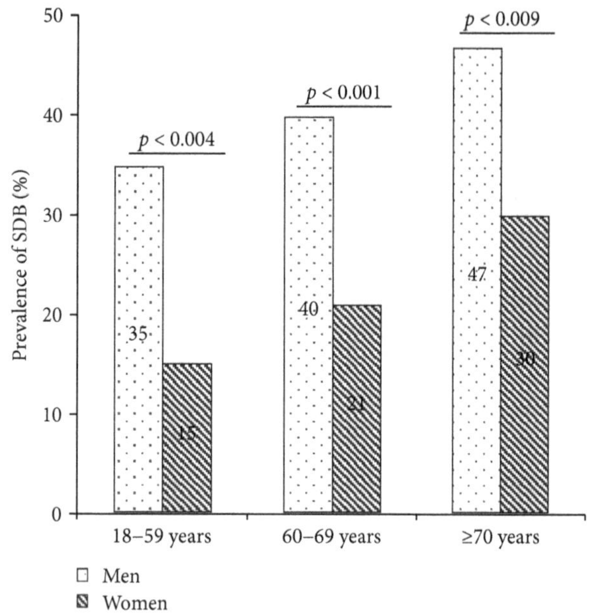

FIGURE 3: Bar charts with the prevalence of sleep-disordered breathing (SDB) in men and women in different age groups (%); p values were assessed by chi-square tests. $n = 679$. SDB was significantly more present in men than in women in each age group.

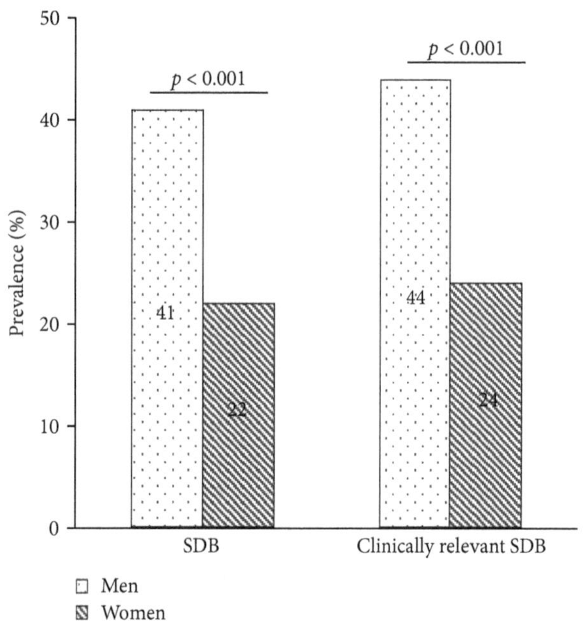

FIGURE 2: Bar charts showing the prevalence of sleep-disordered breathing (SDB) and clinically relevant SDB (AHI ≥5/h + ESS ≥ 11 or AHI ≥ 15/h) in 412 men and 267 women (%); p values assessed by chi-square tests. $n = 679$. SDB as well as clinically relevant SDB was significantly more present in men than in women.

1.5, 3.0, $p < 0.001$), only male sex was independently associated with SDB (OR 2.57, 95% CI 1.7, 3.8, $p < 0.001$). WHR ≥ 0.85, systolic blood pressure ≥ 130 mmHg, and T2D duration were not significantly associated with SDB in either sex (OR 1.87, 95% CI [0.8, 4.4], $p = 0.156$; OR 1.37, 95% CI [1.0, 2.0], $p = 0.091$; and OR 1.02, 95% CI [0.99, 1.04], $p = 0.106$, resp.).

In regression models with all covariates listed above plus including interaction terms of each of the other covariates with sex, no interaction with sex was detected (interaction terms for age ≥ 70 years, BMI ≥ 30 kg/m^2, WHR ≥ 0.85, systolic blood pressure ≥ 130 mmHg, and T2D duration: $p = 0.527$, $p = 0.333$, $p = 0.999$, $p = 0.128$, and $p = 0.280$, resp.). Thus, modulators for SDB seem to be similar in men and women.

3.5. Modulators Associated with AHI in Patients with Type 2 Diabetes. Linear regression analysis (Table 3) showed that a higher AHI was independently associated with higher age, higher BMI, and higher waist-hip ratio in women. In men, only age and BMI, but not waist-hip ratio, were significantly associated with AHI.

In the entire sample, male sex, age, BMI, and waist-hip ratio were associated with a higher AHI independent of the other covariates. Systolic blood pressure and T2D duration showed no significant association with AHI in either sex.

Adding an interaction term of waist-hip ratio with sex to the regression model stated above, no interaction with sex was detected (interaction $p = 0.503$). Thus, modulators for a higher AHI seem to be similar in men and women.

Both, metabolic syndrome and SDB are known to promote cardiovascular disease and arrhythmia [28–30]. Due to this, we added metabolic syndrome to the multivariable analysis and it appeared as a significant modulator of AHI in the whole sample ($B = 5.139$; 95% CI 2.913, 7.364; $p < 0.001$) as well as in women ($B = 5.099$; 95% CI 1.422,

TABLE 3: Linear regression analysis: factors associated with AHI in the total population, in 267 women and in 412 men.

Variable	*Univariable analysis* B (95% CI)	p value	*Multivariable analysis* B (95% CI)	p value
Total population ($n = 679$)				
Female sex	−4.75 (−6.74, −2.76)	**<0.001**	−3.54 (−6.06, −1.02)	**0.006**
Age [per 10 years]	1.70 (0.59, 2.81)	**0.003**	2.55 (1.40, 3.70)	**<0.001**
BMI [per 5 units]	2.99 (2.10, 3.88)	**<0.001**	3.48 (2.53, 4.44)	**<0.001**
Waist-hip ratio [per 0.1 unit]	4.48 (3.25, 5.71)	**<0.001**	2.35 (0.77, 3.94)	**0.004**
Systolic BP	0.08 (0.03, 0.13)	**0.004**	0.02 (−0.04, 0.07)	0.508
T2D duration	0.09 (−0.04, 0.21)	0.165	−0.004 (−0.13, 0.12)	0.952
Women ($n = 267$)				
Age [per 10 years]	1.92 (0.49, 3.35)	**0.009**	2.35 (0.83, 3.87)	**0.003**
BMI [per 5 units]	2.00 (0.87, 3.13)	**0.001**	2.05 (0.88, 3.21)	**0.001**
Waist-hip ratio [per 0.1 units]	3.24 (1.13, 5.35)	**0.003**	2.29 (0.18, 4.40)	**0.034**
Systolic BP	0.08 (0.01, 0.16)	**0.037**	0.03 (−0.05, 0.11)	0.446
T2D duration	0.06 (−0.13, 0.25)	0.527	−0.02 (−0.02, 0.17)	0.826
Men ($n = 412$)				
Age [per 10 years]	1.41 (−0.19, 3.01)	0.084	2.76 (1.09, 4.43)	**0.001**
BMI [per 5 units]	4.75 (3.45, 6.06)	**<0.001**	5.25 (3.73, 6.77)	**<0.001**
Waist-hip ratio [per 0.1 units]	4.92 (2.71, 7.12)	**<0.001**	1.59 (−0.77, 3.94)	0.185
Systolic BP	0.06 (−0.01, 0.14)	0.091	0.01 (−0.06, 0.09)	0.739
T2D duration	0.07 (−0.09, 0.23)	0.393	0.01 (−0.15, 0.17)	0.882

AHI = apnoea-hypopnoea index; B = unstandardized regression coefficient; 95% CI = 95% confidence interval; BMI = body mass index; T2D duration = duration of type 2 diabetes; BP = blood pressure.

8.776; $p = 0.007$) and in men ($B = 5.186$; 95% CI 2.350, 8.022; $p < 0.001$).

4. Discussion

The present study investigating SDB in 679 patients with T2D obtained several key findings. First, moderate to severe SDB, defined as AHI ≥ 15/h, is present in more than a third of our patients with T2D. Second, the prevalence of moderate to severe SDB increases with age and is more common in men than in women yielding a prevalence of 40% and 21% in our sample of 60 to 69-year-old men or women, respectively. Third, age, BMI, and waist-hip ratio are significant and independent modulators were associated with higher AHI. There were no significant differences of these effects between men and women.

The prevalence of SDB in community samples was modestly lower than in samples of patients with T2D. In obese participants of the same age group with a BMI (30.0 to 39.9 kg/m^2) as seen in our sample, 29% of men and 14% of women have SDB [5].

Our results of 34% of patients with T2D with SDB are consistent with the seven prior studies including more than 150 patients with T2D and using polysomnography or SDB monitoring devices for diagnosis of SDB (Table 4). Differences in prevalence could be explained by differences in participant recruiting, patient characteristics, definitions of sleep apnoea, or methods of monitoring for SDB (Table 4 and online Supplement Table S2).

Some studies showed higher prevalence estimates than our study [12, 31] (Table 4). The reason for these higher prevalence estimates might be explained by a higher BMI of participants (Foster et al. BMI = 36.5 ± 5.8 kg/m^2, Schober et al. BMI = 32.6 ± 6.7 kg/m^2, and BMI = 31.0 ± 5.4 kg/m^2 in the DIACORE SDB substudy) [12, 31] since obesity is a known risk factor for SDB [1, 32, 33].

Other studies showed lower prevalence estimates. The patient populations of those studies had significantly lower BMI (25.1 ± 3.6 kg/m^2) [34] or were significantly younger [10, 13].

Similar to previous studies [31, 35], we found a higher prevalence of SDB in men than in women.

In previous studies, varied information about the modulators of SDB in patients with diabetes has been presented. Lam et al. found that male sex, higher age as well as BMI, and diastolic blood pressure were independently associated with AHI [35]. In the present study, age, BMI, and waist-hip ratio were significantly associated with AHI.

Even if there were no significant differences in modulators for a higher AHI between the sexes, waist-hip ratio showed an association with AHI in women in the DIACORE substudy. This finding might be explained by the differences in the distribution of bodily fat between the sexes. In women, fat accumulation in the hip region is more common compared to men [36]. Therefore, it is possible that the effect of a pathologically increased waist-hip ratio on AHI could be higher in women than in men.

Table 4: The prevalence and risk factors of SDB in T2D, comparison of existing studies.

Study, year (Ref.), country	Setting	Patients (n)	Source of patients	SDB diagnosis	Female, n (%)	Prevalence of SDB (%)	Modulators of SDB/higher AHI
Resnick et al., 2003 [10][x], USA	Multicenter	470	Sleep Heart Health Study (SDB as risk factor for the development of cardiovascular disease)	Polysomnography (Compumedics PS®, Melbourne, Australia)	254 (54)	24	AHI: age, BMI, male sex
Einhorn et al., 2007 [11], USA	Single center	279	Diabetes clinic (T2D)	SDB monitoring device (ApneaLink, ResMed Corp., San Diego, CA, USA)	133 (48)	36	SDB: age $\geq$ 62 yrs, male sex, BMI $\geq$ 30 kg/m^2, snoring, reports of stopping breathing during sleep
Laaban et al., 2009 [13], France	Single center	303	Department of Diabetology (hospitalized for poorly controlled T2D)	SDB monitoring device (CID® 102, Cidelec, Angers, France)	147 (49)	29	—
Foster et al., 2009 [12], USA	Multicenter	305	Obese patients with T2D (Sleep AHEAD = Sleep Apnea in Look AHEAD—Action for Health in Diabetes)	Polysomnography (Compumedics®, Abbotsville, Australia)	183 (60)	53[#]	AHI/obstructive sleep apnoea [*]: waist circumference
Lam et al., 2010 [35], China	Single center	165	DM clinic	Polysomnography (Alice 5 Diagnostics System®, Respironics, Murrysville, PA, USA)	62 (38)	33[#]	AHI: age, BMI, diastolic BP, male sex[†]
Schober et al., 2011 [31], Germany	Multicenter	498	Primary care centers and medical department (endocrinology, metabolism)	SDB monitoring device (ApneaLink Oxi®, ResMed, Sydney, Australia)	237 (48)	41	—
Zhang et al., 2016 [34], China	Multicenter	880	Endocrinology ward (hospitalized)	SDB monitoring device (ApneaLink, ResMed, San Diego, CA, USA)	391 (44)	26	—
Kroner et al. (DIACORE), Germany	Multicenter	679	Outpatients	SDB monitoring device (ApneaLink, ResMed, Sydney, Australia)	267 (39)	34	AHI: age, BMI, waist-hip ratio

[*] At cut-off AHI $\geq$ 5/h. [†] n = 162 (3 subjects with central sleep apnoea were excluded). [#] Prevalence of obstructive sleep apnoea. [x] It is not apparent which kind of diabetes sample was used. In other publications, it is interpreted as a sample of patients with type 2 diabetes [37]. Modulators of SDB/higher AHI were assessed in multivariable regression analysis. SDB = sleep-disordered breathing; BMI = body mass index; T2D = type 2 diabetes; AHI = apnoea-hypopnoea index; BP = blood pressure; RDI = respiratory disturbance index.

There is evidence that diabetes and its level of severity could contribute to the development of SDB and its worsening [38, 39]. Although this was only a cross-sectional analysis, our data do not support this hypothesis, since HbA_{1c}, HOMA-IR, and the duration of diabetes were not associated with the presence or severity of SDB.

On the other hand, there is evidence that SDB may contribute to impaired glucose metabolism [40]. Studies investigating the effects of treatment of obstructive sleep apnoea with continuous positive airway pressure show different results. In a randomized controlled trial, this therapy significantly improved glucose tolerance [41]. However, other studies did not find any changes in glycaemic control [42, 43].

Particularly, T2D results in very high economic and social costs [1]. Due to the evidence of a mutual impact of T2D and SDB, the high proportion of SDB in patients with T2D, and the clinical relevance, monitoring for SDB might be profitable as this proportion of patients could benefit from SDB therapy.

Especially patients with typical symptoms like daytime sleepiness, heavy snoring or already occurring apnoeas should be tested for SDB [33, 44], because treatment of SDB with continuous positive airway pressure improves quality of life and daytime sleepiness, even in patients with mild SDB-related symptoms [9, 45]. Additionally, physicians treating patients with SDB should also consider the possibility of T2D and should initiate appropriate tests or measures [33].

The strengths of our study are the large sample size and high-resolution phenotyping of a T2D outpatient cohort with a comparable number of men and women (61%/$n = 412$ versus 39%/$n = 267$), thus enabling us to investigate effects specific to sex and using multivariable modelling. It expands on the knowledge from previous studies that were restricted to a clinically more severe diabetes status.

There are also some limitations that warrant discussion: first, although the use of portable respiratory devices instead of inpatient overnight polysomnography is well established and validated for assessment of SDB [18, 19], we cannot distinguish between obstructive and central sleep apnoea due to simplified monitoring. Second, left ventricular ejection fraction and heart failure were not evaluated in DIACORE, so we cannot report on their implications on the present study. Third, our sample might not be fully representative of an overall T2D patient group, because we did not standardize prevalence estimates to a specific population.

5. Conclusions

More than one-third of patients with T2D had moderate to severe sleep-disordered breathing, which was more common in men than in women. Higher age, higher BMI, and higher waist-hip ratio were associated with higher AHI. Modulators for higher AHI were similar in men and in women. Testing for SDB in patients with type 2 diabetes is recommended and vice versa.

Conflicts of Interest

M. Arzt received research grants from ResMed, Philips Respironics, and the ResMed Foundation and also received lecture fees from Philips Respironics and ResMed. C. A. Böger has received funding from the KfH Stiftung Präventivmedizin e.V., the Else Kröner-Fresenius-Stiftung, and the Dr. Robert Pfleger Stiftung. All other authors declare that there is no conflict of interest regarding the publication of this article.

Authors' Contributions

T. Kroner, S. Stadler, and M. Arzt were involved in the conception, hypotheses delineation, design of the study, analysis and interpretation of obtained information, writing of the article, and its revision prior to submission. C. A. Böger is the DIACORE study PI and was involved in the design of this substudy, acquisition and interpretation of the data, and critical revision of the article prior to submission. T. Kroner and M. Rheinberger were involved in the acquisition and interpretation of the data and critical revision of the article prior to submission. M. Gorski and I. M. Heid helped in statistical analysis and drafting of the manuscript. All authors read and approved the final manuscript. S. Stadler is the guarantor of this work and, as such, had full access to all the data in the study and takes responsibility for the integrity of the data and the accuracy of the data analysis. T. Kroner and M. Arzt contributed equally to this work.

Acknowledgments

The authors thank all participating patients of the DIACORE study. The authors thank the physicians and health insurance companies for supporting the DIACORE study: Axel Andreae, Gerhard Haas, Sabine Haas, Jochen Manz, Johann Nusser, Günther Kreisel, Gerhard Bawidamann, Frederik Mader, Susanne Kißkalt, Johann Hartl, Thomas Segiet, Christiane Gleixner, Christian Scholz, Monika Schober (Chief of Supply Management, Allgemeine Ortskrankenkasse Bayern), Cornelia Heinrich (Communication Manager, Allgemeine Ortskrankenkasse Bayern), Thomas Bohnhoff (Disease Management, Techniker Krankenkasse), Thomas Heilmann (Head of Disease Management, Techniker Krankenkasse), Stefan Stern (Consulting Physician, Allgemeine Ortskrankenkasse Bayern), Andreas Utz (Department Head, Allgemeine Ortskrankenkasse Bayern), Georg Zellner (Chief of Supply Management, Deutsche Angestellten Krankenkasse), Werner Ettl (Barmer-GEK), Thomas Buck (Barmer-GEK), Rainer Bleek (IKK classic), and Ulrich Blaudzun (IKK classic). The authors further thank the study nurses for their expert work in performing the study visits: Simone Neumeier, Sarah Hufnagel, Isabel Haller, Petra Jackermeier, Sabrina Obermüller, Christiane Ried, Ulrike Hanauer, Bärbel Sendtner, and Natalia Riewe-Kerow. Konstantin Dumann and Britta Hörmann (PhD students) are also thanked for their expert work in performing the study visits.

References

[1] International Diabetes Federation, *IDF Diabetes*International Diabetes Federation, Brussels, Belgium, 7 editionJune 2016, http://www.diabetesatlas.org/.

[2] L. Chen, D. J. Magliano, and P. Z. Zimmet, "The worldwide epidemiology of type 2 diabetes mellitus—present and future perspectives," *Nature Reviews Endocrinology*, vol. 8, no. 4, pp. 228–236, 2011.

[3] H. F. Becker, A. Jerrentrup, T. Ploch et al., "Effect of nasal continuous positive airway pressure treatment on blood pressure in patients with obstructive sleep apnea," *Circulation*, vol. 107, no. 1, pp. 68–73, 2003.

[4] G. Mayer, M. Arzt, B. Braumann et al., "S3-Leitlinie Nicht erholsamer Schlaf/Schlafstörungen - Kapitel, Schlafbezogene Atmungsstörungen," *Somnologie*, vol. 20, Supplement 2, pp. 97–180, 2017.

[5] P. E. Peppard, T. Young, J. H. Barnet, M. Palta, E. W. Hagen, and K. M. Hla, "Increased prevalence of sleep-disordered breathing in adults," *American Journal of Epidemiology*, vol. 177, no. 9, pp. 1006–1014, 2013.

[6] T. Young, P. E. Peppard, and D. J. Gottlieb, "Epidemiology of obstructive sleep apnea: a population health perspective," *American Journal of Respiratory and Critical Care Medicine*, vol. 165, no. 9, pp. 1217–1239, 2002.

[7] N. McArdle and N. J. Douglas, "Effect of continuous positive airway pressure on sleep architecture in the sleep apnea-hypopnea syndrome: a randomized controlled trial," *American Journal of Respiratory and Critical Care Medicine*, vol. 164, no. 8, pp. 1459–1463, 2001.

[8] A. Hetzenecker, T. Roth, C. Birner, L. S. Maier, M. Pfeifer, and M. Arzt, "Adaptive servo-ventilation therapy of central sleep apnoea and its effect on sleep quality," *Clinical Research in Cardiology*, vol. 105, no. 3, pp. 189–195, 2016.

[9] S. E. Craig, M. Kohler, D. Nicoll et al., "Continuous positive airway pressure improves sleepiness but not calculated vascular risk in patients with minimally symptomatic obstructive sleep apnoea: the MOSAIC randomised controlled trial," *Thorax*, vol. 67, no. 12, pp. 1090–1096, 2012.

[10] H. E. Resnick, S. Redline, E. Shahar et al., "Diabetes and sleep disturbances: findings from the Sleep Heart Health Study," *Diabetes Care*, vol. 26, no. 3, pp. 702–709, 2003.

[11] D. Einhorn, D. A. Stewart, M. Erman, N. Gordon, A. Philis-Tsimikas, and E. Casal, "Prevalence of sleep apnea in a population of adults with type 2 diabetes mellitus," *Endocrine Practice*, vol. 13, no. 4, pp. 355–362, 2007.

[12] G. D. Foster, M. H. Sanders, R. Millman et al., "Obstructive sleep apnea among obese patients with type 2 diabetes," *Diabetes Care*, vol. 32, no. 6, pp. 1017–1019, 2009.

[13] J. P. Laaban, S. Daenen, D. Léger et al., "Prevalence and predictive factors of sleep apnoea syndrome in type 2 diabetic patients," *Diabetes & Metabolism*, vol. 35, no. 5, pp. 372–377, 2009.

[14] T. Young, R. Hutton, L. Finn, S. Badr, and M. Palta, "The gender bias in sleep apnea diagnosis. Are women missed because they have different symptoms?," *Archives of Internal Medicine*, vol. 156, no. 21, pp. 2445–2451, 1996.

[15] O. K. Basoglu and M. S. Tasbakan, "Gender differences in clinical and polysomnographic features of obstructive sleep apnea: a clinical study of 2827 patients," *Sleep & Breathing*, vol. 22, no. 1, pp. 241–249, 2018.

[16] S. Stadler, T. Zimmermann, F. Franke et al., "Association of sleep-disordered breathing with diabetes-associated kidney disease," *Annals of Medicine*, vol. 49, no. 6, pp. 487–495, 2017.

[17] L. Dörhöfer, for the DIACORE Study Group, A. Lammert et al., "Study design of DIACORE (DIAbetes COhoRtE) - a cohort study of patients with diabetes mellitus type 2," *BMC Medical Genetics*, vol. 14, no. 1, p. 25, 2013.

[18] M. K. Erman, D. Stewart, D. Einhorn, N. Gordon, and E. Casal, "Validation of the ApneaLink for the screening of sleep apnea: a novel and simple single-channel recording device," *Journal of Clinical Sleep Medicine*, vol. 3, no. 4, pp. 387–392, 2007.

[19] M. Arzt, H. Woehrle, O. Oldenburg et al., "Prevalence and predictors of sleep-disordered breathing in patients with stable chronic heart failure: the SchlaHF registry," *JACC: Heart Failure*, vol. 4, no. 2, pp. 116–125, 2016.

[20] B. A. Stuck and H. G. Weeß, "The new "international classification of sleep disorders". A critical acclaim of diagnostic criteria for sleep disordered breathing," *Somnologie - Schlafforschung und Schlafmedizin*, vol. 19, no. 2, pp. 126–132, 2015.

[21] G. Weinreich, J. Armitstead, V. Topfer, Y.-M. Wang, Y. Wang, and H. Teschler, "Validation of ApneaLink as screening device for Cheyne-Stokes respiration," *Sleep*, vol. 32, no. 4, pp. 553–557, 2009.

[22] M. W. Johns, "A new method for measuring daytime sleepiness: the Epworth sleepiness scale," *Sleep*, vol. 14, no. 6, pp. 540–545, 1991.

[23] D. R. Matthews, J. P. Hosker, A. S. Rudenski, B. A. Naylor, D. F. Treacher, and R. C. Turner, "Homeostasis model assessment: insulin resistance and beta-cell function from fasting plasma glucose and insulin concentrations in man," *Diabetologia*, vol. 28, no. 7, pp. 412–419, 1985.

[24] R. Marfella, C. Sardu, P. Calabrò et al., "Non-ST-elevation myocardial infarction outcomes in patients with type 2 diabetes with non-obstructive coronary artery stenosis: effects of incretin treatment," *Diabetes, Obesity and Metabolism*, vol. 20, no. 3, pp. 723–729, 2018.

[25] R. Marfella, C. Sardu, M. L. Balestrieri et al., "Effects of incretin treatment on cardiovascular outcomes in diabetic STEMI-patients with culprit obstructive and multivessel non obstructive-coronary-stenosis," *Diabetology & Metabolic Syndrome*, vol. 10, no. 1, p. 1, 2018.

[26] Third Report of the National Cholesterol Education Program (NCEP) Expert Panel on Detection, "Evaluation, and treatment of high blood cholesterol in adults (adult treatment panel III) final report," *Circulation*, vol. 106, no. 25, pp. 3143–3421, 2002.

[27] World Health Organization, *Waist Circumference and Waist-Hip Ratio: Report of a WHO Expert Consultation*, Geneva, 2008June 23, 2016, http://apps.who.int/iris/bitstream/10665/44583/1/9789241501491_eng.pdf?ua=1.

[28] C. Sardu, M. Santamaria, S. Funaro et al., "Cardiac electrophysiological alterations and clinical response in cardiac resynchronization therapy with a defibrillator treated patients affected by metabolic syndrome," *Medicine*, vol. 96, no. 14, article e6558, 2017.

[29] C. Sardu, G. Carreras, S. Katsanos et al., "Metabolic syndrome is associated with a poor outcome in patients affected by outflow tract premature ventricular contractions treated by catheter ablation," *BMC Cardiovascular Disorders*, vol. 14, no. 1, p. 176, 2014.

[30] R. H. Eckel, S. M. Grundy, and P. Z. Zimmet, "The metabolic syndrome," *Lancet*, vol. 365, no. 9468, pp. 1415–1428, 2005.

[31] A. K. Schober, M. F. Neurath, and I. A. Harsch, "Prevalence of sleep apnoea in diabetic patients," *The Clinical Respiratory Journal*, vol. 5, no. 3, pp. 165–172, 2011.

[32] T. Young, M. Palta, J. Dempsey, J. Skatrud, S. Weber, and S. Badr, "The occurrence of sleep-disordered breathing among middle-aged adults," *The New England Journal of Medicine*, vol. 328, no. 17, pp. 1230–1235, 1993.

[33] International Diabetes Federation, *The IDF Consensus Statement on Sleep Apnoea and Type 2 Diabetes*International Diabetes Federation, Brussels, BelgiumJune 2016, http://www.idf.org/webdata/docs/APNOEA_final.pdf.

[34] P. Zhang, R. Zhang, F. Zhao et al., "The prevalence and characteristics of obstructive sleep apnea in hospitalized patients with type 2 diabetes in China," *Journal of Sleep Research*, vol. 25, no. 1, pp. 39–46, 2016.

[35] D. C. Lam, M. M. Lui, J. C. Lam, L. H. Y. Ong, K. S. L. Lam, and M. S. M. Ip, "Prevalence and recognition of obstructive sleep apnea in Chinese patients with type 2 diabetes mellitus," *Chest*, vol. 138, no. 5, pp. 1101–1107, 2010.

[36] H. Guo, L. Zhang, C. Zhu et al., "A single nucleotide polymorphism in the FADS1 gene is associated with plasma fatty acid and lipid profiles and might explain gender difference in body fat distribution," *Lipids in Health and Disease*, vol. 16, no. 1, p. 67, 2017.

[37] S. Pamidi and E. Tasali, "Obstructive sleep apnea and type 2 diabetes: is there a link?," *Frontiers in Neurology*, vol. 3, p. 126, 2012.

[38] J. H. Ficker, S. H. Dertinger, W. Siegfried et al., "Obstructive sleep apnoea and diabetes mellitus: the role of cardiovascular autonomic neuropathy," *The European Respiratory Journal*, vol. 11, no. 1, pp. 14–19, 1998.

[39] P. Bottini, M. L. Dottorini, M. Cristina Cordoni, G. Casucci, and C. Tantucci, "Sleep-disordered breathing in nonobese diabetic subjects with autonomic neuropathy," *The European Respiratory Journal*, vol. 22, no. 4, pp. 654–660, 2003.

[40] K. A. Stamatakis and N. M. Punjabi, "Effects of sleep fragmentation on glucose metabolism in normal subjects," *Chest*, vol. 137, no. 1, pp. 95–101, 2010.

[41] E. Martínez-Cerón, B. Barquiel, A. M. Bezos et al., "Effect of continuous positive airway pressure on glycemic control in patients with obstructive sleep apnea and type 2 diabetes. A randomized clinical trial," *American Journal of Respiratory and Critical Care Medicine*, vol. 194, no. 4, pp. 476–485, 2016.

[42] J. E. Shaw, N. M. Punjabi, M. T. Naughton et al., "The effect of treatment of obstructive sleep apnea on glycemic control in type 2 diabetes," *American Journal of Respiratory and Critical Care Medicine*, vol. 194, no. 4, pp. 486–492, 2016.

[43] S. D. West, D. J. Nicoll, T. M. Wallace, D. R. Matthews, and J. R. Stradling, "Effect of CPAP on insulin resistance and HbA1c in men with obstructive sleep apnoea and type 2 diabetes," *Thorax*, vol. 62, no. 11, pp. 969–974, 2007.

[44] G. Mayer, M. Arzt, B. Braumann et al., "German S3 guideline nonrestorative sleep/sleep disorders, chapter "sleep-related breathing disorders in adults," short version," *Somnologie*, vol. 21, no. 4, pp. 290–301, 2017.

[45] R. D. McEvoy, N. A. Antic, E. Heeley et al., "CPAP for prevention of cardiovascular events in obstructive sleep apnea," *The New England Journal of Medicine*, vol. 375, no. 10, pp. 919–931, 2016.

19

Extracellular Vesicles: A Novel Target for Exercise-Mediated Reductions in Type 2 Diabetes and Cardiovascular Disease Risk

Natalie Z. M. Eichner,[1] Uta Erdbrügger,[2] and Steven K. Malin[1,3,4]

[1]*Department of Kinesiology, University of Virginia, Charlottesville, VA, USA*
[2]*Division of Nephrology, University of Virginia, Charlottesville, VA, USA*
[3]*Division of Endocrinology and Metabolism, University of Virginia, Charlottesville, VA, USA*
[4]*Robert M. Berne Cardiovascular Research Center, University of Virginia, Charlottesville, VA, USA*

Correspondence should be addressed to Steven K. Malin; skm6n@virginia.edu

Academic Editor: Rosa Fernandes

Regular exercise is important for reducing type 2 diabetes (T2D) and/or cardiovascular disease (CVD) risk. However, only about 40–50% of this CVD risk reduction is accounted for by adiposity, hyperglycemia, hypertension, and dyslipidemia. Herein, we present the novel hypothesis that extracellular vesicles (EVs) are candidate biomarkers that may relate to impaired endothelial function and insulin resistance independent of obesity risk factors. EVs are small membrane-bound particles that are generated by cells following stimulation, stress, or activation. They carry markers of their parent cell and are thought to be potent bioactivators and communicators. We discuss the underlying physiology of specific cell type EVs, as well as examine how acute and chronic exercise interventions impact EV count and phenotype. We also propose that current gaps in the field are in part related to use of different detection techniques and the lack of standardized measurements of EV affecting the pre- and postanalytical phase. Ultimately, improving the understanding of how EVs impact cardiometabolic health and their function will lead to improved approaches for enhancing diagnostic options as well as designing exercise interventions that treat and/or prevent T2D and CVD.

1. Introduction

Nearly 33% of all deaths globally each year are attributed to cardiovascular disease (CVD) [1]. In fact, CVD mortality has increased from 12.59 to 17.82 million between 1990 and 2015 [2]. Individuals with type 2 diabetes (T2D) are 2-3 times more likely to have CVD than their healthy counterparts, indicating that abnormalities in glucose metabolism share a CVD pathogenic root [3]. However, glucose alone may not be a primary driver of CVD in people with T2D given recent interventions focused on lowering glucose alone have failed to significantly lower CVD risk and mortality [4]. As such, it is not surprising that elevated blood pressure and dyslipidemia in people with hyperglycemia are considered critical drivers of CVD that are linked together by insulin resistance [5]. Insulin resistance can be defined as the reduced responsiveness of skeletal muscle, liver, adipose, and vasculature to insulin for the maintenance of nutrient delivery and utilization. Although the exact cause of insulin resistance is unclear, endothelial dysfunction is a leading candidate for promoting these nutrient disturbances [6]. Endothelial function is the ability of the endothelium to respond to both metabolic mediators (e.g., insulin and nitric oxide) and/or shear stress that enhance blood flow. Recently, the American Heart Association suggested that current biomarkers (e.g., blood pressure and lipids) do not account for the majority of adverse outcomes and may account for only 40–50% of CVD risk [7]. Thus, there is an urgent need to identify new treatment targets for T2D and CVD that mediate health and well-being.

Extracellular vesicles (EVs) have emerged as novel biomarkers of T2D and CVD [8, 9]. EVs belong to a heterogeneous population of vesicles summarized with the generic term "Extracellular Vesicles" (EVs). Interestingly, most of

Table 1: Acute effects of exercise on circulating extracellular vesicles.

Author	*Exercise dose*	*Subtype EV*	*Preanalytical phase*	*Collection time*	*Response*
Harrison et al. [76]	Cycling for 90 min at 70% VO_2peak followed by ten 1 min sprints interspersed with 1 min of recovery in young, recreationally active men.	CD31+/CD42b-	1600 g for 15 min at 4°C	Morning following exercise bout	No change
Mobius-Winkler et al. [63]	4 hr cycling at 70% IAT in young, healthy men.	$CD42b^-CD42b^-/CD62E^+$	11,000*g* for 2 min	16 predefined time points during and after finishing cycling.	No change
Jenkins et al. [74]	Exercise at 70% of VO_2peak until 598 kcal was expended in recreationally, healthy active men.	$CD31^+/CD42b^-CD62E^+$	Double centrifugation of 1500*g* for 20 min at room temperature	(i) Pre-meal (ii) 1, 2, 3, and 4 hr postprandial	↓$CD31^+/CD42b^-$ ↓$CD62E^+$ Unaffected by high-fat meal
Guiraud et al. [60]	Single session of HIIE: 15-second intervals at 100% of PPO and 15-second passive recovery intervals or isocaloric MICE in men with coronary heart disease.	$CD31^+$ $CD62E^+$ $CD42b^-$ $CD42b^+$	1500*g* for 15 min followed by a single centrifugation at 13,000*g* for 2 min	(i) 10 min pre-ex (ii) 20 min post-ex (iii) 24 hr post-ex (iv) 72 hr post-ex	No change
Ross et al. [62]	3 sets of 6 resistance exercises at 15 RM w/o rest in young, trained men.	$CD144^+$ $CD146^+$ $CD105^+$	1500*g* for 15 min followed by 13,000*g* for 2 min	(i) Pre-ex (ii) 10 min post-ex (iii) 2 hr post-ex (iv) 24 hr post-ex	No change
Wahl et al. [67]	(1) HVT; 130 min at 55% PPO, (2) 4 × 4 min at 95% PPO, and (3) 4 × 30 sec all-out in healthy male, triathletes.	$CD31^+/CD42b^-$ CD31/CD42b CD14/CD16	1.861*g* for 10 min at 4°C	(i) Pre-ex (ii) Immediately post-ex (iii) 60 min post-ex (iv) 180 min post-ex	↓$CD31^+/CD42b^-$ ↓CD31/CD42b ↓CD14/CD16
Chanda et al. [61]	Acute strenuous exercise (treadmill running VO_2peak) versus. moderate (75% HR_{max} for 45 min) in healthy females.	Total EVs CD41a	2500 rpm for 5 min at 4°C	(i) Pre-ex (ii) Immediately post-ex (iii) 45 min post-ex	↑Total EVs ↑CD41a Only after strenuous ex; No moderate ex change
Durrer et al. [72]	(1) HICE 20 min cycling at just above VT. (2) HIIE 10 × 1 min at 90% peak aerobic power in young, overweight, inactive males and females.	$CD62E^+$ $CD31^+/CD42b^-$	Double centrifugation of 1500*g* for 15 min at room temperature	(i) Pre-ex (ii) Immediate post-ex (iii) Morning post-ex	↑$CD62E^+$ (females only) No change $CD31^+/CD42b^-$ ↓$CD62E^+$ (males only) ↓$CD31^+/CD42b^-$
Lansford et al. [69]	Acute bout at 60–75% VO_2peak in healthy, active individuals	$CD62E^+$, $CD34^+$ $CD31^+/CD42b^-$	Double centrifugation of 1500*g* for 20 min at room temperature	(i) Pre-ex (ii) Post-ex	↑$CD62E^+$ in men ↑$CD34^+$ in women No change $CD31^+/CD42b^-$
Wilhelm et al. [65]	1 h of moderate- (46 ± 2% VO_2peak) or heavy- (67 ± 2% VO_2peak) intensity semirecumbent cycling in healthy, young men.	$CD62E^+$ $CD41^+$	17,500*g* for 1 hr at 4°C	(i) Pre-ex (ii) Post-ex	↑$CD41^+$ following heavy exercise No $CD62E^+$ change

Table 1: Continued.

Author	*Exercise dose*	*Subtype EV*	*Preanalytical phase*	*Collection time*	*Response*
Bei et al. [114]	Exercise stress test in middle-aged, overweight men and women.	$CD63^+$	1000*g* for 10 min and 2500*g* for 15 min at room temperature	(i) Rest (ii) Peak-ex (iii) Recovery (15 min after completion	↑EV count
Whitham et al. [66]	1 hr (30 min at 55%, 20 min at 70%, and ~10 min at 80% of VO_2peak) in healthy males.	ACTN4, ADAM10, ALIX, ANAX11, and CD81	20,000*g* for 2x at 60 min	(i) Pre-ex (ii) Exercise (iii) 4 hr post-ex	↑EV count

IAT: individual anaerobic threshold; HIIE: high-intensity interval exercise; MICE: moderate-intensity continuous exercise; RM: repetition max; HVT: high-volume training; PPO: peak power output; HICE: high-intensity continuous exercise; VT: ventilatory threshold.

TABLE 2: Chronic effects of exercise on circulating extracellular vesicles.

Author (year)	*Exercise dose*	*Subtype EV*	*Preanalytical phase*	*Collection time*	*Response*
La Vignera et al. [87]	150 min aerobic activity/wk for 3 mo in individuals with and without erectile dysfunction.	$CD45^-/CD34^-/CD144^+$	Specifics not reported	(i) Baseline (ii) 3 mo	$\downarrow CD45^-/CD34^-/CD144^+$
Babbitt et al. [90]	24 wk aerobic training, 3x/wk, 40 min at 65% VO_2peak in sedentary, middle-aged African American adults.	$CD62E^+$	2000*g* for 20 min at 4°C	(i) Baseline (ii) 6 mo	$\downarrow CD62E^+$
Kretzschmar et al. [89]	6 mo aerobic training, 3x/wk, 40 min at 65% VO_2peak in pre- and postmenopausal African American women.	$CD62E^+$ $CD31^+/CD42b^-$	Double centrifugation at 1500*g* for 20 min at 24°C	(i) Baseline (ii) 6 mo	$\downarrow CD62E^+$ $\downarrow CD31^+/CD42b^-$ in the premenopausal group only
Bruyndonckx et al. [86]	10 months of 3 supervised sessions/wk combined with diet intervention in obese children between the ages of 12 and 18.	$CD31^+/CD42b^-$	Double centrifugation of 1525*g* for 20 min	(i) Baseline (ii) 5 mo (iii) 10 mo	$\downarrow CD31^+/CD42b^-$
Kim et al. [88]	3 days/wk for 6 mo of 40 min at 65% of predicted HR_{peak} in adults with prehypertension.	$CD31^+/CD42b^-$, $CD62E^-$	Double centrifugation of 1500*g* for 20 min	(i) Baseline (ii) 6 mo	$\downarrow CD31^+/CD42a^-$ $\downarrow CD62E^+$
Pitha et al. [91]	6 mo of supervised training on a cycle ergometer in renal transplant recipients.	$CD34^+$ $CD45^+$	ELISA	(i) Baseline (ii) Median of 6 mo	No change
Van Craenenbroeck et al. [95]	12 wk, 3x/wk aerobic continuous training (70–75% HR_{peak}) or aerobic interval training (four 4 min intervals 90–95% of HR_{peak} with 3 min recovery at 50–70% of HR_{peak}) adults with coronary artery disease.	$CD31^+/CD42b^-$	Double centrifugation at 1550*g*	(i) Baseline (ii) 12 wk	No change

the studies analyzing EVs in metabolic diseases have focused on larger EVs (>100–1000 nm) (Tables 1 and 2, resp.), called microparticles/microvesicles, generated by the low centrifugation speed of up to 20,000 Gs, but our own data [10] and that of others [11–13] indicate that we also see smaller EVs (<100 nm, called exosomes) in these EV preps. As these studies have likely analyzed a mix of larger and smaller EVs of different densities, we will only use the term EV. EVs are unique biomarkers as they are also believed to carry and transfer proteins, lipids, and nucleic acids, and they facilitate communication between cells. How EVs regulate vascular health remains to be fully determined, but obesity-related insulin resistance might be a potential reason through oxidative stress and inflammatory-related mechanisms [14]. Interestingly, physical inactivity also increases EV levels in association with worsening of insulin resistance and endothelial dysfunction, suggesting that muscle contraction alters disease risk in an EV-mediated manner [15]. However, there is limited research regarding the effects of physical activity and/or exercise on EVs in healthy and disease populations. In particular, we propose that EVs may be a novel mediator of T2D and CVD risk. First, we highlight the biogenesis of EVs and the purported mechanism relating EV to insulin resistance and endothelial function. Next, we examine the gaps in knowledge regarding the effectiveness of acute and chronic exercise on EVs. We also discuss the mechanistic role of cell-specific EVs related to leukocytes, platelets, and the endothelium as mediators of cardiometabolic risk. Lastly, we analyze how current EV methodologies could play a role in discrepancies seen across exercise studies and discuss new methodology to advance understanding of EVs and exosomes that could improve diagnostic and treatment options for T2D and CVD.

2. Extracellular Vesicle Biogenesis

First described as merely "cell dust" by Wolf in 1967, EVs are now recognized as cell bioactivators and communicators of cardiometabolic health [16]. Smaller EVs (<100 nm, also called exosomes) are thought to derive from multivesicular bodies inside the cells that are then secreted into different body fluids, whereas larger EVs (>100–100 nm, also called microparticles/microvesicles) are believed to be shed from cells into body fluids/tissue upon stimulation or activation. These larger EVs are likely the product of outward membrane budding through cytoskeletal rearrangement and a loss of calcium-dependent membrane phospholipid asymmetry [17]. These vesicles consist of membrane proteins and cytosolic material from the cell they originate from. Indeed, EVs are derived from cells in circulation (i.e., endothelial, platelet, and leukocyte), erythrocytes [18], as well as progenitor cell populations [19] (Table 3). Additionally, EVs are found in many other body fluids besides blood, including urine [20], which increase the potential for clinical collection sites. EVs are released during conditions of stress that initiate cell activation and/or apoptosis [21]. In particular, proinflammatory stimuli (e.g., oxidative stress/cytokines), bioactive lipids [22], and hyperglycemia [23] are considered key stimuli that impact EV release, phenotype, and function. In particular, hyperglycemia increases endothelium-derived EV formation, size, and reduces surface

Table 3: Most commonly used extracellular vesicles.

EV origin	Surface markers
Endothelium	**CD31 $^+$/CD41 $^-$ (PECAM $^+$/ITGA2B $^-$)** CD31$^+$/CD42$^-$ (PECAM$^+$/GPIb$^-$) **CD31 (PECAM (platelet cell adhesion molecule))** CD144 (VE cadherin (vascular endothelial cadherin)) CD146 (MCAM (melanoma cell adhesion molecule)) CD105 (endoglin) CD106 (VCAM (vascular cell adhesion molecule)) **CD62E (E-selectin (endothelial-selectin))**
Platelet	**CD41 (ITGA2B (integrin alpha 2b))** CD42 (GPIb (glycoprotein Ib)) CD31 (PECAM (platelet cell adhesion molecule))
Leukocyte	CD45 (PTPRC (protein tyrosine phosphate receptor type C)) CD11b (ITGAM (integrin alpha M)) CD14 (coreceptor of lipopolysaccharide) CD16 (on surface of neutrophils, monocytes, and macrophages) CD62L (L-selectin (leukocyte selectin))
Red blood cell	CD235 (glycophorin A)

charge that collectively prompt greater procoagulant activity [24]. Moreover, high glucose conditions increase NADPH oxidase activity in endothelial EVs that work to amplify the effects of oxidative stress-mediated inflammation on the endothelium [23] that decrease endothelial nitric oxide synthase (eNOS) [25], thereby potentially impairing vascular function and raising CVD risk. There is also work suggesting that EVs may not only release inflammatory cytokines [26] but also act as deliverers of bioactive lipids [22], protein, and genetic material [10] between cells. Taken together, EVs represent a potentially novel paradigm in cell-to-cell communications between various organs important for T2D and CVD. For a comprehensive discussion of biogenesis of EVs, we will refer the reader to other review papers [27].

3. Extracellular Vesicles in The Pathogenesis of T2D and CVD

EVs are composed of parental proteins, nucleic acids, and cytoplasm based on the stimuli [10]. This is physiologically important because carrying markers of the parent cell allows for specific subpopulation identification (e.g., endothelium- or leukocyte-derived) [10] that can influence crosstalk between tissues and cells [28]. Indeed, elevated endothelial EVs are thought to reflect vascular injury, whereas increased leukocyte and platelet EVs signify proinflammation and coagulation, respectively. This notion is consistent with literature reporting that different subtypes of EVs are elevated in people with prediabetes [29], T2D, and CVD [8, 9] as well as hypertension [30], chronic kidney disease [31], and heart failure [32]. Even obesity, independent of comorbidities, presents with elevated platelet EV levels [33] in relation to reduced fibrinolytic ability. Subsequently, these observations

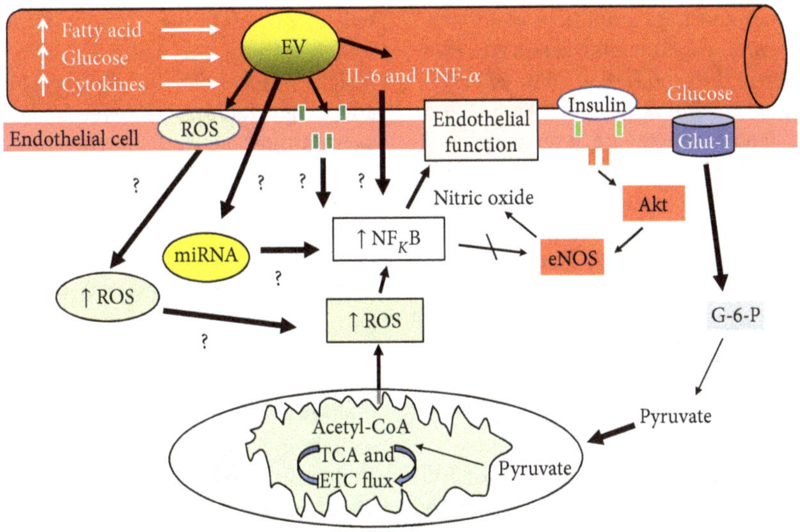

(a) Sedentary condition

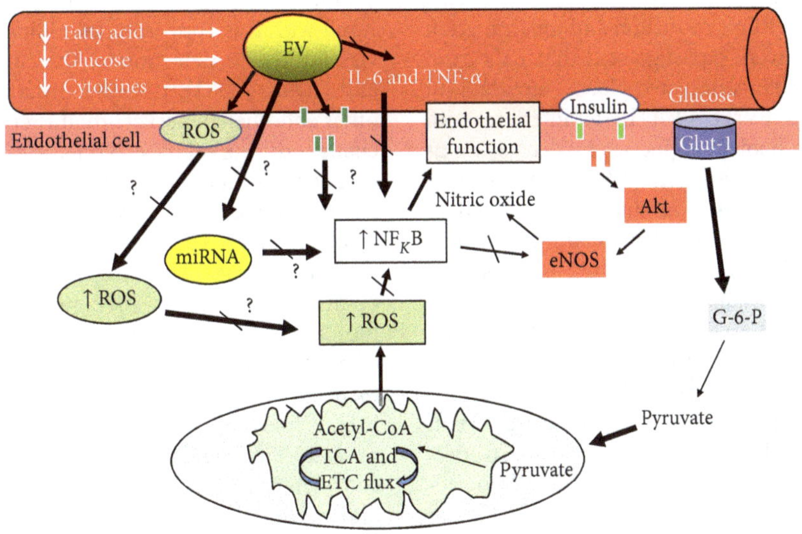

(b) Physical activity/exercise condition

FIGURE 1: Working hypothesis by which extracellular vesicles (EVs) interact with exercise to influence vascular function and insulin sensitivity. Reactive oxygen species (ROS) are generated by EVs in response to bioactive lipids, glucose, and inflammatory cytokines and act as important cellular regulators in cell health. In addition, EVs may bind to cells and interfere with receptor-related mechanisms and/or release microRNA (miRNA) to influence cell activity. Lastly, EVs may release inflammatory cytokines and impact cell NFκB activity, which influences cell vascular function. Exercise (b) decreases circulatory lipids, glucose, and cytokines, thereby improving EV levels and function. We hypothesize herein that EVs not only serve as a biomarker of type 2 diabetes and cardiovascular disease but also regulate vascular function independent of traditional obesity-related risk factors. Future work should consider studying the interaction of EV and exercise doses in order to identify optimal treatment plans for preventing type 2 diabetes and cardiovascular disease.

support that EVs likely play a key physiologic role above and beyond a biomarker.

Circulating EVs are believed to play an important physiologic role in vascular physiology [34] (Figure 1(a)). Werner et al. reported that elevated endothelial EVs ($CD31^+$/Annexin V^+) are correlated with reduced endothelium-dependent vasorelaxation [35]. This is consistent with others reporting that elevations in these same endothelial EVs are related to reduced flow-mediated dilation as well as increased pulse wave velocity and carotid intima-media thickness [36, 37]. Together, these findings suggest that higher levels of EVs relate to poor blood flow and arterial stiffness.

There are several putative mechanisms that may explain how EVs promote dysregulation of blood flow, although most data exists from *in vitro* experiments and more human work is needed. EVs are thought to directly produce reactive oxygen species (ROS). Endothelial EVs (CD144, Annexin V^{+ve}) increase production of superoxide anion and hydrogen peroxide in cultured endothelial cells through NADPH oxidase and mitochondria [38, 39], although others suggest that xanthine oxidase may contribute in endothelial (CD144-PE) [40], lymphocytic (CD4, $CD3^+$, CD8, CD11a, Fas, and FasL) [41], and monocyte-derived EVs [42]. Additionally, EVs are hypothesized to promote *in vivo* inflammation through stimulation of proinflammatory cytokines and the recruitment of inflammatory cells [26]. In *in vitro* experiments, leukocyte EVs ($CD14^+$) promote the release of IL-6 and IL-8 in cultured endothelial cells [43]. In addition, T-cell EVs promote TNF-α and IL-1b by monocytes [44] and promote the interaction and adhesion of leukocytes to endothelial cells [22]. These later findings are consistent with work by Mastronardi et al. [45] demonstrating that injection of EVs from blood of patients with sepsis into mice promotes increased expression of iNOS, COX-2, and NFκB in the heart and lung, thereby supporting a direct role of EVs at producing inflammation. Lastly, circulating EVs express the functionally active eNOS protein [25]. This is clinically germane as patients with endothelial dysfunction have EVs with reduced expression and release of nitric oxide [25].

Another possible mechanism by which EVs contribute to T2D and CVD relates to the interaction and transfer of EV contents to the cell (Figure 1(a)). EVs have been proposed to physically alter cell target receptors that modify signal transmission. For example, blocking EGF receptors in endothelial cells inhibits EV-mediated ROS production and inflammation [38]. Additionally, other work has suggested that EVs from obese subjects reduce insulin-stimulated glucose uptake [46] and macrophage-derived EVs (M0 THP-1) interfere with GLUT-4 translocation in human adipocytes by decreasing p-Akt, thereby inducing insulin resistance [47]. The exact cause of this insulin resistance remains to be elucidated, but activation of NFκB was noted, suggesting that inflammation may play a role. Indeed, it is also possible that miRNA transcripts from EVs also play an important role in communicating signals to local and systemic tissues for the alteration of cell activity [48]. For instance, Rautou et al. [18] demonstrated that EVs ($CD31^+$) derived from apoptotic plaques transferred ICAM-1 to endothelial cells, suggesting that EVs play an important inflammatory response mechanism in atherosclerosis. In addition to ICAM-1, other studies have reported adipocyte-derived EVs ($CD14^+$) to interfere with insulin signaling in both the liver [49] and skeletal muscle [50] via transfer of adipokine content, thereby inducing insulin resistance [46]. However, not all studies support the observation that EVs fuse and transfer content to cells [51], as there are different ways in which EVs promote cell-to-cell communication or even EV uptake [52]. In either case, EVs appear to mediate angiogenesis and induce endothelial repair [34, 53–55] by at least partially [56] vascular endothelial growth factor-A [57] or eNOS [25]. In this way, EVs may promote increased angiogenesis and blood flow via cargo such as eNOS-induced nitric oxide. In turn, this compensatory response of increased blood flow may allow nutrient delivery to tissue, thereby contributing to insulin-mediated GLUT-4 translocation. Given the literature linking oxidative stress and inflammation to the pathogenesis of insulin resistance and endothelial dysfunction [58], the identification of how EVs may be modified or targeted for metabolic health warrants attention.

4. Effects of Acute Exercise Bouts on Extracellular Vesicles

A majority of the chronic exercise training induced an effect on insulin resistance and endothelial function is considered to be the result of the last bout of exercise [59]. Subsequently, understanding the acute exercise effect on EVs provides insight independent of cardiorespiratory fitness adaptation and weight/fat loss. However, to date there are limited studies examining the effects of acute aerobic [60, 61] or resistance exercise [62] on EVs (Table 1). For instance, Mobius-Winkler et al. tested the effect of a 4 hr cycling protocol at 70% of the anaerobic threshold in 18 young, lean, healthy males [63] and found no change in endothelial EVs ($CD42b^-$, $CD42b^-/CD62E^+$) in the immediate postexercise period, despite increases in cytokine IL-6. It was speculated that the lack of exercise effect might have been due to the population studied (healthy versus diseased) or the low to moderate intensity exercise prescribed. We add to this by speculating that the lack of EV differences following exercise could also be related to technical differences of EV detection. Blood was collected and EV pellet was enriched from platelet-poor plasma using conventional flow cytometry. Smaller EVs (e.g., <500 nm) might not have also been captured with this approach. In addition, targeted phenotyping was limited to detection of the surface marker for CD62E and CD42. CD62E is found on activated endothelium, but other endothelial markers might reflect better the endothelial changes during exercise. Nonetheless, these findings are consistent with Guiraud et al. who showed that there was no change in endothelial EVs ($CD31^+$, $CD62E^+$, and $CD42b^-$) or platelet EVs ($CD42b^+$) in 19 male coronary heart disease patients when measured up to 72 hr following either high-intensity interval or moderate-intensity cycling exercise [60]. In contrast, Chanda et al. reported that a maximal bout of exercise (defined as a VO_2max test) elicited an approximate 40% increase in platelet (CD41a) EVs in healthy adults [61]. While these later findings suggest that exercise intensity raises EV, it should be noted that maximal exercise would be considered a stressful perturbation to the system and it is known that high-intensity exercise raises oxidative stress and inflammation in the immediate postexercise period, thereby conferring a stimulus for metabolic adaptation [64]. Indeed, *in vitro* experiments by Wilhelm et al. demonstrate that EVs generated after intense exercise in healthy young men enhanced endothelial proliferation, migration, and tubule formation compared with EV derived from the rest [65]. Interestingly, platelet EVs ($CD41^+$) from the same patients were elevated during 1 hr of high (67% VO_2max), but not moderate (46% VO_2max), intensity exercise. These later findings are of potential significance as they suggest that exercise intensity promotes angiogenesis for improved blood flow and nutrient delivery. Whether EVs from people with T2D or CVD respond to exercise comparably to lean healthy people remains to be seen. This is particularly of interest given recent work highlighting that single bouts of exercise increase EVs (ACTN4, ADAM10, ALIX, ANAX11, and CD81) and miRNA to potentially coordinate communication of nutrient homeostasis between muscle, endothelium, as well as liver [66, 67].

Another possible reason explaining why acute exercise has yielded equivocal EV results may relate to sex differences. Toth et al. reported elevated total Annexin V EV, platelet EV (CD63, P-selectin-exposing), and endothelial EV (CD62,

E-selectin-exposing) in 27 young healthy women compared to men while at rest. It was reported that elevated EVs (Annexin V-binding EV, CD61, P-selectin-exposing EV, and E-selectin-exposing EV) in women were related to the menstrual luteal cycle [68]. However, no significant sex- or menstrual cycle-dependent differences were observed in the endothelial EV ($CD144^+$). Lansford et al. [69] recently tested the effect of an acute bout of exercise (60–75% VO_2max) on endothelial EVs ($CD62E^+$, $CD31^+/CD42b^-$, $CD34^+$) in recreationally active men and women and demonstrated that endothelial EV ($CD62E^+$) increased by 107% in men but not in women. Conversely, women displayed a 253% elevation in mononuclear EVs ($CD34^+$). Based on previous research [70, 71], these results suggest that increased levels may prime $CD34^+$ peripheral blood mononuclear cells for paracrine angiogenic effects in females. Interestingly, the endothelial EVs ($CD31^+/CD42b^-$) remained unchanged following exercise in either sex. These results suggest that only certain phenotypes of endothelial EVs ($CD62E^+$) or other not yet tested EV phenotypes may be affected by sex and exercise. In another study, Durrer et al. examined the effects of high-intensity continuous versus interval exercise on EVs in young, overweight inactive adults and reported that both exercises lowered EVs in men ($n = 6$), but endothelial EV counts ($CD31^+/CD42b^-$) were unaffected in females ($n = 7$) [72]. However, high-intensity continuous exercise increased endothelial EVs ($CD62E^+$) in females. Although this was a relatively small sample size, the data suggest that sex may be an important factor explaining differential EV responses to exercise. Further work is needed to elucidate the mechanism by which men and women differ in EV profiles in order to individualize exercise to treat and/or prevent disease.

It reasons that dietary intake may also influence EV responses postexercise since circulating bioactive lipids are considered a stimulus for EV biogenesis. In fact, high-fat meals induce endothelial dysfunction in healthy and T2D individuals [73]. Although Jenkins et al. reported that a high-fat meal had no independent effect on endothelial EVs, acute exercise at 70% VO_2max lowered endothelial EVs ($CD62E^+$ and $CD31^+/CD42b^-$) by 55% and 30%, respectively (both $P < 0.05$) compared to a sedentary control in healthy, recreationally active men [74]. Interestingly, the lowering of endothelial EVs ($CD62E^+$ and $CD31^+/CD42b^-$) postexercise was associated with blunted ROS production during postprandial lipemia. This finding supports the notion that EVs may induce vascular dysfunction through an oxidative stress-mediated mechanism. The modulation of oxidative stress postexercise may also be clinically relevant since it relates to fasting and postprandial endothelial dysfunction in obese individuals with prediabetes [75]. In addition, a lowering of endothelial EVs ($CD31^+$, $CD31^+/CD42b^-$), which may be indicative of endothelial activation and apoptosis, suggests that exercise confers cardiovascular protection through modulation of the EV phenotype. However, Harrison et al. reported that high-intensity exercise performed at ~70% VO_2max for 90 min had no effect on high-fat-fed-induced elevations in endothelial EVs ($CD31^+/CD42b^-$) in recreationally active young men [76]. This observation is in stark contrast to Jenkins et al. [74]. Despite both studies prescribing exercise at 70% VO_2max, Harrison et al. included ten 1 min sprints. This subtle difference in exercise protocols may be of relevance since high-intensity exercise could have promoted greater vascular injury and prohibited the lowering of EVs. Additionally, differences in EV preparation and analysis, such as centrifugation at 1500*g* for 20 min at room temperature [74] as opposed to 1600*g* for 15 min at 4°C [76], may account for differences between the two studies. In either case, additional work is required to determine if exercise restores diet-induced EV levels to optimize exercise prescription for disease prevention in men and women given that postprandial metabolism is a strong predictor of CVD [77].

5. Effects of Chronic Exercise Training on Extracellular Vesicles

Exercise training improves whole body insulin sensitivity [78, 79] and glucose tolerance [80, 81] in adults with prediabetes and T2D. Additionally, chronic exercise enhances endothelial function in healthy individuals [82] and those at risk for [83] or with CVD [84, 85]. Therefore, it would be expected that long-term exercise training would also have favorable effects on EV phenotype and count. Bruyndonckx et al. recently demonstrated that 10 months of exercise training significantly decreased endothelial EVs ($CD31^+/CD42b^-$) as measured by conventional flow cytometry in 33 overweight children [86]. In addition to decreasing endothelial EVs, exercise training significantly improved microvascular function (measured via pulse amplitude tonometry), increased circulating adiponectin, and reduced body fat and high-sensitivity C-reactive protein. These findings are consistent with other work reporting that 12–24 weeks of aerobic exercise with weight loss significantly lowered endothelial EVs ($CD31^+/CD41a$; $CD62E^+$) in middle-aged men with erectile dysfunction [87] or prehypertensive men and women [88], as well as in African American women [89, 90] (Table 2). Interestingly, changes in endothelial EVs ($CD62E^+$), IL-6, and IL-10 accounted for nearly 11% of the improvements in flow-mediated dilation following exercise training in the later studies [89, 90].

Although exercise training appears to favorably lower endothelial EVs ($CD31^+/CD41a$; $CD62E^+$), not all individuals appear to respond the same [91]. Kretzschmar et al. [89] demonstrated that endothelial EVs ($CD31^+/CD42b$) only decreased in premenopausal compared with postmenopausal women following exercise training. It is not clear why postmenopausal women did not respond to exercise, but it is consistent with work suggesting some individuals are "exercise resistant" [75]. Another plausible reason may relate to the notion that estrogen provides protective heart effects and lowers CVD risk in women [93]. Notwithstanding these hormonal differences across the lifespan in women or compared with men, fitness may be an additional determinant of EV improvement posttraining. Indeed, recent work by our group [94], following minimal requirements of EV detection and functional studies established by the International Society of Extracellular Vesicles [12], as well as advanced imaging flow cytometry (*see below for details*), showed that EVs correlate with aerobic fitness and other cardiometabolic health factors in obese adults, highlighting again the potential role of fitness in modulating EVs. Furthermore, Van Craenenbroeck et al. reported that preintervention endothelial EVs ($CD31^+/CD42b$) count significantly predicted improvements in VO_2max despite no effect of a 12-week training program on these EVs in 200 individuals with coronary artery disease [95]. Together, these later findings suggest that EV may modulate training responses through a yet to be defined mechanism.

As exercise training promotes weight loss and decreases adipose-derived inflammation [96, 97], it is reasonable to expect that habitual exercise improves EVs originating from platelets and leukocytes. Murakami et al. reported that platelet EVs ($CD41^+$) were significantly correlated with a subcutaneous fat area in 49 obese, nondiabetic subjects following 12 weeks of a restricted caloric diet or a restricted caloric diet plus exercise [33]. Although EVs did not correlate with visceral fat, which is considered a chief site for inflammatory production, this finding is reasonable since subcutaneous tissue is a primary supplier of free fatty acids, and elevated free fatty acids may act as a bioactive lipid that stimulates coagulation and platelet recruitment [98]. Whether exercise or exercise plus diet alter free fatty acid mediated EV levels or function waits to be tested. In either case, in the only studies to investigate exercise on leukocyte EVs ($CD16^+$, $CD14^+$), it was shown that training decreases neutrophil- and monocyte-derived EVs ($CD16^+$, $CD14^+$). This observation highlights that exercise has multicell EV effects that may favor improvement in cardiometabolic health [99, 100].

6. Extracellular Vesicle Analysis and Gaps

To date, most exercise studies lack sensitivity to optimally enrich and phenotype EVs. A leading challenge in doing so is the lack of consensus on the nomenclature of EVs as well as the precise detection method or sample preparation (i.e., the preanalytical phase) [12, 101]. In fact, the preanalytical phase includes several important steps that could impact the clarity and precision of results, including but not limited to blood collection technique (e.g., needle size or blood draw rate that impacts shear stress), sample centrifugation, timing of sample processing, sample freezing, thawing, and storage [102]. Generally speaking, EVs collected from fresh blood is considered more accurate and reflective true *in vivo* EV levels when compared with frozen samples [101, 103], but plasma frozen for only 24 hr may yield comparable counts when compared to fresh sample [104]. In either case, it is suggested that samples should be analyzed after the same "freezing period" [105] to enhance accuracy of sample analysis. Centrifugation speed crucially affects the type of EV population isolated. Most of the studies analyzing EVs in exercise interventions have utilized low centrifugation speeds (Tables 1 and 2, resp.). As different speeds are used, they have likely isolated different EV populations. In addition, they might have enriched for larger EVs and therefore used the term microparticles. However, this topic is still in debate and our work [10, 94] and that of others [11–13] indicates that we also see smaller EVs (e.g., exosomes, <100 nm) in these preparations, thereby making it difficult to distinguish between various types of EVs [11].

Conventional flow cytometry is the most commonly used technique for phenotyping and enumeration of EVs [106]. However, many older flow cytometer models limit the detection of smaller EVs, thereby contributing to potential gaps in our understanding of all subtypes of EVs [10]. Indeed, recent evidence suggests that while >80% of EVs are <500 nm, most conventional flow cytometers have a detection threshold greater than 500 nm, suggesting that a vast majority of EVs may not be quantified [107] with this technique. To address this discrepancy, an alternative approach has been developed, combining flow cytometry with imaging (called imaging flow cytometry). Erdbrügger et al. found that by adding imaging to flow cytometry, EVs can be clearly differentiated from the beads and cells, as well as debris. It also provides the advantage of confirming the presence of these vesicles based not only on fluorescence but also on scatter and morphology as well [108]. By detection of EV fluorescence only, even smaller EVs can be detected. The detection threshold is likely down to 100–200 nm. To date though, no prospective exercise research exists utilizing this approach to assess EV phenotypes. As interest in the role of EVs as mediators and markers of disease continues to grow, implementation of standardized EV approaches will be needed to elucidate the exact role of EVs in chronic disease. One approach to close this method gap is that future studies consider using established guidelines by the EV-TRACK Consortium to improve transparency in reporting EV research [106] and follow minimal experimental requirements for definition of EVs and their functions, as published by the International Society for Extracellular Vesicles [12]. Finally, implementation of these minimal experimental requirements described [12] is crucial in moving forward with functional studies combined with content analysis (genetic, proteomic, and metabolomics) in order to better advance our understanding preventing/treating chronic disease in relation to EVs.

7. Analysis of Smaller Extracellular Vesicles

Most of the studies discussed so far have used low centrifugation speeds to enrich for EVs, but likely analyzed a mix of large and smaller vesicles in their preparations. A few studies have focused on use of high centrifugation speed of 100,000 G to enrich for smaller EVs called exosomes. It is important to study all subtypes of EVs given that they play roles in immune modulation [109, 110], activating tissue repair [111], and angiogenesis as the following studies demonstrate. Interestingly, Fruhbeis et al. was one of them to report that cycling exercise increased smaller EVs (called exosomes, positive for Flot1, Hsp/Hsc70, and IntαIIb) to a greater extent when compared to treadmill exercise, but the rise in these smaller EVs (exosomes) remained elevated for a longer period of time into recovery with treadmill exercise [112]. The reason for these differential responses between treadmill and cycling exercise is not clear, but it might relate to the higher heart rate and eccentric muscle contraction associated with running. This would be consistent with prior work [65], suggesting that EVs are important for vascular repair and adaptation. Moreover, recent work from Safdar et al. has suggested that smaller EVs (exosomes) may be essential following endurance-oriented exercise as a means to treat metabolic disease [113]. This assertion is supported by evidence from Bei et al. who demonstrated that exercise-induced increases in circulating EVs enhanced the protective effects of endogenous EVs against cardiac ischemia/reperfusion injury [114]. These later findings are consistent with new work highlighting that exosomes play critical roles in interorgan crosstalk during exercise to regulate energy homeostasis [66]. Taken together, these preliminary data suggest more work is needed to characterize all subtypes of EVs, including smaller (exosomes) and larger (microparticle) EVs in people with T2D and CVD following different doses of exercise, with or without diet modification, to improve clinical practice for patient care.

8. Conclusion and Clinical Perspectives

The precise mechanism by which exercise lowers CVD is unclear, as only 40–50% of the reduction in CVD risk in subjects reporting >1500 kcal/week of exercise is attributed to nontraditional CVD risk factors [115]. EVs have emerged as novel markers of T2D and CVD that have potential functional and therapeutic benefit by transferring proteins, lipids, and nucleic acids. In fact, EV physiology appears critical towards the production of oxidative stress [54], inflammation [23], and/or physical contact/release of signaling molecules (i.e., miRNA) that modulate endothelial function [116]. Herein, we present evidence that suggests EVs represent a potentially novel mechanism by which exercise could fill a "cardio-protection risk gap." Exercise may impact EVs by not only reducing substrates thought to drive EV functional responses but also altering the release of oxidative stress, inflammatory cytokines, and miRNA (Figure 1). Indeed, the acute effects of exercise on EVs are limited to endothelium-derived EVs ($CD62E^+$, $CD31^+/CD42b^-$, $CD144^+$) with little change or slight increases and few to no work on platelet- or leukocyte-derived EVs (Table 1). In contrast, exercise training appears to have more robust effects on decreasing endothelium-, platelet-, and leukocyte-derived EVs in men and women (Table 2). However, these studies are limited in that conventional flow cytometry has been used, thereby providing less sensitivity to detecting a variety of EV sizes (<500 nm) as well as distinguishing EVs from small cells/debris. Further work is needed using various tools including imaging or high-resolution flow cytometry, tunable resistive pulse sensing, or nanoparticle tracking device and electron microscopy before and after exercise interventions in order to ascertain a comprehensive EV profile in adults at risk for and with T2D or CVD. Knowledge of EV content and function may ultimately lead to improved patient care by enabling health care providers to provide bioengineered agents that mitigate "cargo" released from these EVs and/or deliver exercise-derived EVs as therapeutic options for optimization of T2D and CVD management.

Abbreviations

EVs: Extracellular vesicles
T2D: Type 2 diabetes
CVD: Cardiovascular disease.

Conflicts of Interest

All authors declare that they have no competing interests.

Authors' Contributions

Natalie Z. M. Eichner and Steven K. Malin were primarily responsible for writing the manuscript. Uta Erdbrügger reviewed and edited the manuscript.

Acknowledgements

The authors thank members of the Applied Metabolism & Physiology Laboratory for helpful discussion on the manuscript.

References

[1] Centers for Disease Control and Prevention (CDC), *National Diabetes Fact Sheet: National Estimates and General Information on Diabetes and Prediabetes in the United States, 2011, vol. 201*, US Department of Health and Human Services, Centers for Disease Control and Prevention, Atlanta, GA, USA, 2011.

[2] G. A. Roth, C. Johnson, A. Abajobir et al., "Global, regional, and national burden of cardiovascular diseases for 10 causes, 1990 to 2015," *Journal of the American College of Cardiology*, vol. 70, no. 1, pp. 1–25, 2017.

[3] N. J. Morrish, S.-L. Wang, L. K. Stevens, J. H. Fuller, H. Keen, and WHO Multinational Study Group, "Mortality and causes of death in the WHO Multinational Study of Vascular Disease in Diabetes," *Diabetologia*, vol. 44, Supplement 2, pp. S14–S21, 2001.

[4] W. Duckworth, C. Abraira, T. Moritz et al., "Glucose control and vascular complications in veterans with type 2 diabetes," *New England Journal of Medicine*, vol. 360, no. 2, pp. 129–139, 2009.

[5] M. Abdul-Ghani, R. A. DeFronzo, S. Del Prato, R. Chilton, R. Singh, and R. E. J. Ryder, "Cardiovascular disease and type 2 diabetes: has the dawn of a new era arrived?," *Diabetes Care*, vol. 40, no. 7, pp. 813–820, 2017.

[6] L. Zhang, M. A. Vincent, S. M. Richards et al., "Insulin sensitivity of muscle capillary recruitment in vivo," *Diabetes*, vol. 53, no. 2, pp. 447–453, 2004.

[7] P. M. Ridker, J. E. Buring, N. Rifai, and N. R. Cook, "Development and validation of improved algorithms for the assessment of global cardiovascular risk in women: the Reynolds Risk Score," *JAMA*, vol. 297, no. 6, pp. 611–619, 2007.

[8] N. Amabile, P.-E. Rautou, A. Tedgui, and C. M. Boulanger, "Microparticles: key protagonists in cardiovascular disorders," *Seminars in Thrombosis and Hemostasis*, vol. 36, no. 8, pp. 907–916, 2010.

[9] S. Nomura, "Dynamic role of microparticles in type 2 diabetes mellitus," *Current Diabetes Reviews*, vol. 5, no. 4, pp. 245–251, 2009.

[10] U. Erdbrügger and J. Lannigan, "Analytical challenges of extracellular vesicle detection: a comparison of different techniques," *Cytometry Part A*, vol. 89, no. 2, pp. 123–134, 2016.

[11] K. W. Witwer, E. I. Buzas, L. T. Bemis et al., "Standardization of sample collection, isolation and analysis methods in extracellular vesicle research," *Journal of Extracellular Vesicles*, vol. 2, no. 1, p. 20360, 2013.

[12] J. Lötvall, A. F. Hill, F. Hochberg et al., "Minimal experimental requirements for definition of extracellular vesicles and their functions: a position statement from the International Society for Extracellular Vesicles," *Journal of Extracellular Vesicles*, vol. 3, no. 1, 2014.

[13] J. Kowal, G. Arras, M. Colombo et al., "Proteomic comparison defines novel markers to characterize heterogeneous populations of extracellular vesicle subtypes," *Proceedings of the National Academy of Sciences of the United States of America*, vol. 113, no. 8, pp. E968–E977, 2016.

[14] F. Santilli, R. Liani, P. Di Fulvio et al., "Increased circulating resistin is associated with insulin resistance, oxidative stress and platelet activation in type 2 diabetes mellitus," *Thrombosis and Haemostasis*, vol. 116, no. 12, pp. 1089–1099, 2016.

[15] N. M. Navasiolava, F. Dignat-George, F. Sabatier et al., "Enforced physical inactivity increases endothelial microparticle levels in healthy volunteers," *American journal of Physiology-Heart and Circulatory Physiology*, vol. 299, no. 2, pp. H248–H256, 2010.

[16] P. Wolf, "The nature and significance of platelet products in human plasma," *British Journal of Haematology*, vol. 13, no. 3, pp. 269–288, 1967.

[17] B. Hugel, M. C. Martinez, C. Kunzelmann, and J. M. Freyssinet, "Membrane microparticles: two sides of the coin," *Physiology*, vol. 20, no. 1, pp. 22–27, 2005.

[18] P. E. Rautou, A. S. Leroyer, B. Ramkhelawon et al., "Microparticles from human atherosclerotic plaques promote endothelial ICAM-1-dependent monocyte adhesion and transendothelial migration," *Circulation Research*, vol. 108, no. 3, pp. 335–343, 2011.

[19] M. Pirro, G. Schillaci, F. Bagaglia et al., "Microparticles derived from endothelial progenitor cells in patients at different cardiovascular risk," *Atherosclerosis*, vol. 197, no. 2, pp. 757–767, 2008.

[20] D. M. Smalley, N. E. Sheman, K. Nelson, and D. Theodorescu, "Isolation and identification of potential urinary microparticle biomarkers of bladder cancer," *Journal of Proteome Research*, vol. 7, no. 5, pp. 2088–2096, 2008.

[21] C. M. Boulanger, "Microparticles, vascular function and hypertension," *Current Opinion in Nephrology and Hypertension*, vol. 19, no. 2, pp. 177–180, 2010.

[22] O. P. Barry, D. Pratico, J. A. Lawson, and G. A. FitzGerald-Transcellular activation of platelets and endothelial cells by bioactive lipids in platelet microparticles," *The Journal of Clinical Investigation*, vol. 99, no. 9, pp. 2118–2127, 1997.

[23] F. Jansen, X. Yang, B. S. Franklin et al., "High glucose condition increases NADPH oxidase activity in endothelial microparticles that promote vascular inflammation," *Cardiovascular Research*, vol. 98, no. 1, pp. 94–106, 2013.

[24] D. Burger, M. Turner, F. Xiao, M. N. Munkonda, S. Akbari, and K. D. Burns, "High glucose increases the formation and pro-oxidative activity of endothelial microparticles," *Diabetologia*, vol. 60, no. 9, pp. 1791–1800, 2017.

[25] P. Horn, M. M. Cortese-Krott, N. Amabile et al., "Circulating microparticles carry a functional endothelial nitric oxide synthase that is decreased in patients with endothelial dysfunction," *Journal of the American Heart Association*, vol. 2, no. 1, article e003764, 2012.

[26] G. Y. Chen and G. Nuñez, "Sterile inflammation: sensing and reacting to damage," *Nature Reviews Immunology*, vol. 10, no. 12, pp. 826–837, 2010.

[27] E. R. Abels and X. O. Breakefield, "Introduction to extracellular vesicles: biogenesis, RNA cargo selection, content, release, and uptake," *Cellular and Molecular Neurobiology*, vol. 36, no. 3, pp. 301–312, 2016.

[28] P. Bastos-Amador, B. Perez-Cabezas, N. Izquierdo-Useros et al., "Capture of cell-derived microvesicles (exosomes and apoptotic bodies) by human plasmacytoid dendritic cells," *Journal of Leukocyte Biology*, vol. 91, no. 5, pp. 751–758, 2012.

[29] A. Giannella, C. M. Radu, L. Franco et al., "Circulating levels and characterization of microparticles in patients with different degrees of glucose tolerance," *Cardiovascular Diabetology*, vol. 16, no. 1, p. 118, 2017.

[30] J.-M. Wang, C. Su, Y. Wang et al., "Elevated circulating endothelial microparticles and brachial–ankle pulse wave velocity in well-controlled hypertensive patients," *Journal of Human Hypertension*, vol. 23, no. 5, pp. 307–315, 2009.

[31] N. Amabile, A. P. Guerin, A. Tedgui, C. M. Boulanger, and G. M. London, "Predictive value of circulating endothelial microparticles for cardiovascular mortality in end-stage renal failure: a pilot study," *Nephrology, Dialysis, Transplantation*, vol. 27, no. 5, pp. 1873–1880, 2012.

[32] T. Nozaki, S. Sugiyama, K. Sugamura et al., "Prognostic value of endothelial microparticles in patients with heart failure," *European Journal of Heart Failure*, vol. 12, no. 11, pp. 1223–1228, 2010.

[33] T. Murakami, H. Horigome, K. Tanaka et al., "Impact of weight reduction on production of platelet-derived microparticles and fibrinolytic parameters in obesity," *Thrombosis Research*, vol. 119, no. 1, pp. 45–53, 2007.

[34] F. Dignat-George and C. M. Boulanger, "The many faces of endothelial microparticles," *Arteriosclerosis, Thrombosis, and Vascular Biology*, vol. 31, no. 1, pp. 27–33, 2011.

[35] N. Werner, S. Wassmann, P. Ahlers, S. Kosiol, and G. Nickenig, "Circulating $CD31^+$/annexin V^+ apoptotic microparticles correlate with coronary endothelial function in patients with coronary artery disease," *Arteriosclerosis, Thrombosis, and Vascular Biology*, vol. 26, no. 1, pp. 112–116, 2006.

[36] C.-H. Yun, K. H. Jung, K. Chu et al., "Increased circulating endothelial microparticles and carotid atherosclerosis in obstructive sleep apnea," *Journal of Clinical Neurology*, vol. 6, no. 2, pp. 89–98, 2010.

[37] K. Esposito, M. Ciotola, B. Schisano et al., "Endothelial microparticles correlate with endothelial dysfunction in obese women," *The Journal of Clinical Endocrinology & Metabolism*, vol. 91, no. 9, pp. 3676–3679, 2006.

[38] D. Burger, A. C. Montezano, N. Nishigaki, Y. He, A. Carter, and R. M. Touyz, "Endothelial microparticle formation by angiotensin II is mediated via Ang II receptor type I/NADPH oxidase/Rho kinase pathways targeted to lipid rafts," *Arteriosclerosis, Thrombosis, and Vascular Biology*, vol. 31, no. 8, pp. 1898–1907, 2011.

[39] D. Burger, D. G. Kwart, A. C. Montezano et al., "Microparticles induce cell cycle arrest through redox-sensitive processes in endothelial cells: implications in vascular senescence,"

Journal of the American Heart Association, vol. 1, no. 3, article e001842, 2012.

[40] A. D. Terrisse, N. Puech, S. Allart et al., "Internalization of microparticles by endothelial cells promotes platelet/endothelial cell interaction under flow," *Journal of Thrombosis and Haemostasis*, vol. 8, no. 12, pp. 2810–2819, 2010.

[41] H. A. Mostefai, A. Agouni, N. Carusio et al., "Phosphatidylinositol 3-kinase and xanthine oxidase regulate nitric oxide and reactive oxygen species productions by apoptotic lymphocyte microparticles in endothelial cells," *Journal of Immunology*, vol. 180, no. 7, pp. 5028-5035, 2008.

[42] S. Essayagh, J.-M. Xuereb, A.-D. Terrisse, L. Tellier-Cirioni, B. Pipy, and P. Sié, "Microparticles from apoptotic monocytes induce transient platelet recruitment and tissue factor expression by cultured human vascular endothelial cells via a redox-sensitive mechanism," *Thrombosis and Haemostasis*, vol. 98, no. 10, pp. 831–837, 2007.

[43] M. Mesri and D. C. Altieri, "Endothelial cell activation by leukocyte microparticles," *The Journal of Immunology*, vol. 161, no. 8, pp. 4382–4387, 1998.

[44] A. Scanu, N. Molnarfi, K. J. Brandt, L. Gruaz, J. M. Dayer, and D. Burger, "Stimulated T cells generate microparticles, which mimic cellular contact activation of human monocytes: differential regulation of pro- and anti-inflammatory cytokine production by high-density lipoproteins," *Journal of Leukocyte Biology*, vol. 83, no. 4, pp. 921-927, 2008.

[45] M. L. Mastronardi, H. A. Mostefai, F. Meziani, M. C. Martinez, P. Asfar, and R. Andriantsitohaina, "Circulating microparticles from septic shock patients exert differential tissue expression of enzymes related to inflammation and oxidative stress," *Critical Care Medicine*, vol. 39, no. 7, pp. 1739–1748, 2011.

[46] J. Mleczko, F. J. Ortega, J. M. Falcon-Perez, M. Wabitsch, J. M. Fernandez-Real, and S. Mora, "Extracellular Vesicles from Hypoxic Adipocytes and obese subjects reduce Insulin-Stimulated Glucose Uptake," *Molecular Nutrition & Food Research*, vol. 62, no. 5, 2018.

[47] Y. Zhang, L. Shi, H. Mei et al., "Inflamed macrophage microvesicles induce insulin resistance in human adipocytes," *Nutrition & Metabolism*, vol. 12, no. 1, p. 21, 2015.

[48] P. Diehl, A. Fricke, L. Sander et al., "Microparticles: major transport vehicles for distinct microRNAs in circulation," *Cardiovascular Research*, vol. 93, no. 4, pp. 633-644, 2012.

[49] M. E. G. Kranendonk, D. P. V. de Kleijn, E. Kalkhoven et al., "Extracellular vesicle markers in relation to obesity and metabolic complications in patients with manifest cardiovascular disease," *Cardiovascular Diabetology*, vol. 13, no. 1, p. 37, 2014.

[50] Y. Choi, Y. Kwon, D. K. Kim et al., "Gut microbe-derived extracellular vesicles induce insulin resistance, thereby impairing glucose metabolism in skeletal muscle," *Scientific Reports*, vol. 5, no. 1, p. 15878, 2015.

[51] D. Faille, F. el-Assaad, A. J. Mitchell et al., "Endocytosis and intracellular processing of platelet microparticles by brain endothelial cells," *Journal of Cellular and Molecular Medicine*, vol. 16, no. 8, pp. 1731–1738, 2012.

[52] L. A. Mulcahy, R. C. Pink, and D. R. F. Carter, "Routes and mechanisms of extracellular vesicle uptake," *Journal of Extracellular Vesicles*, vol. 3, no. 1, 2014.

[53] A. S. Leroyer, P. E. Rautou, J. S. Silvestre et al., "CD40 ligand microparticles from human atherosclerotic plaques stimulate endothelial proliferation and angiogenesis: a potential mechanism for intraplaque neovascularization," *Journal of the American College of Cardiology*, vol. 52, no. 16, pp. 1302–1311, 2008.

[54] A. Mezentsev, R. M. H. Merks, E. O'Riordan et al., "Endothelial microparticles affect angiogenesis in vitro: role of oxidative stress," *American Journal of Physiology-Heart and Circulatory Physiology*, vol. 289, no. 3, pp. H1106–H1114, 2005.

[55] H. K. Kim, K. S. Song, J. H. Chung, K. R. Lee, and S. N. Lee, "Platelet microparticles induce angiogenesis in vitro," *British Journal of Haematology*, vol. 124, no. 3, pp. 376–384, 2004.

[56] C. Yang, B. R. Mwaikambo, T. Zhu et al., "Lymphocytic microparticles inhibit angiogenesis by stimulating oxidative stress and negatively regulating VEGF-induced pathways," *American Journal of Physiology-Regulatory, Integrative and Comparative Physiology*, vol. 294, no. 2, pp. R467–R476, 2008.

[57] F. R. Formiga, B. Pelacho, E. Garbayo et al., "Sustained release of VEGF through PLGA microparticles improves vasculogenesis and tissue remodeling in an acute myocardial ischemia–reperfusion model," *Journal of Controlled Release*, vol. 147, no. 1, pp. 30–37, 2010.

[58] A. Ceriello and E. Motz, "Is oxidative stress the pathogenic mechanism underlying insulin resistance, diabetes, and cardiovascular disease? The common soil hypothesis revisited," *Arteriosclerosis, Thrombosis, and Vascular Biology*, vol. 24, no. 5, pp. 816–823, 2004.

[59] E. J. Henriksen, "Invited review: effects of acute exercise and exercise training on insulin resistance," *Journal of Applied Physiology*, vol. 93, no. 2, pp. 788–796, 2002.

[60] T. Guiraud, M. Gayda, M. Juneau et al., "A single bout of high-intensity interval exercise does not increase endothelial or platelet microparticles in stable, physically fit men with coronary heart disease," *Canadian Journal of Cardiology*, vol. 29, no. 10, pp. 1285–1291, 2013.

[61] M. Chanda, D. Nantakomol, D. Suksom, and A. Palasuwan, "Cell-derived microparticles after exercise in individuals with G6PD Viangchan," *Clinical Hemorheology and Microcirculation*, vol. 60, no. 2, pp. 241–251, 2015.

[62] M. D. Ross, A. L. Wekesa, J. P. Phelan, and M. Harrison, "Resistance exercise increases endothelial progenitor cells and angiogenic factors," *Medicine and Science in Sports and Exercise*, vol. 46, no. 1, pp. 16–23, 2014.

[63] S. Mobius-Winkler, T. Hilberg, K. Menzel et al., "Time-dependent mobilization of circulating progenitor cells during strenuous exercise in healthy individuals," *Journal of Applied Physiology*, vol. 107, no. 6, pp. 1943–1950, 2009.

[64] S. K. Powers, L. L. Ji, A. N. Kavazis, and M. J. Jackson, "Reactive oxygen species: impact on skeletal muscle," *Comprehensive Physiology*, vol. 1, pp. 941–969, 2011.

[65] E. N. Wilhelm, J. Gonzalez-Alonso, C. Parris, and M. Rakobowchuk, "Exercise intensity modulates the appearance of circulating microvesicles with proangiogenic potential upon endothelial cells," *American Journal of Physiology-Heart and Circulatory Physiology*, vol. 311, no. 5, pp. H1297–H1310, 2016.

[66] M. Whitham, B. L. Parker, M. Friedrichsen et al., "Extracellular vesicles provide a means for tissue crosstalk during

exercise," *Cell Metabolism*, vol. 27, no. 1, pp. 237–251.e4, 2018.

[67] P. Wahl, U. F. Wehmeier, F. J. Jansen et al., "Acute effects of different exercise protocols on the circulating vascular microRNAs -16, -21, and -126 in trained subjects," *Frontiers in Physiology*, vol. 7, p. 643, 2016.

[68] B. Toth, K. Nikolajek, A. Rank et al., "Gender-specific and menstrual cycle dependent differences in circulating microparticles," *Platelets*, vol. 18, no. 7, pp. 515–521, 2007.

[69] K. A. Lansford, D. D. Shill, A. B. Dicks, M. P. Marshburn, W. M. Southern, and N. T. Jenkins, "Effect of acute exercise on circulating angiogenic cell and microparticle populations," *Experimental Physiology*, vol. 101, no. 1, pp. 155–167, 2016.

[70] S. Sahoo, E. Klychko, T. Thorne et al., "Exosomes from human $CD34^+$ stem cells mediate their proangiogenic paracrine activity," *Circulation Research*, vol. 109, no. 7, pp. 724–728, 2011.

[71] T. Asahara, T. Murohara, A. Sullivan et al., "Isolation of putative progenitor endothelial cells for angiogenesis," *Science*, vol. 275, no. 5302, pp. 964–966, 1997.

[72] C. Durrer, E. Robinson, Z. Wan et al., "Differential impact of acute high-intensity exercise on circulating endothelial microparticles and insulin resistance between overweight/obese males and females," *PLoS One*, vol. 10, no. 2, article e0115860, 2015.

[73] A. Fard, C. H. Tuck, J. A. Donis et al., "Acute elevations of plasma asymmetric dimethylarginine and impaired endothelial function in response to a high-fat meal in patients with type 2 diabetes," *Arteriosclerosis, Thrombosis, and Vascular Biology*, vol. 20, no. 9, pp. 2039–2044, 2000.

[74] N. T. Jenkins, J. Padilla, L. J. Boyle, D. P. Credeur, M. H. Laughlin, and P. J. Fadel, "Disturbed blood flow acutely induces activation and apoptosis of the human vascular endothelium," *Hypertension*, vol. 61, no. 3, pp. 615–621, 2013.

[75] S. K. Malin, Z. Liu, E. J. Barrett, and A. Weltman, "Exercise resistance across the prediabetes phenotypes: impact on insulin sensitivity and substrate metabolism," *Reviews in Endocrine and Metabolic Disorders*, vol. 17, no. 1, pp. 81–90, 2016.

[76] M. Harrison, R. P. Murphy, P. L. O'Connor et al., "The endothelial microparticle response to a high fat meal is not attenuated by prior exercise," *European Journal of Applied Physiology*, vol. 106, no. 4, pp. 555–562, 2009.

[77] D. R. Blake, J. B. Meigs, D. C. Muller, S. S. Najjar, R. Andres, and D. M. Nathan, "Impaired glucose tolerance, but not impaired fasting glucose, is associated with increased levels of coronary heart disease risk factors: results from the Baltimore Longitudinal Study on Aging," *Diabetes*, vol. 53, no. 8, pp. 2095–2100, 2004.

[78] B. H. Goodpaster, D. E. Kelley, R. R. Wing, A. Meier, and F. L. Thaete, "Effects of weight loss on regional fat distribution and insulin sensitivity in obesity," *Diabetes*, vol. 48, no. 4, pp. 839–847, 1999.

[79] S. K. Malin, R. Gerber, S. R. Chipkin, and B. Braun, "Independent and combined effects of exercise training and metformin on insulin sensitivity in individuals with prediabetes," *Diabetes Care*, vol. 35, no. 1, pp. 131–136, 2012.

[80] S. K. Malin, J. M. Haus, T. P. J. Solomon, A. Blaszczak, S. R. Kashyap, and J. P. Kirwan, "Insulin sensitivity and metabolic flexibility following exercise training among different obese insulin-resistant phenotypes," *American journal of Physiology-Endocrinology and Metabolism*, vol. 305, no. 10, pp. E1292–E1298, 2013.

[81] T. P. J. Solomon, S. K. Malin, K. Karstoft, J. M. Haus, and J. P. Kirwan, "The influence of hyperglycemia on the therapeutic effect of exercise on glycemic control in patients with type 2 diabetes mellitus," *JAMA Internal Medicine*, vol. 173, no. 19, pp. 1834–1836, 2013.

[82] P. Clarkson, H. E. Montgomery, M. J. Mullen et al., "Exercise training enhances endothelial function in young men," *Journal of the American College of Cardiology*, vol. 33, no. 5, pp. 1379–1385, 1999.

[83] D. L. Swift, J. Y. Weltman, J. T. Patrie et al., "Predictors of improvement in endothelial function after exercise training in a diverse sample of postmenopausal women," *Journal of Women's Health*, vol. 23, no. 3, pp. 260–266, 2014.

[84] N. Gokce, J. A. Vita, D. S. Bader et al., "Effect of exercise on upper and lower extremity endothelial function in patients with coronary artery disease," *The American Journal of Cardiology*, vol. 90, no. 2, pp. 124–127, 2002.

[85] R. Hambrecht, A. Wolf, S. Gielen et al., "Effect of exercise on coronary endothelial function in patients with coronary artery disease," *New England Journal of Medicine*, vol. 342, no. 7, pp. 454–460, 2000.

[86] L. Bruyndonckx, V. Y. Hoymans, A. De Guchtenaere et al., "Diet, exercise, and endothelial function in obese adolescents," *Pediatrics*, vol. 135, no. 3, pp. e653–e661, 2015.

[87] S. La Vignera, R. Condorelli, E. Vicari, R. D'agata, and A. Calogero, "Aerobic physical activity improves endothelial function in the middle-aged patients with erectile dysfunction," *The Aging Male*, vol. 14, no. 4, pp. 265–272, 2011.

[88] J. S. Kim, B. Kim, H. Lee et al., "Shear stress-induced mitochondrial biogenesis decreases the release of microparticles from endothelial cells," *American Journal of Physiology-Heart and Circulatory Physiology*, vol. 309, no. 3, pp. H425–H433, 2015.

[89] J. Kretzschmar, D. M. Babbitt, K. M. Diaz et al., "A standardized exercise intervention differentially affects premenopausal and postmenopausal African-American women," *Menopause*, vol. 21, no. 6, pp. 579–584, 2014.

[90] D. M. Babbitt, K. M. Diaz, D. L. Feairheller et al., "Endothelial activation microparticles and inflammation status improve with exercise training in African Americans," *International Journal of Hypertension*, vol. 2013, Article ID 538017, 8 pages, 2013.

[91] J. Pitha, I. Kralova Lesna, P. Stavek et al., "Effect of exercise on markers of vascular health in renal transplant recipients," *Physiological Research*, vol. 64, no. 6, pp. 945–949, 2015.

[92] I. Y. Oh, C. H. Yoon, J. Hur et al., "Involvement of E-selectin in recruitment of endothelial progenitor cells and angiogenesis in ischemic muscle," *Blood*, vol. 110, no. 12, pp. 3891–3899, 2007.

[93] M. E. Mendelsohn, "Protective effects of estrogen on the cardiovascular system," *The American Journal of Cardiology*, vol. 89, no. 12, pp. 12–17, 2002.

[94] N. Z. M. Eichner, N. M. Gilbertson, J. M. Gaitan et al., "Low cardiorespiratory fitness is associated with higher microparticle counts in obese adults," *Physiological Reports*, vol. 6, no. 10, article e13701, 2018.

[95] E. M. Van Craenenbroeck, G. Frederix, N. Pattyn et al., "Effects of aerobic interval training and continuous training on cellular markers of endothelial integrity in coronary artery disease: a SAINTEX-CAD substudy," *American Journal of Physiology-Heart and Circulatory Physiology*, vol. 309, no. 11, pp. H1876–H1882, 2015.

[96] I. J. Kullo, M. Khaleghi, and D. D. Hensrud, "Markers of inflammation are inversely associated with $VO_{2\ max}$ in asymptomatic men," *Journal of Applied Physiology*, vol. 102, no. 4, pp. 1374–1379, 2007.

[97] X. Wang, T. You, K. Murphy, M. F. Lyles, and B. J. Nicklas, "Addition of exercise increases plasma adiponectin and release from adipose tissue," *Medicine and Science in Sports and Exercise*, vol. 47, no. 11, pp. 2450–2455, 2015.

[98] A. Silveira, F. Karpe, H. Johnsson, K. A. Bauer, and A. Hamsten, "In vivo demonstration in humans that large postprandial triglyceride-rich lipoproteins activate coagulation factor VII through the intrinsic coagulation pathway," *Arteriosclerosis, Thrombosis, and Vascular Biology*, vol. 16, no. 11, pp. 1333–1339, 1996.

[99] Y. C. Chen, C. W. Ho, H. H. Tsai, and J. S. Wang, "Interval and continuous exercise regimens suppress neutrophil-derived microparticle formation and neutrophil-promoted thrombin generation under hypoxic stress," *Clinical Science*, vol. 128, no. 7, pp. 425–436, 2015.

[100] J. S. Wang, Y. L. Chang, Y. C. Chen, H. H. Tsai, and T. C. Fu, "Effects of normoxic and hypoxic exercise regimens on monocyte-mediated thrombin generation in sedentary men," *Clinical Science*, vol. 129, no. 4, pp. 363–374, 2015.

[101] Y. Yuana, R. M. Bertina, and S. Osanto, "Pre-analytical and analytical issues in the analysis of blood microparticles," *Thrombosis and Haemostasis*, vol. 105, no. 03, pp. 396–408, 2011.

[102] S. H. van Ierssel, E. M. Van Craenenbroeck, V. M. Conraads et al., "Flow cytometric detection of endothelial microparticles (EMP): effects of centrifugation and storage alter with the phenotype studied," *Thrombosis Research*, vol. 125, no. 4, pp. 332–339, 2010.

[103] F. Mobarrez, J. Antovic, N. Egberg et al., "A multicolor flow cytometric assay for measurement of platelet-derived microparticles," *Thrombosis Research*, vol. 125, no. 3, pp. e110–e116, 2010.

[104] A. G. Kriebardis, M. H. Antonelou, H. T. Georgatzakou, V. L. Tzounakas, K. E. Stamoulis, and I. S. Papassideri, "Microparticles variability in fresh frozen plasma: preparation protocol and storage time effects," *Blood Transfusion*, vol. 14, no. 2, pp. 228–237, 2016.

[105] E. Dey-Hazra, B. Hertel, T. Kirsch et al., "Detection of circulating microparticles by flow cytometry: influence of centrifugation, filtration of buffer, and freezing," *Vascular Health and Risk Management*, vol. 6, pp. 1125–1133, 2010.

[106] EV-TRACK Consortium, J. van Deun, P. Mestdagh et al., "EV-TRACK: transparent reporting and centralizing knowledge in extracellular vesicle research," *Nature Methods*, vol. 14, no. 3, pp. 228–232, 2017.

[107] N. Arraud, R. Linares, S. Tan et al., "Extracellular vesicles from blood plasma: determination of their morphology, size, phenotype and concentration," *Journal of Thrombosis and Haemostasis*, vol. 12, no. 5, pp. 614–627, 2014.

[108] U. Erdbrügger, C. K. Rudy, M. E. Etter et al., "Imaging flow cytometry elucidates limitations of microparticle analysis by conventional flow cytometry," *Cytometry Part A*, vol. 85, no. 9, pp. 756–770, 2014.

[109] C. Théry, M. Ostrowski, and E. Segura, "Membrane vesicles as conveyors of immune responses," *Nature Reviews Immunology*, vol. 9, no. 8, pp. 581–593, 2009.

[110] D. W. Greening, S. K. Gopal, R. Xu, R. J. Simpson, and W. Chen, "Exosomes and their roles in immune regulation and cancer," *Seminars in Cell & Developmental Biology*, vol. 40, pp. 72–81, 2015.

[111] G. Camussi, M. C. Deregibus, S. Bruno, V. Cantaluppi, and L. Biancone, "Exosomes/microvesicles as a mechanism of cell-to-cell communication," *Kidney International*, vol. 78, no. 9, pp. 838–848, 2010.

[112] C. Fruhbeis, S. Helmig, S. Tug, P. Simon, and E. M. Kramer-Albers, "Physical exercise induces rapid release of small extracellular vesicles into the circulation," *Journal of Extracellular Vesicles*, vol. 4, no. 1, article 28239, 2015.

[113] A. Safdar, A. Saleem, and M. A. Tarnopolsky, "The potential of endurance exercise-derived exosomes to treat metabolic diseases," *Nature Reviews Endocrinology*, vol. 12, no. 9, pp. 504–517, 2016.

[114] Y. Bei, T. Xu, D. Lv et al., "Exercise-induced circulating extracellular vesicles protect against cardiac ischemia–reperfusion injury," *Basic Research in Cardiology*, vol. 112, no. 4, p. 38, 2017.

[115] S. Mora, N. Cook, J. E. Buring, P. M. Ridker, and I. M. Lee, "Physical activity and reduced risk of cardiovascular events: potential mediating mechanisms," *Circulation*, vol. 116, no. 19, pp. 2110–2118, 2007.

[116] S. el Andaloussi, I. Mäger, X. O. Breakefield, and M. J. A. Wood, "Extracellular vesicles: biology and emerging therapeutic opportunities," *Nature Reviews Drug Discovery*, vol. 12, no. 5, pp. 347–357, 2013.

20

Identification of Potential Therapeutic Targets in the Liver of Pioglitazone-Treated Type 2 Diabetes Sprague-Dawley Rats via Expression Profile Chip and iTRAQ Assay

Zhong-Xia Lu,[1] Wen-Jun Xu,[1] Yang-Sheng Wu,[2] Chang-Yu Li,[2] and Yi-Tao Chen[1]

[1]College of Life Sciences, Zhejiang Chinese Medical University, Hangzhou 310053, China
[2]College of Pharmacy, Zhejiang Chinese Medical University, Hangzhou 310053, China

Correspondence should be addressed to Chang-Yu Li; lcyzcmu@sina.com and Yi-Tao Chen; cytworld@zcmu.edu.cn

Academic Editor: Secundino Cigarran

The aim of the present study was to identify key antidiabetic nodes in the livers of pioglitazone-treated type 2 diabetes mellitus Sprague-Dawley rats by transcriptomic and proteomic analysis. Rats were randomly divided into the control, the diabetes model, and the pioglitazone-treated groups. After treatment with pioglitazone for 11 weeks, the effects on fasting blood glucose, body weight, and blood biochemistry parameters were evaluated. Microarray and iTRAQ analysis were used to determine the differentially expressed genes/proteins in rat livers. 1.5-fold changes in gene expression and 1.2-fold changes in protein were set as the screening criteria. After treatment with pioglitazone for 11 weeks, fasting blood glucose in pioglitazone-treated rats was significantly lower than that in the model group. There was a tendency for pioglitazone to reduce TC, TG, TP, ALB, BUN, and HDL-c levels. Kyoto Encyclopedia of Genes and Genomes (KEGG) and gene ontology (GO) were applied to analyze differentially expressed genes/proteins. Furthermore, Western blotting and RT-qPCR were used to validate the results of microarray and iTRAQ. In conclusion, *Cyp7a1*, *Cp*, and *RT1-EC2* are differentially expressed genes/proteins since they showed a similar trend in rats in the model group and the pioglitazone-treated group.

1. Introduction

Diabetes mellitus (DM) is a chronic metabolic disease affecting more than 400 million people worldwide [1]. Type 2 diabetes mellitus (T2DM) is caused by insulin resistance and/or insulin deficiency and constitutes almost 95 percent of all diabetes cases [2]. Previous studies have shown that several drugs, including metformin, rosiglitazone, and pioglitazone, can control high blood glucose levels and protect patients from diabetes-related complications [3].

Pioglitazone belongs to the thiazolidinedione class of drugs and was deemed as an insulin sensitizer for the therapy of T2DM [4]. As a highly selective agonist for peroxisome proliferator-activated receptor γ (PPAR-γ), pioglitazone regulates the transcription of several genes and proteins involved in glucose and lipid metabolism [5]. Shannon et al. reported that pioglitazone inhibited pyruvate-driven ATP synthesis and hepatocellular glucose production as well as suppressing mitochondrial pyruvate transport regulators, MPC1 and MPC2 [6]. Moreover, the expression of adiponectin is upregulated by pioglitazone [7]. Furthermore, the phosphorylation of AKT is decreased in T2DM mice while receiving pioglitazone treatment [8]. Therefore, it is obvious that pioglitazone is a multitarget and multipathway compound involved in antidiabetic efficacy. However, the key nodes involved in the multitarget antidiabetic effect of pioglitazone still need to be elucidated.

Network pharmacology, which is based on the concept that many drugs act on multiple rather than a single therapeutic target, is recognized as a kind of system biology and network analysis methodology and technology [9, 10]. Key molecular networks involved in biochemical networks, bioinformatics, and systems biology have been reconstructed, which are helpful in predicting novel targets with high efficiency [11–13]. For many drugs, including metformin, morin, and curcumin, several novel candidate targets were identified through network pharmacology assays [14–16].

In the present study, we established type 2 diabetes mellitus rats by injection of streptozotocin (STZ), and the potential therapeutic target nodes in the liver of pioglitazone-treated rats were screened by expression profile chip and iTRAQ assay. Furthermore, metabolic pathways regulated by pioglitazone were also explored.

2. Materials and Methods

2.1. Drugs and Reagents. Pioglitazone hydrochloride tablets were purchased from Takeda Pharmaceutical Industry (Osaka, Japan), rat GE 4x44K v3 microarrays and a Gene Expression Hybridization Kit were from Agilent Technologies (Shanghai, China), and QIAGEN RNeasy® Mini Kit was from QIAGEN (Shanghai, China). A prime Script RT Reagent Kit was from TaKaRa Biotechnology (Dalian, China).

2.2. Groups and Treatments. Male SD rats (three per cage, 200 g average body weight), 8 weeks of age, were obtained from the Animal Center of Zhejiang Chinese Medical University (Hangzhou, China). All animal experiments were carried out in Zhejiang Chinese Medical University Laboratory Animal Research Center (rodent license number SCXK 2013-0115). The experimental protocol was approved by the Ethics Committee of Zhejiang Chinese Medical University.

Before the experimental test, all animals were fed with the basic diet (Zhejiang Academy of Medical Sciences, Hangzhou, China) for 3 weeks. Subsequently, a type 2 diabetes model was established by injection of freshly prepared STZ (30 mg/kg) dissolved in ice-cold citrate buffer (0.1 M, pH 4.2). To obtain diabetic symptoms, T2DM rats were fed with high-glucose/high-fat diet, consisting of 69.75% basic diet, 10% lard, 10% yolk powder, 0.25% cholesterol, and 10% sucrose (Zhejiang Academy of Medical Sciences, Hangzhou, China), whereas 10 normal rats in the control group were fed with basic diet. Rats with blood glucose at 15–25 mmol/l were used in the experimental test, which were randomly divided into two groups, the diabetes model group (DM, $n = 12$) and the pioglitazone-treated group ($n = 12$). Rats in the control and the model group were given 0.25% CMC-Na (10 ml/kg, China National Pharmaceutical Group, Shanghai, China), whereas rats in the treated groups received pioglitazone (5 mg/kg, in 0.25% CMC-Na) via gavage once a day for 11 weeks. All animals were housed at 25°C with 50~70% humidity and a 12 h light/12 h dark cycle with free access to food and water.

2.3. Sample Collection and Index Detection. At the starting (0 week) and in the end (11th week) of the experiment, blood was collected from the orbital veins of the rats. The blood was used for the determination of biochemistry parameters, using commercially available kits in a semiauto analyzer (Photometer 5010 V5+, Berlin, Germany). Moreover, after an eight-hour fasting period, blood glucose levels were measured every two weeks using a glucose meter (Accu-Chek Performa, Roche Diagnostics GmbH, Mannheim, Germany). Body weights were recorded every two weeks. At the end of the experiment, rats were euthanized and livers were quickly dissected on ice. The livers were washed with DEPC water, frozen in liquid nitrogen, and stored at −80°C.

2.4. Microarray and iTRAQ Assay. A total of 18 samples ($n = 6$ samples per group) were used for microarray and iTRAQ assay. Total RNA was extracted from liver tissues using the MiniRNeasy Kit based on the manufacturer's instructions (QIAGEN, Shanghai, China). After the determination of the RNA integrity (Agilent Bioanalyzer 2100), RNA was hybridized to a Whole Rat Genome Oligo 4x44 K microarray (Agilent Technologies, Shanghai, China). The significantly differentially expressed genes were screened with a >1.5-fold differential expression, and $P < 0.05$ was considered statistically significant.

Total liver protein (100 μg) from each sample was digested with trypsin, dried, and labeled with different tags per group. Control group samples labeled 114 tags, model group samples labeled 116, and pioglitazone-treated samples labeled 121. The labeled peptides were purified with a strong cation exchange chromatography (SCX) column (Phenomenex, California, USA) and separated by liquid chromatography (LC) using the LC-20AB HPLC Pump system (Shimadzu, Kyoto, Japan). Proteomic data collection was performed using a Triple TOF 5600 system (AB SCIEX, ON, USA) and a pulled quartz tip as the emitter (New Objectives, MA, USA). Proteins that were significantly different were screened with a >1.2-fold differential expression, and $P < 0.05$ cut-off in statistical analyses.

2.5. GO Enrichment and KEGG Analysis. The GO platform is a bioinformatics resource describing gene product attributes which have three categories, namely, biological process (BP), molecular function (MF), and cellular component (CC) [17]. We defined the significance of GO enrichment according to a P value, with a cut-off value of 0.05. The KEGG was applied to investigate if target genes were involved in multiple pathways. The top 10 pathway candidates that were potentially related to treatment were selected.

2.6. Reverse Transcription Quantitative Polymerase Chain Reaction (RT-qPCR) Assay. RT-qPCR was used to verify experimental data. Total RNA was extracted as described above, and double-strand cDNA was synthesized according to the manufacturer's instructions (TaKaRa Biotechnology, Shanghai, China). Primers were purchased from Sangon Biological Technology (Shanghai, China), of which the *Cyp7a1* former primer was 5′-GCATCTCAAGCAAACACCAT-3′, the downstream primer was 5′-TCCACTCACTTCTTCA GAGGC-3′, and the amplified fragment was 98 bp. Besides, the former primer of *Cp* was 5′-TGATGGCTATGGGC AATGA-3′, the downstream primer was 5′- GGTTTGG TATGTTCCAGGGA-3′, and the amplified fragment was 125 bp. Data were normalized to the expression level of a *β-actin* reference gene, in which upstream primer was 5′-GCTCTCTTCCAGCCTTCCTT-3′ and the downstream primer was 5′-GGTCTTTACGGATGTCAACG-3′. And its amplified fragment was 105 bp. RT-qPCR was performed with a Real Time PCR Machine (Eppendorf Realplex-4, Eppendorf, Germany).

2.7. Western Blotting Assay. Proteins (20 μg) were separated by 12% SDS-PAGE and transferred onto PVDF membranes (Immobilon-FL membrane, Millipore Company, Massachusetts, USA). Then, the membranes were incubated with 5% milk in TBST (Tris-buffered saline and 0.5% Tween 20) and incubated overnight with antibodies against *Cyp7a1*, *Cp*, or *β-actin* (1 : 1000 Cell Signaling Technology, American) at 4°C, followed by incubation with goat anti-rabbit IgG HRP (Sangon Biological Technology, Shanghai, China) for 2 h. Finally, the membranes were visualized with a gel documentation system (Aplegen Omega Lum G, American).

2.8. Statistical Analysis. Data are expressed as the mean ± standard deviation (SD). SPSS software version 16.0 (Chicago, USA) was used for statistical analyses. Results of fasting blood glucose level, body weight, and biochemistry parameters were subjected to one-way analysis of variance (ANOVA). Western blotting results were quantitated by ImageJ software and analyzed by ANOVA. $P < 0.05$ was considered statistically significant.

3. Results

3.1. Effect of Pioglitazone on the Fasting Blood Glucose Level of Rats. To examine the influence of pioglitazone *in vivo*, we administered pioglitazone to STZ-induced T2DM rats for a period of 11 weeks. As shown in Figure 1, the fasting blood glucose levels of DM rats and pioglitazone-treated rats were significantly higher compared to those of rats in the control groups at week 0 ($P < 0.01$). Moreover, after 11 weeks of treatment with pioglitazone, fasting blood glucose levels of pioglitazone-treated rats were significantly lower compared to those of rats in the DM model group ($P < 0.05$).

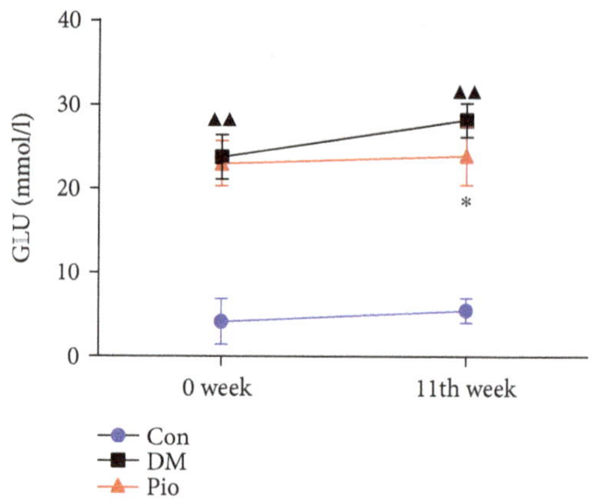

FIGURE 1: Pioglitazone reduces the fasting blood glucose level of DM rats. The fasting blood glucose levels in rats were significantly reduced after treatment with pioglitazone. ▲▲$P < 0.01$, the DM model group compared with the control group; *$P < 0.05$, the DM model group compared with the pioglitazone-treated group.

3.2. Effect of Pioglitazone on Body Weight of Rats. Body weight of rats in the control group, the DM model group, and the pioglitazone-treated group was also recorded in 0, 1st, 3rd, 5th, 7th, 9th, and 11th weeks. In the control group, the body weight of rats showed an upward trend from 435.83 ± 12.97 g in 0 week to 532.75 ± 23.18 g in the 11th week. However, rats in the DM model group demonstrated a significant loss in the body weight during the 11 weeks. Treatment with pioglitazone slightly increased the body weight of pioglitazone-treated rats and was significantly different compared with the body weights of rats in the DM model group (Figure 2, $P < 0.05$).

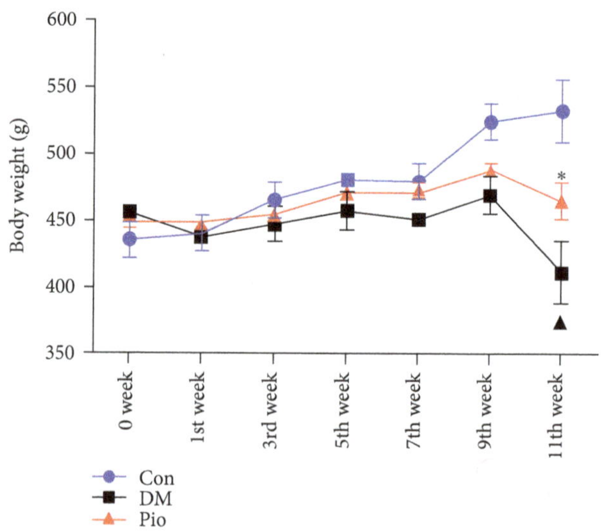

FIGURE 2: Pioglitazone alters the body weight of rats. The body weight of rats was recorded in 0, 1st, 3rd, 5th, 7th, 9th, and 11th weeks. ▲$P < 0.05$, the DM model group compared with the control group; *$P < 0.05$, the DM model group compared with the pioglitazone-treated group.

3.3. Effect of Pioglitazone on Biochemistry Parameters of Rats. Rats' plasma lipids were used for the evaluation of biochemistry parameters, including blood urea nitrogen (BUN), total cholesterol (TC), triglyceride (TG), high-density lipoprotein cholesterol (HDL-c), total protein (TP), and albumin (ALB). As shown in Figure 3, levels of the TC, TG, and HDL-c were significantly elevated in response to a high-glucose/high-fat diet ($P < 0.01$). After 11 weeks of pioglitazone treatment, TC, TG, TP, and HDL-c levels significantly decreased compared with rats in the DM model group ($P < 0.05$; $P < 0.01$). In previous studies, BUN and ALB measurements were commonly used to determine the liver function and renal function, respectively [18]. We found that levels of BUN and ALB were significantly decreased after pioglitazone treatment ($P < 0.01$), suggesting that pioglitazone has a protective effect on the kidney and liver.

3.4. Differentially Expressed Genes Screened by Expression Profile Chip. By using a 1.5-fold change as the screening criteria for differentially expressed genes, a total of 322 genes were screened in the DM model group and the pioglitazone-

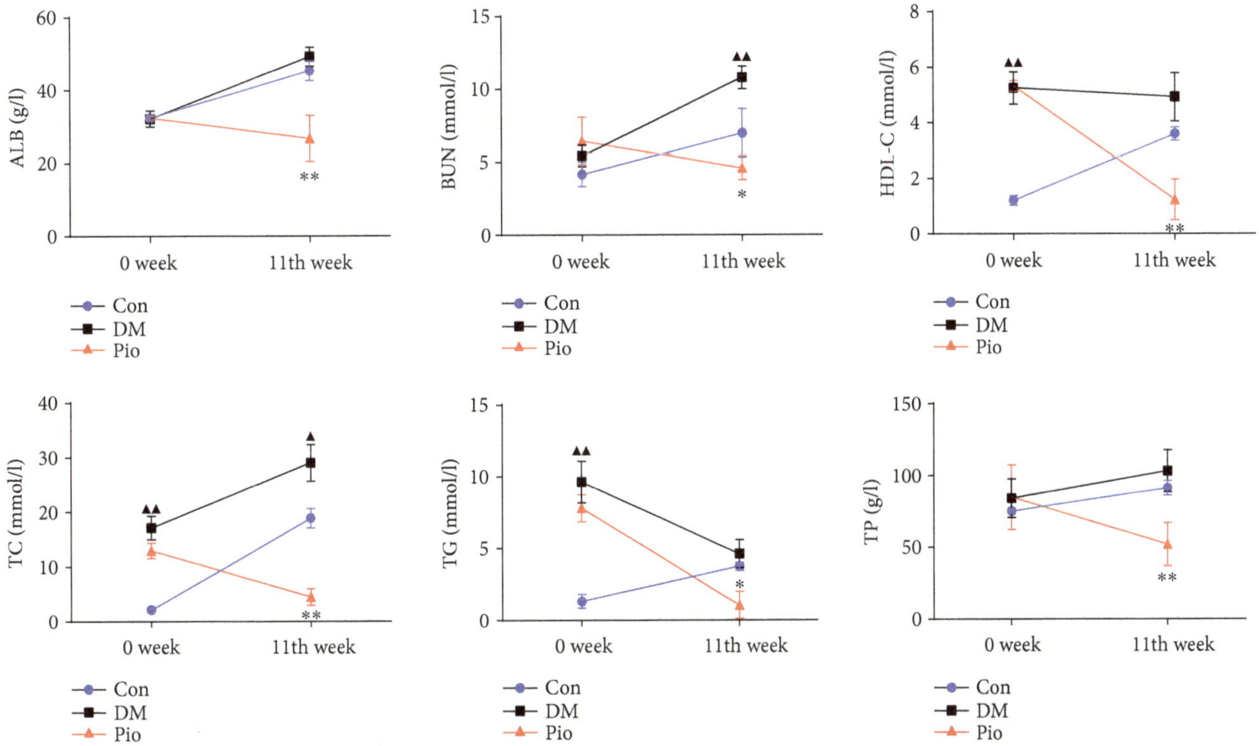

FIGURE 3: Pioglitazone changes blood biochemistry parameters. After treatment with pioglitazone for 11 weeks, the levels of TC, TG, TP, ALB, BUN, and HDL-c were significantly decreased. ▲$P < 0.05$; ▲▲$P < 0.01$, the DM model group compared with the control group; and $^{*}P < 0.05$ and $^{**}P < 0.01$, the DM model group compared with the pioglitazone-treated group.

treated group, in which 191 genes were significantly upregulated and 141 genes were significantly downregulated. GO enrichment and KEGG analysis were applied to assay the differentially expressed genes. As shown in Figure 4, pioglitazone treatment had a big impact on the biology process, the molecular function, and the cellular component in the liver. The biology process was affected by pioglitazone treatment, including the response to cAMP, epidermal growth factor receptor signaling pathway, and histone H2A acetylation. The pioglitazone-affected molecular function is involved for example in arginine-tRNA ligase activity, pheromone receptor activity, and unfolded protein binding. The cellular component was associated with keratin filament, melanosome, and cytoskeleton. As shown in Table 1, top 10 signaling pathways enriched by KEGG included ribosome biogenesis in eukaryotes, fatty acid metabolism, and protein processing in endoplasmic.

3.5. Differentially Expressed Proteins Screened by iTRAQ. To explore the differentially expressed proteins in the liver, we applied iTRAQ to select potential targets with 1.2-fold change differences as the screening criteria. A total of 204 proteins were found as differentially expressed proteins in the DM model group and the pioglitazone-treated group, of which 96 proteins were significantly upregulated and 108 proteins were significantly downregulated. KEGG pathway enrichment results are presented in Table 2. Proteins with altered expression were categorized according to KEGG pathway analysis and included the retinol metabolism, steroid hormone biosynthesis, and metabolic pathways. Figure 5 presents the gene ontology results. Cellular components affected by pioglitazone mainly included cellular parts, envelope, and extracellular regions. Using GO analysis, major molecular functions intervened by pioglitazone included antioxidant, auxiliary transport protein, and binding. Biological processes identified by GO assay of proteins are presented in Figure 5. The anatomical structure formation, biological adhesion, and biological regulation were among the main affected biological process.

3.6. Transcriptomic and Proteomic Conjoint Analysis of Potential Therapeutic Targets. Further analysis showed 3 molecules were found with the same trend in the pioglitazone-treated group after transcriptomic and proteomic conjoint analysis, namely, *Cyp7a1*, *Cp*, and *RT1-EC2*. Among these targets, the expression levels of *Cyp7a1* and *Cp* were significantly increased, whereas that of *RT1-EC2* decreased (Table 3). Therefore, *Cyp7a1*, *Cp*, and *RT1-EC2* were identified as potential therapeutic targets in the liver with pioglitazone treatment.

3.7. Validation of Potential Therapeutic Targets. Cyp7a1 (cytochrome P450, family 7, subfamily a, polypeptide I) and *Cp* (Ceruloplasmin) were further validated by qRT-PCR and Western blotting assay. As shown in Figure 6, compared with the DM model group, the gene expressions and protein levels of *Cyp7a1* in the pioglitazone-treated group were significantly decreased, while the gene expression level of

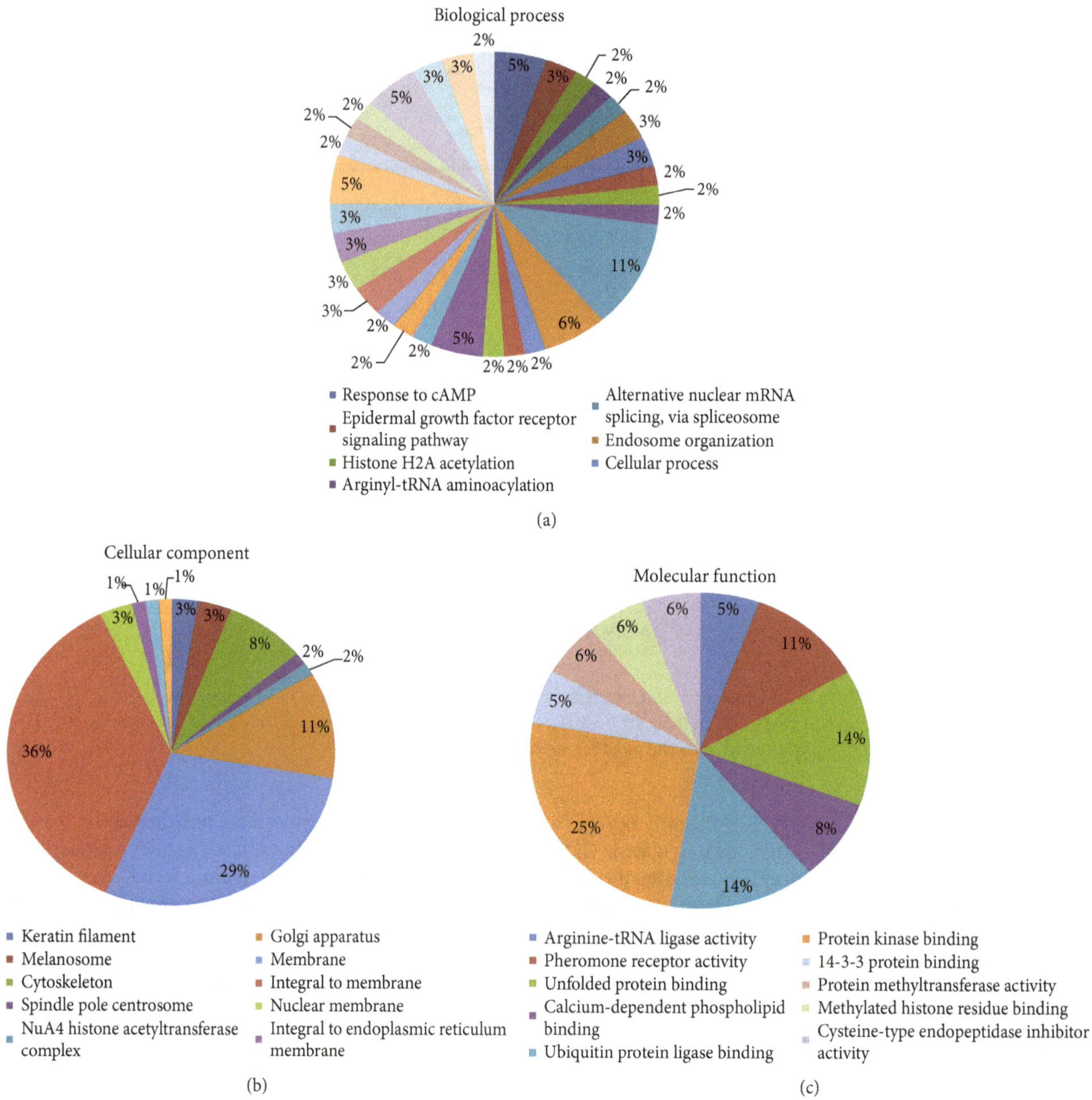

FIGURE 4: GO analysis of differentially expressed genes after treatment with pioglitazone. Microarray assay results of the DM model group and the pioglitazone-treated group. (a) Biological process. (b) Cellular component. (c) Molecular function.

TABLE 1: KEGG pathway enrichment via gene expression profile chip (DM versus Pio).

Number	Pathway ID	Pathway	*P* value
1	ko03008	Ribosome biogenesis in eukaryotes	$2.92E-02$
2	ko04977	Vitamin digestion and absorption	$4.21E-02$
3	ko04141	Protein processing in endoplasmic reticulum	$1.21E-01$
4	ko00051	Fructose and mannose metabolism	$1.48E-01$
5	ko00790	Folate biosynthesis	$1.62E-01$
6	ko00071	Fatty acid metabolism	$1.69E-01$
7	ko00970	Aminoacyl-tRNA biosynthesis	$1.69E-01$
8	ko04960	Aldosterone-regulated sodium reabsorption	$1.69E-01$
9	ko03040	Spliceosome	$1.71E-01$
10	ko04612	Antigen processing and presentation	$1.85E-01$

Table 2: KEGG pathway enrichment via iTRAQ (DM versus Pio).

Number	Pathway ID	Pathway	P value
1	ko00830	Retinol metabolism	$4.44E-09$
2	ko00140	Steroid hormone biosynthesis	$2.49E-06$
3	ko01100	Metabolic pathways	$8.68E-06$
4	ko00980	Metabolism of xenobiotics by cytochrome P450	$1.54E-05$
5	ko00982	Drug metabolism—cytochrome P450	$1.62E-05$
6	ko04976	Bile secretion	$7.75E-05$
7	ko03320	PPAR signaling pathway	$4.96E-04$
8	ko00590	Arachidonic acid metabolism	$6.60E-04$
9	ko00920	Sulfur metabolism	$2.41E-03$
10	ko00983	Drug metabolism—other enzymes	$4.72E-03$

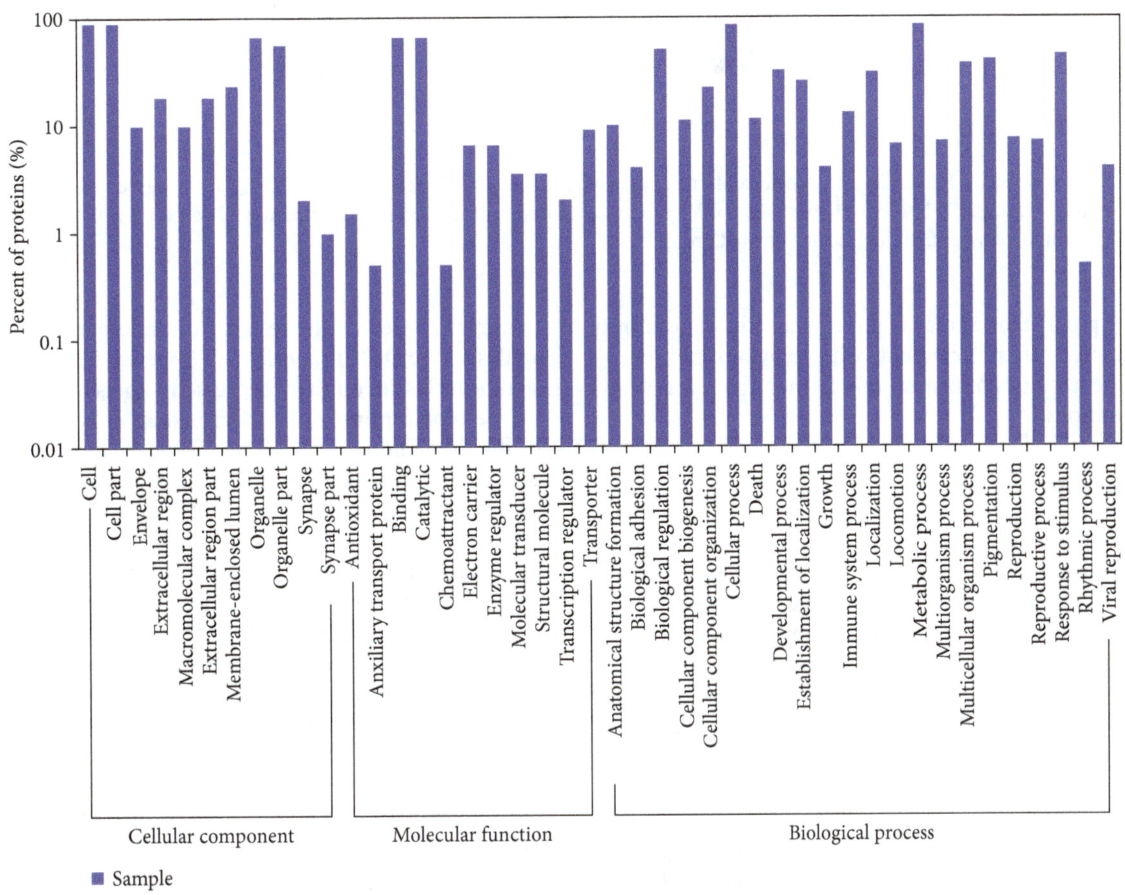

Figure 5: GO analysis of differentially expressed proteins after treatment with pioglitazone. iTRAQ assay results of the DM model group and the pioglitazone-treated group.

Table 3: Transcriptomic and proteomic conjoint analysis of potential targets.

Gene symbol	Transcriptomics		Proteomics		Regulation
	Log (Pio versus DM)	Log (Con versus DM)	Pio versus DM	Con versus DM	
Cyp7a1	−0.06	−1.52	0.488	0.361	Down
Cp	−0.17	−1.15	0.826	0.648	Down
RT1-EC2	0.21	0.24	1.255	1.204	Up

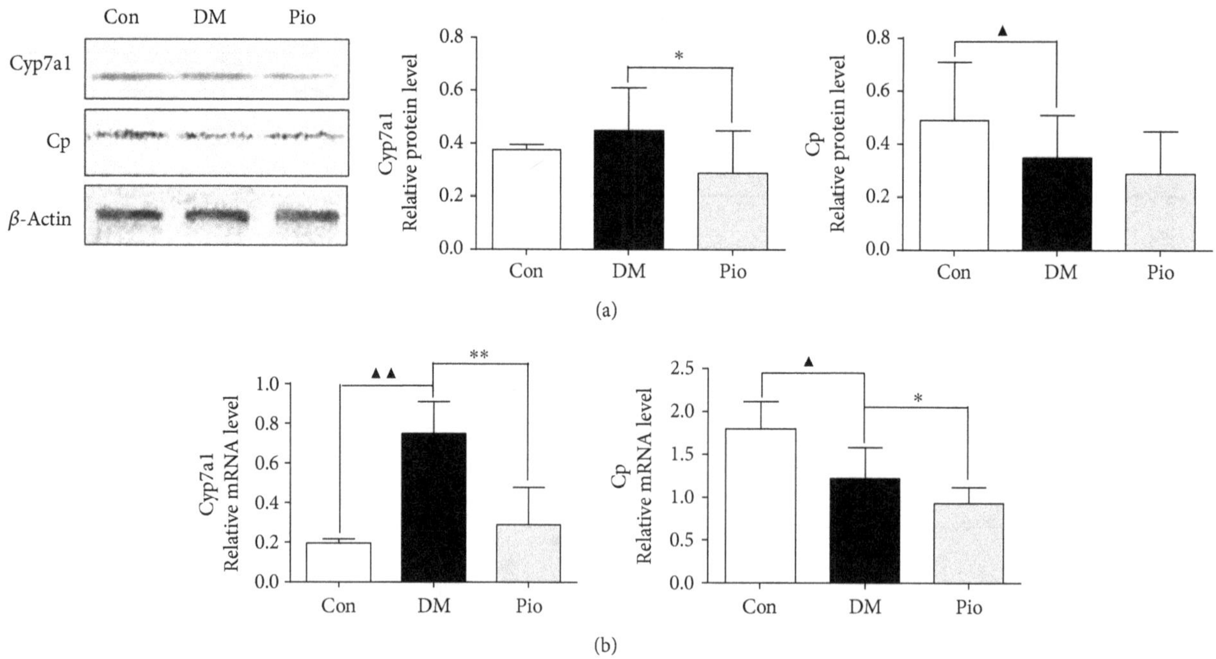

FIGURE 6: Data verified by RT-qPCR and Western blotting. (a) Gene expression detected by RT-qPCR. (b) Protein expression detected by Western blotting. ▲$P < 0.05$; ▲▲$P < 0.01$, the DM model group compared with the control group; and $^*P < 0.05$ and $^{**}P < 0.01$, the DM model group compared with the pioglitazone-treated group.

Cp in the pioglitazone-treated group was also significantly downregulated after treatment with pioglitazone for 11 weeks. The results confirmed the former microarray and iTRAQ findings.

4. Discussion

T2DM is characterized by chronic hyperglycemia due to worsening insulin resistance, which is a hallmark of type 2 diabetes [19]. Practically, insulin resistance exists throughout the course of diabetes; thus, enhancing insulin sensitivity is a key strategy for treatment [20]. Pioglitazone is an antidiabetic drug for the clinical treatment of T2DM and has been used over the past 50 years. It is known to improve insulin sensitivity, glycaemic control, hypertension, dyslipidemia, and microalbuminuria acting on PPAR-γ [21, 22].

In the present study, we established T2DM model rats with STZ and a high-glucose/high-fat diet according to the Reed method [23]. Pioglitazone was given by gavage to treat T2DM rats. After treatment with pioglitazone, fasting blood glucose levels were significantly lower compared to that in the model group. In addition, the levels of TC, TG, TP, ALB, BUN, and HDL-c were also significantly reduced.

Microarray and iTRAQ, high-throughput bioinformatics technologies, are widely used in drug screening, new drug development, and disease diagnosis [24–26]. The liver is regarded as a metabolic center and plays vital important roles in material metabolism and energy metabolism by regulating the metabolism of numerous molecules, such as carbohydrates, lipids, proteins, and hormones [27]. Hence, in the present study, we selected the liver as the target organ to study the changes of genes and proteins after pioglitazone treatment. Based on the results from microarray and iTRAQ analysis, *Cyp7a1*, *Cp*, and *RT1-EC2* were selected as the most significantly differentially expressed targets.

Ceruloplasmin(*Cp*) is a ferroxidase enzyme synthesized in the liver and is involved in carrying copper in the blood and in addition plays a role in iron metabolism [28, 29]. *Cp* is also used as an index to assess hepatic disease; the expression level of *Cp* dropped due to reduced synthesizing capabilities after liver damage [30]. *RT1-EC2* is a class 1b gene of the rat major histocompatibility complex, which is reported to be responsible for the development of diabetes in rats [31, 32]. *Cyp7a1* belongs to the cytochrome P450 family of enzymes and encodes cholesterol 7a-hydroxylase, which is the rate-limiting enzyme in bile acid biosynthesis from cholesterol [33]. Previous studies have reported that *Cyp7a1* is associated with circulating cholesterol concentrations in response to various dietary interventions [34]. Furthermore, numerous studies have reported that *Cyp7a1* plays a vitally important role in modulation of bile acid, lipid, and glucose homeostasis [35–37]. Therefore, *Cyp7a1* may serve as a potential candidate therapeutic node for diabetes.

5. Conclusions

In summary, our study demonstrated that pioglitazone is a multitarget antidiabetic drug affecting numerous genes involved in lipid and cholesterol metabolism pathways. Through microarray and iTRAQ analyses, *Cyp7a1*, *Cp*, and *RT1-EC2* were the most differentially expressed molecules in the DM group and the pioglitazone-treated group. Moreover, our study provides valuable data that may help in elucidating the underlying mechanism of pioglitazone in T2DM.

Abbreviations

TC: Total cholesterol
TG: Triglyceride
TP: Total protein
ALB: Albumin
BUN: Blood urea nitrogen
HDL-c: High-density lipoprotein cholesterol
DM: Diabetes mellitus
T2DM: Type 2 diabetes mellitus
GO: Gene ontology
KEGG: Kyoto Encyclopedia of Genes and Genomes
Cyp7a1: Cytochrome P450, family 7, subfamily a, polypeptide I
Cp: Ceruloplasmin
RT1-EC2: RT1 class Ib, locus EC2.

Conflicts of Interest

The authors declare that they have no conflicts of interest.

Acknowledgments

The present study was supported by grants from National Great New Drug Research and Development (no. 2012ZX09503001-001) and Traditional Chinese Medicine Open Funds of Zhejiang Chinese Medical University (no. 752223A00201/005/019).

References

[1] L. Luo, W. H. Zhou, J. J. Cai et al., "Gene expression profiling identifies downregulation of the neurotrophin-MAPK signaling pathway in female diabetic peripheral neuropathy patients," *Journal of Diabetes Research*, vol. 2017, Article ID 8103904, 11 pages, 2017.

[2] J. S. Skyler, G. L. Bakris, E. Bonifacio et al., "Differentiation of diabetes by pathophysiology, natural history, and prognosis," *Diabetes*, vol. 66, no. 2, pp. 241–255, 2017.

[3] Y. Luo, S. K. Paul, X. Zhou et al., "Design, and baseline characteristics of Beijing prediabetes reversion program: a randomized controlled clinical trial to evaluate the efficacy of lifestyle intervention and/or pioglitazone in reversion to normal glucose tolerance in prediabetes," *Journal of Diabetes Research*, vol. 2017, Article ID 7602408, 2017.

[4] J. Zhang, X. J. Wang, X. Liu et al., "Design, sythesis and evaluation of a series of 3- or 4-alkoxy substituted phenoxy derivatives as PPARs agonists," *Oncotarget*, vol. 8, no. 13, pp. 20766–20783, 2017.

[5] Y. Zhang, J. Yu, V. Grachtchouk et al., "Genomic binding of PAX8-PPARG fusion protein regulates cancer-related pathways and alters the immune landscape of thyroid cancer," *Oncotarget*, vol. 8, no. 4, pp. 5761–5773, 2017.

[6] C. E. Shannon, G. Daniele, C. Galindo, M. A. Abdul-Ghani, R. A. DeFronzo, and L. Norton, "Pioglitazone inhibits mitochondrial pyruvate metabolism and glucose production in hepatocytes," *FEBS Journal*, vol. 284, no. 3, pp. 451–465, 2017.

[7] S. Yandrapalli and W. S. Aronow, "Cardiovascular benefits of the newer medications for treating type 2 diabetes mellitus," *Journal of Thoracic Disease*, vol. 9, no. 7, pp. 2124–2134, 2017.

[8] L. Zhao, Y. Pan, K. Peng et al., "Inhibition of 11β-HSD1 by LG13 improves glucose metabolism in type 2 diabetic mice," *Journal of Molecular Endocrinology*, vol. 55, no. 2, pp. 119–131, 2015.

[9] A. L. Hopkins, "Network pharmacology: the next paradigm in drug discovery," *Nature Chemical Biology*, vol. 4, no. 11, pp. 682–690, 2008.

[10] A. L. Hopkins, "Network pharmacology," *Nature Biotechnology*, vol. 25, no. 10, pp. 1110-1111, 2007.

[11] J. Fang, L. Wang, T. Wu et al., "Network pharmacology-based study on the mechanism of action for herbal medicines in Alzheimer treatment," *Journal of Ethnopharmacology*, vol. 196, pp. 281–292, 2017.

[12] C. Perrino, A. L. Barabasi, G. Condorelli et al., "Epigenomic and transcriptomic approaches in the post-genomic era: path to novel targets for diagnosis and therapy of the ischaemic heart? Position paper of the European Society of Cardiology Working Group on cellular biology of the heart," *Cardiovascular Research*, vol. 113, no. 7, pp. 725–736, 2017.

[13] F. Sun, S. Chai, L. Li et al., "Effects of glucagon-like peptide-1 receptor agonists on weight loss in patients with type 2 diabetes: a systematic review and network meta-analysis," *Journal of Diabetes Research*, vol. 2015, Article ID 157201, 9 pages, 2015.

[14] B. Li, X. Jin, H. Meng et al., "Morin promotes prostate cancer cells chemosensitivity to paclitaxel through miR-155/GATA3 axis," *Oncotarget*, vol. 8, no. 29, pp. 47849–47860, 2017.

[15] H. Cao, H. Yu, Y. Feng, L. Chen, and F. Liang, "Curcumin inhibits prostate cancer by targeting PGK1 in the FOXD3/miR-143 axis," *Cancer Chemotherapy and Pharmacology*, vol. 79, no. 5, pp. 985–994, 2017.

[16] A. Madsen, O. Bozickovic, J. I. Bjune, G. Mellgren, and J. V. Sagen, "Metformin inhibits hepatocellular glucose, lipid and cholesterol biosynthetic pathways by transcriptionally suppressing steroid receptor coactivator 2 (SRC-2)," *Scientific Reports*, vol. 5, no. 1, article 16430, 2015.

[17] Y. S. Wu, Y. T. Chen, Y. T. Bao et al., "Identification and verification of potential therapeutic target genes in Berberine-treated Zucker diabetic fatty rats through bioinformatics analysis," *PLoS One*, vol. 11, no. 11, article e0166378, 2016.

[18] J. A. Messana, S. S. Schwartz, and R. R. Townsend, "An evidence-based practice-oriented review focusing on canagliflozin in the management of type 2 diabetes," *Vascular Health and Risk Management*, vol. 13, pp. 43–54, 2017.

[19] P. Zizkova, M. Stefek, L. Rackova, M. Prnova, and L. Horakova, "Novel quercetin derivatives: from redox properties to promising treatment of oxidative stress related diseases," *Chemico-Biological Interactions*, vol. 265, pp. 36–46, 2017.

[20] X. T. Feng, S. Y. Tang, Y. X. Jiang, and W. Zhao, "Anti-diabetic effects of Zhuoduqing formula, a Chinese herbal decoction, on a rat model of type 2 diabetes," *African Journal of Traditional Complementary and Alternative Medicines*, vol. 14, no. 3, pp. 42–50, 2017.

[21] X. Z. Zhang, H. Imachi, J. Y. Lyu et al., "Prolactin regulatory element-binding protein is involved in suppression of the adiponectin gene in vivo," *Journal of Endocrinological Investigation*, vol. 40, no. 4, pp. 437–445, 2017.

[22] H. W. Liao, J. L. Saver, Y. L. Wu, T. H. Chen, M. Lee, and B. Ovbiagele, "Pioglitazone and cardiovascular outcomes in patients with insulin resistance, pre-diabetes and type 2 diabetes: a systematic review and meta-analysis," *BMJ Open*, vol. 7, no. 1, article e013927, 2017.

[23] M. J. Reed, K. Meszaros, L. J. Entes et al., "A new rat model of type 2 diabetes: the fat-fed, streptozotocin-treated rat," *Metabolism*, vol. 49, no. 11, pp. 1390–1394, 2000.

[24] J. Yu, X. Li, C. Zhong et al., "High-throughput proteomics integrated with gene microarray for discovery of colorectal cancer potential biomarkers," *Oncotarget*, vol. 7, no. 46, pp. 75279–75292, 2016.

[25] H. Lu, Y. Yang, E. M. Allister, N. Wijesekara, and M. B. Wheeler, "The identification of potential factors associated with the development of type 2 diabetes: a quantitative proteomics approach," *Molecular & Cellular Proteomics*, vol. 7, no. 8, pp. 1434–1451, 2008.

[26] C. H. White, H. E. Johnston, B. Moesker et al., "Mixed effects of suberoylanilide hydroxamic acid (SAHA) on the host transcriptome and proteome and their implications for HIV reactivation from latency," *Antiviral Research*, vol. 123, pp. 78–85, 2015.

[27] H. Yoshida, R. Tsuhako, T. Atsumi et al., "Naringenin interferes with the anti-diabetic actions of pioglitazone via pharmacodynamic interactions," *Journal of Natural Medicines*, vol. 71, no. 2, pp. 442–448, 2017.

[28] M. G. Skalnaya, A. V. Skalny, and A. A. Tinkov, "Serum copper, zinc, and iron levels, and markers of carbohydrate metabolism in postmenopausal women with prediabetes and type 2 diabetes mellitus," *Journal of Trace Elements in Medicine and Biology*, vol. 43, pp. 46–51, 2017.

[29] C. Gluhovschi, G. Gluhovschi, L. Petrica et al., "Urinary biomarkers in the assessment of early diabetic nephropathy," *Journal of Diabetes Research*, vol. 2016, Article ID 4626125, 13 pages, 2016.

[30] R. Squitti, A. J. Mendez, I. Simonelli, and C. Ricordi, "Diabetes and Alzheimer's disease: can elevated free copper predict the risk of the disease?," *Journal of Alzheimers Disease*, vol. 56, no. 3, pp. 1055–1064, 2017.

[31] E. Rothermel, L. Heine, W. Wurst, and E. Gunther, "Characterization of a class Ib gene of the rat major histocompatibility complex," *Immunogenetics*, vol. 38, no. 2, pp. 82–91, 1993.

[32] N. Yokoi, C. Hayashi, Y. Fujiwara, H. Y. Wang, and S. Seino, "Genetic reconstitution of autoimmune type 1 diabetes with two major susceptibility genes in the rat," *Diabetes*, vol. 56, no. 2, pp. 506–512, 2007.

[33] Q. Wu, X. Zhang, M. Zhong et al., "Effects of bariatric surgery on serum bile acid composition and conjugation in a diabetic rat model," *Obesity Surgery*, vol. 26, no. 10, pp. 2384–2392, 2016.

[34] Y. Wang, S. V. Harding, P. Eck et al., "High-molecular-weight beta-glucan decreases serum cholesterol differentially based on the CYP7A1 rs3808607 polymorphism in mildly hypercholesterolemic adults," *Journal of Nutrition*, vol. 146, no. 4, pp. 720–727, 2016.

[35] M. Zhou, J. Luo, M. Chen et al., "Mouse species-specific control of hepatocarcinogenesis and metabolism by FGF19/FGF15," *Journal of Hepatology*, vol. 66, no. 6, pp. 1182–1192, 2017.

[36] D. Y. Saad, M. M. Soliman, A. A. Baiomy, M. H. Yassin, and H. B. El-Sawy, "Effects of karela (bitter melon; *Momordica charantia*) on genes of lipids and carbohydrates metabolism in experimental hypercholesterolemia: biochemical, molecular and histopathological study," *BMC Complementary and Alternative Medicine*, vol. 17, no. 1, p. 319, 2017.

[37] J. S. Bae, J. M. Park, J. Lee et al., "Amelioration of non-alcoholic fatty liver disease with NPC1L1-targeted IgY or n-3 polyunsaturated fatty acids in mice," *Metabolism*, vol. 66, pp. 32–44, 2017.

21

Alpinia oxyphylla Miq. Extract Prevents Diabetes in Mice by Modulating Gut Microbiota

Yiqiang Xie,[1] Man Xiao,[2] Yali Ni,[1] Shangfei Jiang,[2] Guizhu Feng,[2] Shenggang Sang,[1] and Guankui Du[2]

[1]*First Affiliated Hospital of Hainan Medical University, Haikou 571199, China*
[2]*Department of Biochemistry and Molecular Biology, Hainan Medical University, Haikou 571101, China*

Correspondence should be addressed to Guankui Du; duguankui@163.com

Academic Editor: Pedro M. Geraldes

Recently, the role of gut microbiota in the development of obesity and type 2 diabetes mellitus (T2DM) has been highlighted. We performed an 8-week administration protocol on T2DM (C57BL/6J db-/db-) mice and fecal samples were collected. Comparisons of fecal bacterial communities were performed between db-/db- mice and normal mice (DB/DB) and between the db-/db mice treated and untreated with AOE using next-generation sequencing technology. Our results showed that the db-/db-AOE group had improved glycemic control and renal function compared with the db-/db-H_2O group. Compared with the db-/db-H_2O group, AOE administration resulted in significantly increased ratio of Bacteroidetes-to-Firmicutes in db-/db- mice. In addition, the abundance of *Akkermansia* was significantly increased, while *Helicobacter* was significantly suppressed in the db-/db-AOE group compared with the db-/db-H_2O group. Our data suggest that AOE treatment decreased blood glucose levels and significantly reduced damage of renal pathology in the T2DM mice by modulating gut microbiota composition.

1. Introduction

Diabetes mellitus (DM) is a metabolic disease whose principal cause is obesity-linked insulin resistance. This disease is becoming a major public health challenge, and the incidence of DM is projected to rise to 439 million by 2030, while 90% patients have type 2 diabetes mellitus (T2DM) [1]. The main clinical methods in DM therapy have involved alleviating hyperglycemia, hypertension, and dyslipidemia [2]. A mutation in the leptin receptor gene in db/db mice is a rodent model of genetic diabetes, and the development of glomerular hypertrophy is evident early in response to hyperglycemia [3].

In recent years, the role of gut microbiota in host physiology, disease, and behavior has been generally recognized [4]. Next-generation sequencing technology provides a new perspective of the role of microbiota in human health, including shaping our immune system, metabolism, and energy balance [5]. Altered gut microbiota is related to multiple diseases, such as T2DM and obesity [5]. Recently, growing evidence has shown that gut microbiota during clinical T2DM results in compositional changes between patients and healthy controls, including an obesity-related change in the abundance ratio of Bacteroidetes : Firmicutes [6, 7] and a decreased abundance of mucin-degrading *Akkermansia muciniphila* in overweight children and pregnant women [8]. Notably, reduced levels of *Akkermansia* have been observed in patients with inflammatory bowel diseases and metabolic disorders [9]. It has been reported that fruits and vegetables, such as bamboo shoot fiber [10], capsaicin [11], and polyphenol [12, 13], the consumption of which is strongly associated with a healthy lifestyle, prevented diet-induced obesity in association with a remarkable change of gut microbiota, especially increase in the abundance of *Akkermansia* [14, 15]. Therefore, understanding the alteration of gut microbiota under different situations will be beneficial for the diagnosis and treatment of different diseases.

Alpinia oxyphylla (*A. oxyphylla*) can be used for different purposes. In China, *A. oxyphylla* is traditionally used as a dietary supplement. The herb is used in traditional Chinese medicine and has been widely used to treat diarrhea, abdominal pain, intestinal disorders, dementia, and inflammatory conditions [16–18]. Component isolates from *A. oxyphylla* show antioxidative stress properties, such as protocatechuic acid [19, 20]. Previous studies have shown that *A. oxyphylla* can promote the migration and proliferation of human adipose tissue-derived stromal cells [21, 22]. In our previous study, we found that *A. oxyphylla* extract (AOE) exhibits an antioxidant and anti-T2DM capacity [23, 24]. However, the mechanism of AOE-mediated anti-T2DM function remains largely unknown. Moreover, because of the importance of gut microbiota in the development of T2DM and obesity, we investigated the alteration of gut microbiota in db-/db- mice treated with AOE.

2. Material and Methods

2.1. Preparation of the Plant Extract. The ripe fruits of *A. oxyphylla* were collected from herb market (Haikou, China) and were identified by Dr. Qiang Liu (Department of Pharmacognosy, Hainan Medical College). Briefly, the ripe fruits were extracted with water for 16 hours at 90°C two times, and then the extract was lyophilized. The dry yield was 8% (*w*/*w*).

2.2. Animals. For this study, we performed experiments strictly in accordance with protocols approved by the Ethics Committee of Hainan Medical College for Animal Care and Use. The animals were monitored twice per week, and none of the animals showed severe illness, died, or appeared moribund during any of the experiments.

All mice purchased from the Model Animal Research Center of Nanjing University, China. Mice were housed in an environmentally controlled room at 22 ± 1°C with a relative humidity of 50 ± 5% under a light cycle of 12 h light/12 h dark. Specific pathogen-free hygienic status was approved by a health certificate according to the Federation of European Laboratory Animal Science Associations guidelines [25]. They had free access to standard rodent diet (GMLAC, Guangdong) and water, unless stated otherwise in substudies. Mice were maintained in polycarbonate individually ventilated cages with corncob bedding (GMLAC, Guangdong). Body weights were monitored weekly during the studies.

A total of 30 male mice (3 to 4 weeks old), including 6 DB/DB mice and 24 db-/db- mice (i.e., mice carrying a mutation in the leptin receptor gene) with a C57BL/Ks background (BKS.Cg-Dock7$^{m+/+}$Lepr^{db}/Nju, NBRI 2B051), were divided into 5 groups, with 6 animals in each group. Mice were allowed to acclimatize for 1 week before experiment. The DB/DB mice group and db-/db-H_2O group were given saline only, and the AOE-treated group received 100 mg/kg (db-/db-AOE100), 300 mg/kg (db-/db-AOE300), or 500 mg/kg (db-/db-AOE500) of AOE via the intragastric route once a day for 8 weeks (approximately, 0.2 mL in volume), respectively.

At 8th week, 24 h urine collection and feces were obtained. Then, the mice were euthanized by chloral hydrate anesthesia. Blood and kidney samples were taken for further analysis. Blood samples were collected from the hepatic portal vein into tubes containing EDTA anticoagulation and centrifuged (3000 rpm for 15 minutes at 4°C) for separating the plasma, which was then frozen at −70°C for biochemical analysis.

2.3. Measurement of Concentration of Glucose and Albumin. Glucose was measured using commercial kits (glucose (F006)) (Nanjing Jiancheng Bioengineering Institute, Nanjing, China), according to the manufacturer's instructions. Glucose concentration was assayed by the glucose oxidase method [26]. HbA1c levels were evaluated using commercial kits (Beijing HOMA Biologicals, China). Urine albumin was measured using an Albumin Mouse ELISA kit (ab108792), which was purchased from Abcam (Cambridge, UK). The absorbance was read using an automated microplate ELISA reader (BioTek Instruments Inc., Winooski, VT, USA), and concentrations were calculated by the standard curve run on each assay plate. All samples were measured in duplicate.

2.4. Glucose Tolerance Test. The oral glucose tolerance test (OGTT) was performed after 6 weeks of AOE administration. After an overnight fast, the animals were administered glucose (1.0 g/kg) solution orally. After 0, 30, 60, 90, and 120 minutes, Blood samples were collected via the tail vein and measured for blood glucose concentration.

2.5. Histological Examination. For histological analysis, animals were perfused with phosphate-buffered saline and 4% paraformaldehyde in phosphate-buffered saline. Organs were dissected and kept in the same fixation solution overnight at 4°C. Samples were embedded in paraffin following dehydration in ethanol. Tissues were cut into 6 μm sections and stored for staining. For hematoxylin-eosin (Sigma) staining, sections were freed of paraffin and stained. The slides were evaluated by blinded visual inspection including an experienced pathologist. All biopsies were analyzed quantitatively to determine the percentages of glomeruli with (1) segmental and global sclerosis, (2) mesangial cell proliferation, and/or (3) increase in mesangial matrix. All biopsies were scored semiquantitatively for the percentages of the aforementioned lesioned glomeruli (score 0, 0%; score 1, 1 to 24%; score 2, 25 to 49%; and score 3, ≥50% of all glomeruli) [27]. Scoring of the chronic tubulointerstitial injury was based on the percentage of tubular atrophy and interstitial fibrosis and was graded as mild (1+) if involving <25%, moderate (2+) if involving 25–50%, and severe (3+) if involving ≥50%.

2.6. Microbiota Analysis by 16S rRNA Gene Sequencing. Total fecal DNA was extracted by QIAamp DNA Stool mini kit (Qiagen, Hilden, Germany) according to the manufacturer's instructions. The V3-V4 region (~450 bp) of the 16S rRNA gene was amplified using the universal primers 341F (5′-CCTACGGGNGGCWGCAG-3′) and 802R (5′-TACNVGGGTATCTAATCC-3′). The forward primer 341F contained the sequence of the Roche B adapter for Illumina library construction and the reverse primer 802R attached to the Roche A adapter. Sequencing was carried out on Illumina HiSeq/MiSeq platform, and at least 48,000 reads per sample (mean reads per sample 65,610 ± 1346) was obtained. FLASH

[28] and QIIME (Quantitative Insights Into Microbial Ecology) was used to merge reads. Greengenes database [29] and the UPARSE algorithm [30] were used to group paired-end joined sequences into operational taxonomic units (OTUs) (97% threshold of pairwise identity). The RDP classifier [30] was used to annotate taxonomic information. Alpha diversity (within samples) and beta diversity (among samples) were analyzed by in-house Perl scripts. Unweighted UniFrac for principal coordinate analysis (PCoA) was used to assess the variation between experimental groups.

2.7. Statistics. All data are presented as the mean ± SEM. Statistical analysis of physiological and biochemical data was conducted using the GraphPad Prism version 7.0 (GraphPad Software, San Diego, CA). One-way ANOVA followed by Tukey's test was used to determine significant mean differences. Data was expressed as mean ± SE. *P* values less than 0.05 were considered statistically significant. A two-way nonparametric permutation analysis of variance (perMANOVA) was applied to evaluate the bacterial differences under different treatments. The *P* value from Fisher's exact test was corrected by the Holm-Bonferroni method. Canonical correspondence analysis (CCA) was performed using Canoco software version 4.5 [31].

3. Results

After AOE administration, changes in body weight of db-/db- mice did not differ (Figure 1(a)), while plasma glucose significantly decreased (AOE administration for 4 weeks, 13.2% ($P = 0.0271$) in db-/db-AOE100, 10.6% ($P = 0.0143$) in db-/db-AOE300, and 29.3% ($P = 0.0048$) in db-/db-AOE500) compared with the db-/db-H_2O group in a dose-dependent manner (Figure 1(b)). Meanwhile, urine albumin excretion decreased significantly after AOE administration (23.1% ($P = 0.0176$) in db-/db-AOE100, 35.1% ($P = 0.0077$) in db-/db-AOE300, and 52.9% ($P = 0.0052$) in db-/db-AOE500) for 8 weeks compared with the db-/db-H_2O group in a dose-dependent manner (Figure 1(c)). The effects of the AOE on the glucose intolerance were measured. In oral glucose tolerance test, the db-/db- mice treated with AOE had improved glucose intolerance compared to db-/db-H_2O mice, in which the db-/db-AOE500 mice revealed the lower plasma glucose concentrations and lower area under the curve (AUC) of glucose (19.9%, $P = 0.0386$) (Figures 1(d), 1(e)). Glycated hemoglobin, HbA1c, was tested at the end of AOE treatment. Compared to DB/DB mice, db-/db-H_2O mice displayed elevated HbA1c levels (3.2 fold, $P = 0.0044$). On the 8 weeks of treatment, 300 mg/kg (30.9%, $P = 0.0076$) and 500 mg/kg AOE (30.6%, $P = 0.0082$) both reduced HbA1c levels significantly, indicating efficient glycemic control (Figure 1(f)). Those results showed that 500 mg/kg AOE could effectively decrease blood glucose level and urine albumin excretion.

H&E-stained kidney tissue sections were used to assess renal morphology and pathology. An example of normal kidney structure is illustrated in Figure 2(a), depicting a kidney section from a normal DB/DB mouse. Glomeruli are numerous and distinct with patent capillaries, normal cellularity, and architecture, and their tubules are compact and of normal shape. In comparison, kidney sections from db-/db- mice (Figure 2(b)) exhibited severe disruption of kidney architecture, lesions involving all glomeruli and tubular atrophy. After AOE administration, especially at 500 mg/kg AOE, kidney structure was almost recovered (Figures 2(c)–2(e)). In addition, scores of renal injury (glomeruli and tubulointerstitial injury) in the db-/db-H_2O group were higher than those in the DB/DB group ($P = 2.82E - 10$), while AOE treatment reduced scores of renal injury in a dose-dependent manner ($P = 0.157$ in db-/db-AOE100, $P = 1.58E - 05$ in db-/db-AOE300, and $P = 2.94E$ in db-/db-AOE500 compared with db-/db-H_2O mice) (Figures 2(f), 2(g)). Those results showed that 500 mg/kg AOE was the most effective at attenuating renal injury.

Thus, we assessed changes in the gut microbial community induced by AOE500. 16S ribosomal RNA gene from variable regions V3-V4 of the fecal samples from DB/DB, db-/db-H_2O, and db-/db-AOE500 diet groups was sequenced by Illumina HiSeq/MiSeq platforms, and the results were presented as operational taxonomic units (OTUs) using a 97% homology cutoff value. The phylogenetic differences within the intestinal microbiota were assessed by principal coordinate analysis (PCoA) (Figure 3(a)). The db-/db-H_2O mice had a distinct microbiota composition that clustered separately from the DB/DB mice. The db-/db-AOE500 mice were clearly distinct from the db-/db-H_2O mice. Hierarchical clustering results were consistent with the previous PCoA analysis (Figure 3(b)). To assess intestinal microbial community structure, richness and evenness were calculated (Figures 3(c)–3(e)). Diversity measured by Shannon's richness index decreased slightly in the db-/db-H_2O group compared with the DB/DB group. The db-/db-AOE500 mice had slightly increased values of Shannon's index compared with the db-/db-H_2O group (Figure 3(c)). Diversity measured by Simpson's evenness index and CHAO1 diversity showed slightly increased values in the db-/db-H_2O group compared with the DB/DB group. The values of Simpson's index and CHAO1 diversity in the db-/db-AOE500 group were slightly lower than those in the db-/db-H_2O group (Figures 3(d), 3(e)).

To assess specific changes in the gut microbiota, we compared the relative abundance of the predominant taxa identified from sequencing in the three diet groups (Figure 3). Significant differences in the composition of the gut microbiota were found at all taxonomic levels. At the phylum level, the db-/db-H_2O-associated fecal microbiota community showed a dramatic increase in the relative abundance of Firmicutes ($P = 0.00198$, $Q = 0.00396$) and Cyanobacteria ($P = 0.00014$, $Q = 0.00089$) and a marked decrease in the relative abundance of Bacteroidetes ($P = 0.00121$, $Q = 0.00362$) compared with the DB/DB group (Figure 4(a)). Differing greatly from the db-/db-H2O group, the db-/db-AOE500-associated gut community had a trend toward an increase in the relative abundance of Bacteriodetes and decrease in Firmicutes ($P = 0.04353$, $Q = 0.08706$). On the other hand, the relative abundance of Verrucomicrobia ($P = 0.01305$, $Q = 0.03916$) showed a sharp increase in the db-/db-AOE500 mice (Figure 4(a)).

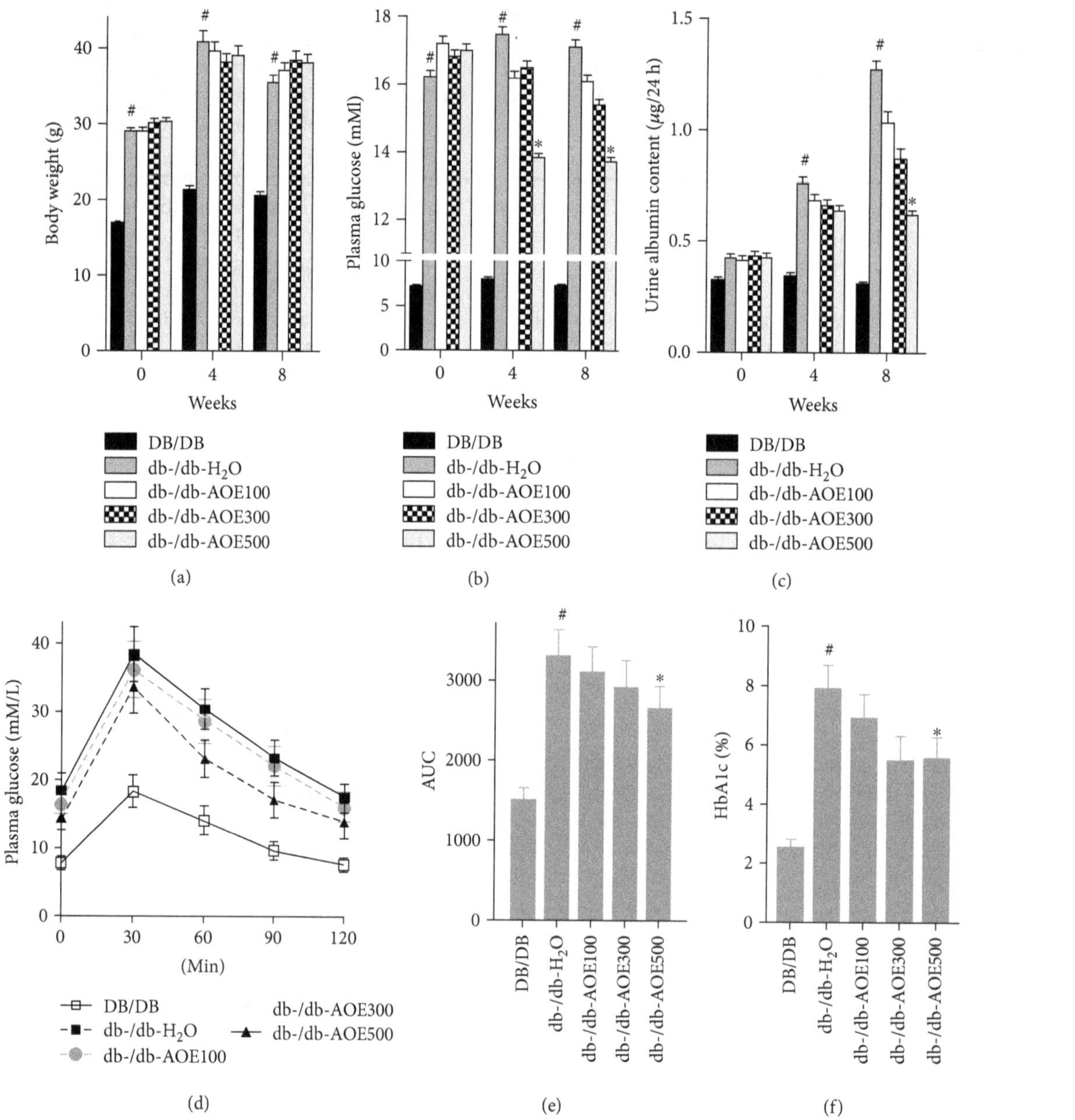

FIGURE 1: Effects of AOE on body weight, blood glucose levels, and renal function. The alteration of body weight (a), blood glucose (b), and urine albumin (c) after AOE treatment for 4 and 8 weeks. $^{*}P < 0.05$ for the db-/db-AOE group compared with the db-/db-H_2O group; $^{\#}P < 0.05$ for db-/db-H_2O-treated compared with DB/DB.

At the family level, the fecal microbiota was dominated by S24-7 followed by Lachnospiraceae in all groups. The db-/db-H_2O-associated fecal microbiota community showed a dramatic increase in the relative abundance of Lachnospiraceae ($P = 0.00912$, $Q = 0.03040$) and Porphyromonadaceae ($P = 0.00023$, $Q = 0.00237$) and a marked decrease in the relative abundance of S24-7 ($P = 0.00121$, $Q = 0.00605$) and Lactobacillaceae ($P = 0.03187$, $Q = 0.07969$) (Figure 4(b)). The db-/db-AOE500 increased the relative abundance of Verrucomicrobiaceae by ninefold ($P = 7.767\text{E}-06$, $Q = 7.767\text{E}-05$), S24-7 33.3% ($P = 0.00106$, $Q = 0.00533$), Bacteroidaceae 34.4% ($P = 0.00158$, $Q = 0.00528$), and Lactobacillaceae 127.2% ($P = 0.01991$, $Q = 0.03983$) and decreased the relative abundance of Rikenellaceae 47.8% (0.00106, $Q = 0.00533$) and Lachnospiraceae 20.6% ($P = 0.02484$, $Q = 0.04141$) (Figure 4(b)).

At the genus level, the db-/db-H_2O-associated fecal microbiota community showed a dramatic increase in the relative abundance of *Blautia* ($P = 0.00032$, $Q = 0.00387$) and Ruminococcaceae ($P = 0.00478$, $Q = 0.01914$) and a marked decrease in the relative abundance of S24-7 ($P < 0.05$). The db-/db-AOE500 resulted in a sharp increase in *Akkermansia* and *Bacteroides* but a decrease in *Helicobacter* and *Blautia* (Figure 4(c)). The db-/db-AOE500 increased *Akkermansia* by ninefold ($P = 3.45\text{E}-05$, $Q = 0.00041$) and *Bacteroides* 34% ($P = 0.00544$, $Q = 0.01633$), while it decreased *Helicobacter* 99.8% ($P = 0.00248$, $Q = 0.00993$) and *Blautia* 43.7% ($P = 7.34\text{E}-05$, $Q = 0.00044$) (Figure 4(c)). For factors with

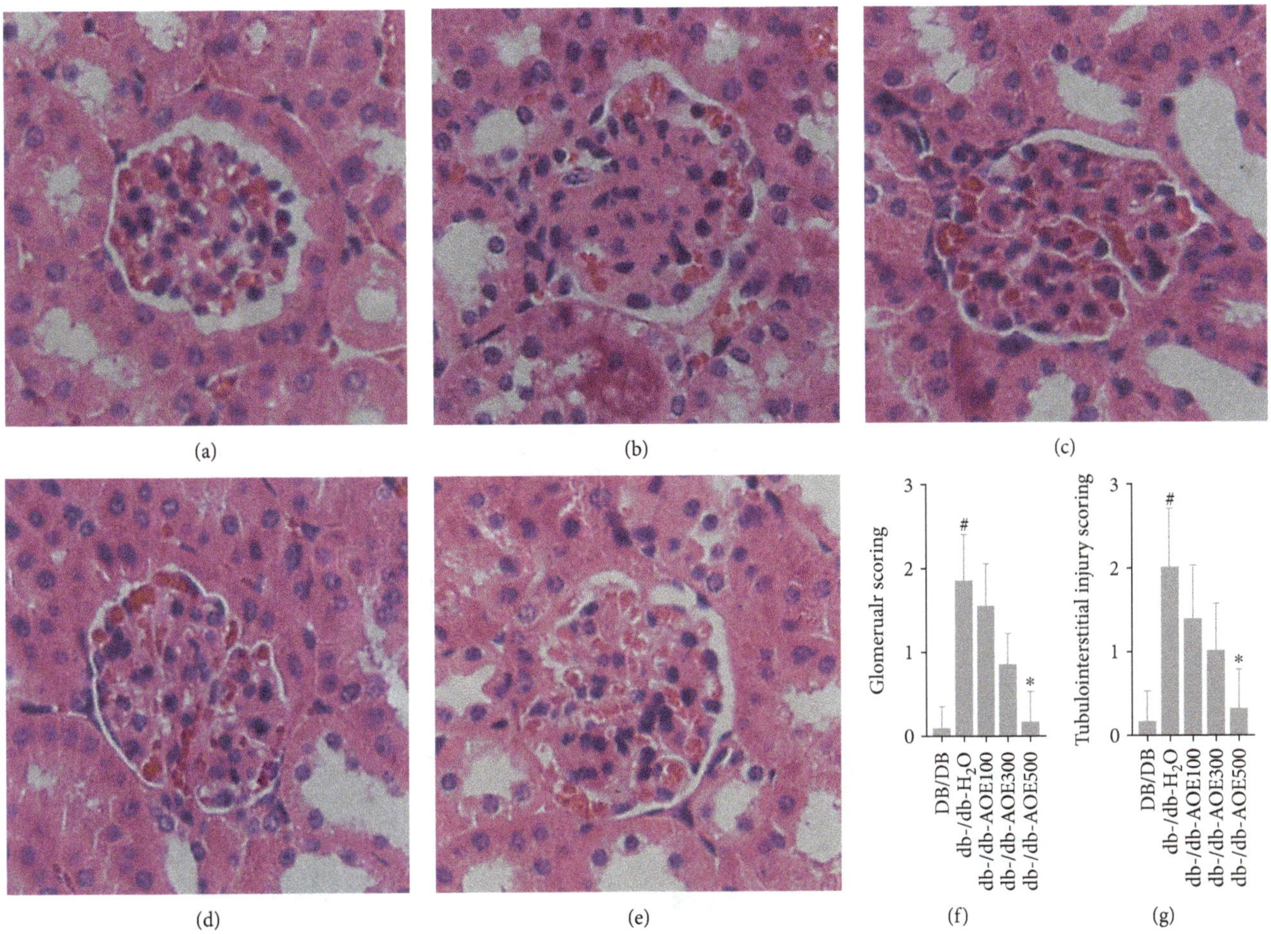

FIGURE 2: HE staining in the kidney of mice after 8 weeks of AOE treatment. Representative HE staining showed the inflammatory cell infiltration in the kidney of DB/DB mice (a), db-/db-H_2O (b), db-/db-AOE100 (c), db-/db-AOE300 (d), and db-/db-AOE500 (e). Bar graphs (f) showed the changes of average infiltration percentage of inflammatory cells in the kidney. Data represent the mean ± SD ($n = 6$). $^*P < 0.05$ for the db-/db-AOE group compared with the db-/db-H_2O group, $^\#P < 0.05$ for db-/db-H_2O-treated compared with DB/DB.

a statistically significant fit, constrained canonical analysis (CCA) was performed at the genus levels. The results showed that *Akkermansia* might be a key target while db-/db- mice treated with AOE (Figure 5). Collectively, these results show that AOE500 modulates the gut microbiota of T2DM mice.

4. Discussion

Gut microbiota play an important role in the development of T2DM and metabolic disorders. Meanwhile, the composition of gut microbiota might be shaped by multiple diets, such as a high-fat diet and high-fiber diet. The alteration of gut microbiota diversity has a profound influence on host metabolism. Studies have shown that hyperglycemia results in overproduction of ROS, which impairs glucose-stimulated insulin secretion and induces insulin resistance [32, 33]. In our previous study, AOE exhibited antioxidative capacity in vitro and in vivo [23]. In addition, the blood glucose levels and urine albumin secretion were significantly reduced after AOE treatment. Antioxidative capacity may partly underlie mechanism in the treatment of diabetes with AOE; however, more information is required to determine the antidiabetic mechanism of AOE. In this study, we found that AOE not only has a hypoglycemic capacity but also modulates gut microbiota composition.

The mouse and human microbiota are similar at the division level, with Firmicutes and Bacteroidetes dominating. Many studies have shown that increased ratios of Firmicutes to Bacteroides are associated with a diabetic phenotype [34, 35]. Geurts et al. observed a significantly higher abundance of Firmicutes in db/db mice [36]. The early gut microbiota composition was found to be different between NOD mice that later in life were classified as diabetic or nondiabetic. Bacteroidetes act in favor of diabetes protection, whereas members of Firmicutes promote diabetes onset, regulatory imbalance, and IFN-gamma level in NOD mice [37]. Various studies have shown that dietary manipulation of gut microbiota may be a novel mechanism to delay diabetes onset [38]. Consumption of acidic water alters the gut microbiome and decreases the risk of diabetes [38]. Sardine-enriched diet interventions altered gut microbiota composition of drug-naive patients with T2DM [39]. Bamboo shoot fiber modulates the gut microbiota and improves host metabolism [10]. In agreement with these findings, we observed that the abundance of Firmicutes in db-/db-AOE mice markedly decreased compared with that in the db-/db-H_2O mice

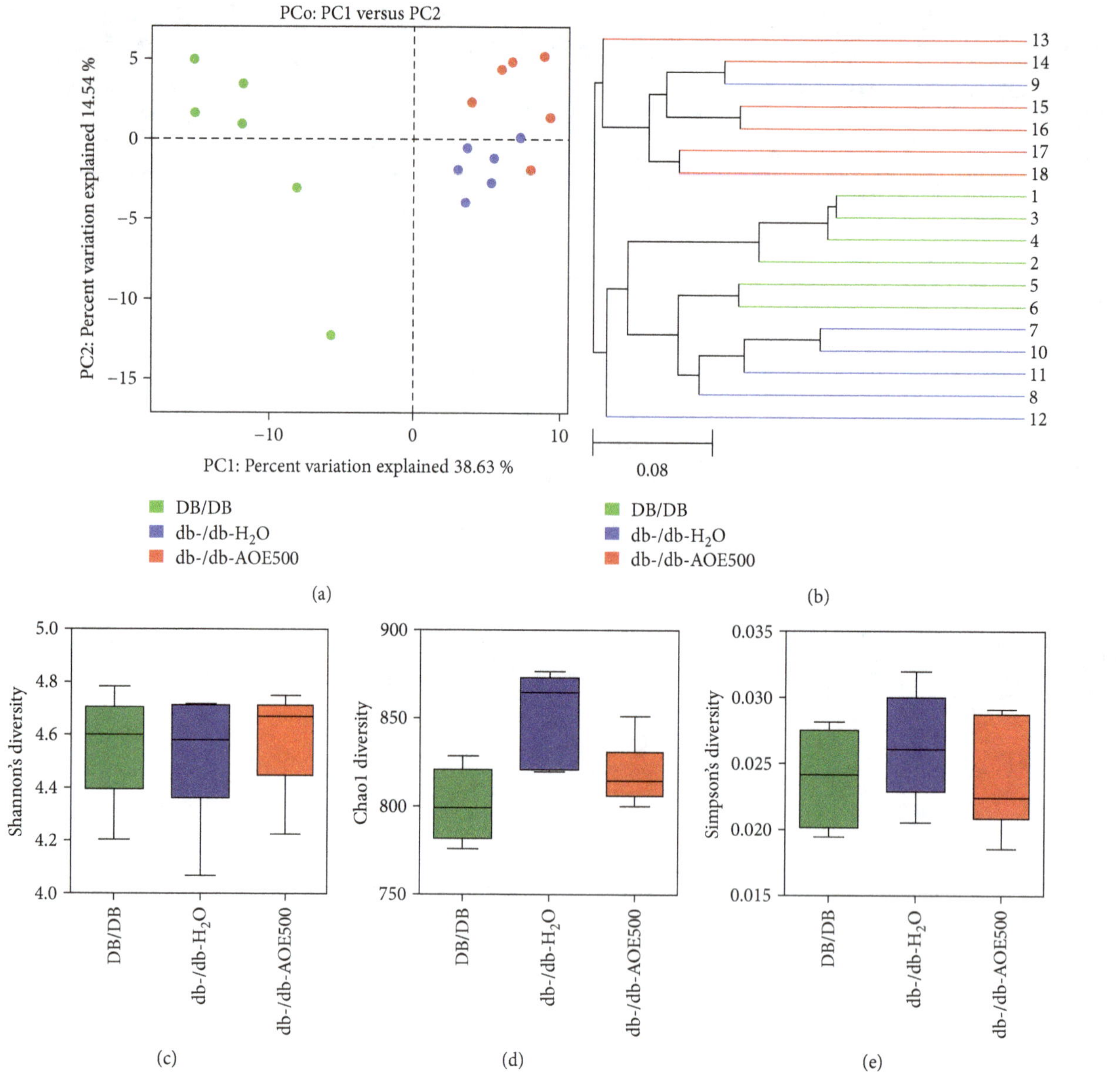

FIGURE 3: AOE modulated the structure and diversity of the gut microbiota. (a) Principal coordinate analysis (PCoA) and (b) sample clustering results of the unweighted UniFrac distances of microbial 16S rRNA sequences from the V3-V4 region in fecal contents at week 8. The alpha diversity analysis, including Shannon diversity (c), Chao1 diversity (d), and Simpson diversity (c). There were six mice in each group.

and was much higher than that in the DB/DB mice. Meanwhile, the abundance of Bacteroidetes in db-/db-AOE500 mice markedly increased compared with that in the db-/db-H_2O mice and was much less than that in the DB/DB mice. These results suggest that AOE selectively promoted growth of Bacteroidetes and inhibited growth of Firmicutes.

Akkermansia is a mucin-degrading bacterium that lives in the mucus layer of the intestine. There has also been growing interest in *Akkermansia* due to its association with health in animals and humans. *Akkermansia* prevented Western diet-induced inflammation in both the circulation and local atherosclerotic lesion [40, 41] and negatively mediated effects of IFN-γ on glucose tolerance [42]. Moreover, calorie restriction [43, 44], metformin treatment [15], or Roux-en-Y gastric bypass surgery [45] showed a higher abundance of *Akkermansia*. The increased amount of *Akkermansia* may be related to elevated GLP-1 secretion, elevated serum insulin, and improved insulin resistance [45]. In agreement with these findings, we found a sharp increase in the relative abundance of *Akkermansia* in db-/db- mice after AOE treatment. Therefore, alteration of *Akkermansia* levels might be important with regard to their functions.

Recent studies have demonstrated the possible existence of an association between infection with *Helicobacter pylori* and metabolic syndrome, such as in insulin resistance and DM [46, 47]. *Helicobacter* can influence the absorption of glucose and lipids in DM [48]. *Helicobacter* is associated with oxidative stress, and there is a cross-relation between *Helicobacter* and T2DM [49]. In the present study, the abundance of *Helicobacter* in db-/db-H_2O mice markedly increased

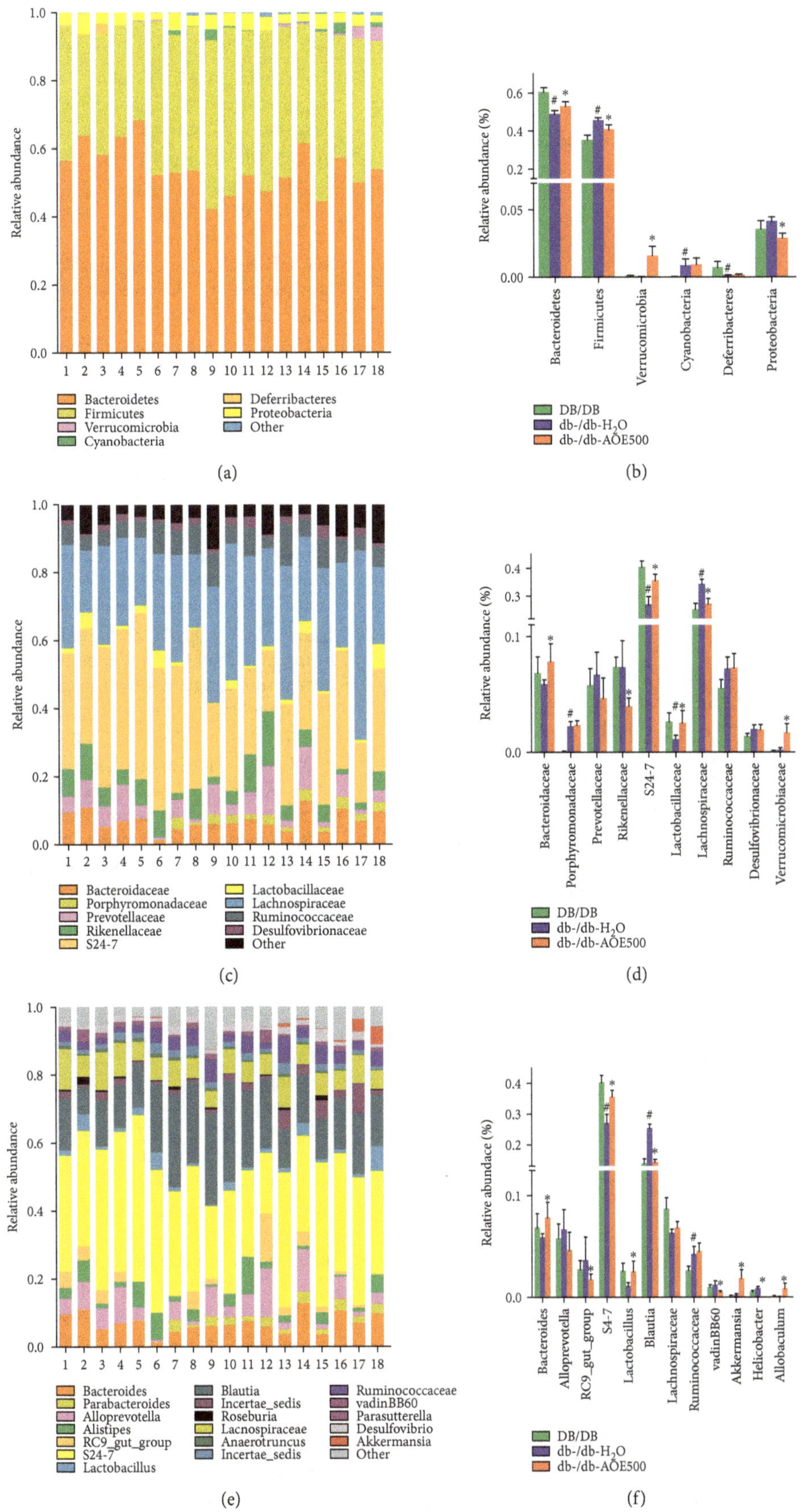

FIGURE 4: AOE modulated the composition of the gut microbiota. (a) Phylum-level, (b) family-level, and (c) genus-level taxonomic distributions of the microbial communities in fecal contents determined by next generation sequencing. Data represent the mean ± SD ($n = 6$). $^*P < 0.05$ for db-/db-AOE group compared with db-/db-H_2O, $^\#P < 0.05$ for db-/db-H_2O treated compared with DB/DB.

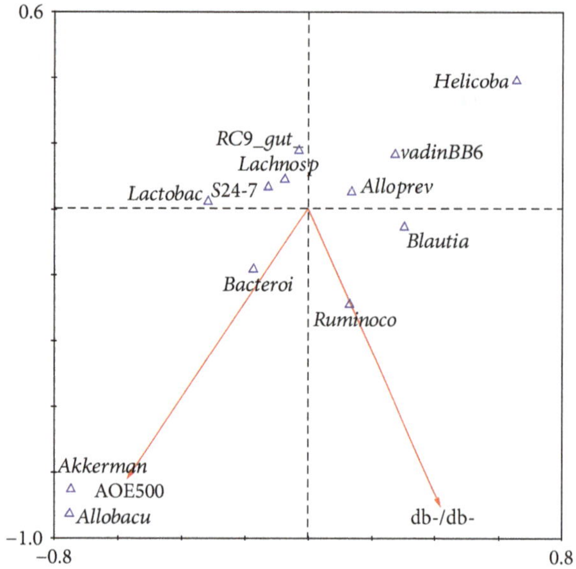

Figure 5: Canonical correspondence analysis (CCA) of bacterial community profiles from mice fecal samples. The length of each line represents the contribution of each variable to the bacterial community structure difference.

compared with that in the DB/DB mice. Meanwhile, AOE treatment significantly inhibited the growth of *Helicobacter*. The abundance of *Helicobacter* in db-/db-AOE500 was significantly less than that both in the db-/db-H_2O and DB/DB mice. Thus, the suppression of *Helicobacter* will also help to elucidate the underlying mechanisms of AOE antidiabetic function. Since AOE was shown to play a role in controlling glucose level, future investigation using humanized mouse models and transfer experiments will provide more details about how AOE differentially modulates gut microbiota across species.

In conclusion, based on the results of the present study, we suggest that AOE treatment decreases blood glucose levels and plays a protective role in renal function in T2DM by modulating gut microbiota composition.

Conflicts of Interest

The authors declare that there are no known competing interests regarding this study.

Authors' Contributions

Yiqiang Xie and Man Xiao contributed equally to this work.

Acknowledgments

The authors thank the Model Animal Research Center of Nanjing University for supplying mice. This study was funded by the National Natural Science Foundation of China (Grant nos. 81473618, 81360586) (Yiqiang Xie).

References

[1] J. E. Shaw, R. A. Sicree, and P. Z. Zimmet, "Global estimates of the prevalence of diabetes for 2010 and 2030," *Diabetes Research and Clinical Practice*, vol. 87, no. 1, pp. 4–14, 2010.

[2] D. LeRoith, "Hyperglycemia, hypertension, and dyslipidemia in type 2 diabetes mellitus: goals for diabetes management," *Clinical Cornerstone*, vol. 9, pp. S8–S16, 2008.

[3] M. Guo, S. D. Ricardo, J. A. Deane, M. Shi, L. Cullen-McEwen, and J. F. Bertram, "A stereological study of the renal glomerular vasculature in the db/db mouse model of diabetic nephropathy," *Journal of Anatomy*, vol. 207, no. 6, pp. 813–821, 2005.

[4] S. Ussar, S. Fujisaka, and C. R. Kahn, "Interactions between host genetics and gut microbiome in diabetes and metabolic syndrome," *Molecular Metabolism*, vol. 5, no. 9, pp. 795–803, 2016.

[5] G. M. Barlow, A. Yu, and R. Mathur, "Role of the gut microbiome in obesity and diabetes mellitus," *Nutrition in Clinical Practice*, vol. 30, no. 6, pp. 787–797, 2015.

[6] M. Sasaki, N. Ogasawara, Y. Funaki et al., "Transglucosidase improves the gut microbiota profile of type 2 diabetes mellitus patients: a randomized double-blind, placebo-controlled study," *BMC Gastroenterology*, vol. 13, no. 1, p. 81, 2013.

[7] J. Graessler, Y. Qin, H. Zhong et al., "Metagenomic sequencing of the human gut microbiome before and after bariatric surgery in obese patients with type 2 diabetes: correlation with inflammatory and metabolic parameters," *The Pharmacogenomics Journal*, vol. 13, no. 6, pp. 514–522, 2013.

[8] L. Wang, C. T. Christophersen, M. J. Sorich, J. P. Gerber, M. T. Angley, and M. A. Conlon, "Low relative abundances of the mucolytic bacterium Akkermansia muciniphila and Bifidobacterium spp. in feces of children with autism," *Applied and Environmental Microbiology*, vol. 77, no. 18, pp. 6718–6721, 2011.

[9] M. Derrien, C. Belzer, and W. M. de Vos, "*Akkermansia muciniphila* and its role in regulating host functions," *Microbial Pathogenesis*, vol. 106, pp. 171–181, 2017.

[10] X. Li, J. Guo, K. Ji, and P. Zhang, "Bamboo shoot fiber prevents obesity in mice by modulating the gut microbiota," *Scientific Reports*, vol. 6, no. 1, p. 32953, 2016.

[11] C. Kang, Y. Zhang, X. Zhu et al., "Healthy subjects differentially respond to dietary capsaicin correlating with specific gut enterotypes," *The Journal of Clinical Endocrinology and Metabolism*, vol. 101, no. 12, pp. 4681–4689, 2016.

[12] F. F. Anhê, D. Roy, G. Pilon et al., "A polyphenol-rich cranberry extract protects from diet-induced obesity, insulin resistance and intestinal inflammation in association with increased *Akkermansia* spp. population in the gut microbiota of mice," *Gut*, vol. 64, no. 6, pp. 872–883, 2015.

[13] D. E. Roopchand, R. N. Carmody, P. Kuhn et al., "Dietary polyphenols promote growth of the gut bacterium Akkermansia muciniphila and attenuate high-fat diet-induced metabolic syndrome," *Diabetes*, vol. 64, no. 8, pp. 2847–2858, 2015.

[14] F. F. Anhe, G. Pilon, D. Roy, Y. Desjardins, E. Levy, and A. Marette, "Triggering Akkermansia with dietary polyphenols: a new weapon to combat the metabolic syndrome?," *Gut Microbes*, vol. 7, no. 2, pp. 146–153, 2016.

[15] N. R. Shin, J. C. Lee, H. Y. Lee et al., "An increase in the Akkermansia spp. population induced by metformin treatment improves glucose homeostasis in diet-induced obese mice," *Gut*, vol. 63, no. 5, pp. 727–735, 2014.

[16] S.-H. Shi, X. Zhao, B. Liu et al., "The effects of sesquiterpenes-rich extract of *Alpinia oxyphylla* Miq. on amyloid-β-induced cognitive impairment and neuronal abnormalities in the cortex and hippocampus of mice," *Oxidative Medicine and Cellular Longevity*, vol. 2014, Article ID 451802, 11 pages, 2014.

[17] S. Wang, Y. Zhao, J. Zhang et al., "Antidiarrheal effect of Alpinia oxyphylla Miq.(Zingiberaceae) in experimental mice and its possible mechanism of action," *Journal of Ethnopharmacology*, vol. 168, pp. 182–190, 2015.

[18] Q. Zhang, C. Cui, C.-Q. Chen et al., "Anti-proliferative and pro-apoptotic activities of Alpinia oxyphylla on HepG2 cells through ROS-mediated signaling pathway," *Journal of Ethnopharmacology*, vol. 169, pp. 99–108, 2015.

[19] L. J. An, S. Guan, G. F. Shi, Y. M. Bao, Y. L. Duan, and B. Jiang, "Protocatechuic acid from Alpinia oxyphylla against MPP+ –induced neurotoxicity in PC12 cells," *Food and Chemical Toxicology*, vol. 44, no. 3, pp. 436–443, 2006.

[20] G.-F. Shi, L.-J. An, B. Jiang, S. Guan, and Y.-M. Bao, "Alpinia protocatechuic acid protects against oxidative damage in vitro and reduces oxidative stress in vivo," *Neuroscience Letters*, vol. 403, no. 3, pp. 206–210, 2006.

[21] H. Wang, T.-Q. Liu, S. Guan, Y.-X. Zhu, and Z.-F. Cui, "Protocatechuic acid from Alpinia oxyphylla promotes migration of human adipose tissue-derived stromal cells in vitro," *European Journal of Pharmacology*, vol. 599, no. 1–3, pp. 24–31, 2008.

[22] H. Wang, T.-Q. Liu, Y.-X. Zhu, S. Guan, X.-H. Ma, and Z.-F. Cui, "Effect of protocatechuic acid from Alpinia oxyphylla on proliferation of human adipose tissue-derived stromal cells in vitro," *Molecular and Cellular Biochemistry*, vol. 330, no. 1-2, pp. 47–53, 2009.

[23] Y. Xie, M. Xiao, D. Li et al., "Anti-diabetic effect of Alpinia oxyphylla extract on 57BL/KsJ db–/db- mice," *Experimental and Therapeutic Medicine*, vol. 13, no. 4, pp. 1321–1328, 2017.

[24] G. Du, M. Xiao, X. Zhang et al., "Alpinia oxyphylla Miq. extract changes miRNA expression profiles in db–/db- mouse kidney," *Biological Research*, vol. 50, no. 1, p. 9, 2017.

[25] W. Nicklas, P. Baneux, R. Boot et al., "Recommendations for the health monitoring of rodent and rabbit colonies in breeding and experimental units," *Laboratory Animals*, vol. 36, no. 1, pp. 20–42, 2002.

[26] J. A. Lott and K. Turner, "Evaluation of Trinder's glucose oxidase method for measuring glucose in serum and urine," *Clinical Chemistry*, vol. 21, no. 12, pp. 1754–1760, 1975.

[27] R. Katafuchi, Y. Kiyoshi, Y. Oh et al., "Glomerular score as a prognosticator in IgA nephropathy: its usefulness and limitation," *Clinical Nephrology*, vol. 49, no. 1, pp. 1–8, 1998.

[28] T. Magoc and S. L. Salzberg, "FLASH: fast length adjustment of short reads to improve genome assemblies," *Bioinformatics*, vol. 27, no. 21, pp. 2957–2963, 2011.

[29] T. Z. DeSantis, P. Hugenholtz, N. Larsen et al., "Greengenes, a chimera-checked 16S rRNA gene database and workbench compatible with ARB," *Applied and Environmental Microbiology*, vol. 72, no. 7, pp. 5069–5072, 2006.

[30] R. C. Edgar, "UPARSE: highly accurate OTU sequences from microbial amplicon reads," *Nature Methods*, vol. 10, no. 10, pp. 996–998, 2013.

[31] T. Braak, J. F. Cajo, and P. Smilauer, "CANOCO reference manual and CanoDraw for Windows user's guide: software for canonical community ordination (version 4.5)," 2002, http://www.canoco.com.

[32] A. P. Rolo and C. M. Palmeira, "Diabetes and mitochondrial function: role of hyperglycemia and oxidative stress," *Toxicology and Applied Pharmacology*, vol. 212, no. 2, pp. 167–178, 2006.

[33] Y. Ihara, S. Toyokuni, K. Uchida et al., "Hyperglycemia causes oxidative stress in pancreatic beta-cells of GK rats, a model of type 2 diabetes," *Diabetes*, vol. 48, no. 4, pp. 927–932, 1999.

[34] N. Larsen, F. K. Vogensen, F. W. J. van den Berg et al., "Gut microbiota in human adults with type 2 diabetes differs from non-diabetic adults," *PLoS One*, vol. 5, no. 2, article e9085, 2010.

[35] M. Murri, I. Leiva, J. M. Gomez-Zumaquero et al., "Gut microbiota in children with type 1 diabetes differs from that in healthy children: a case-control study," *BMC Medicine*, vol. 11, no. 1, p. 46, 2013.

[36] L. Geurts, V. Lazarevic, M. Derrien et al., "Altered gut microbiota and endocannabinoid system tone in obese and diabetic leptin-resistant mice: impact on apelin regulation in adipose tissue," *Frontiers in Microbiology*, vol. 2, p. 149, 2011.

[37] L. Krych, D. S. Nielsen, A. K. Hansen, and C. H. Hansen, "Gut microbial markers are associated with diabetes onset, regulatory imbalance, and IFN-γ level in NOD mice," *Gut Microbes*, vol. 6, no. 2, pp. 101–109, 2015.

[38] K. J. Wolf, J. G. Daft, S. M. Tanner, R. Hartmann, E. Khafipour, and R. G. Lorenz, "Consumption of acidic water alters the gut microbiome and decreases the risk of diabetes in NOD mice," *Journal of Histochemistry and Cytochemistry*, vol. 62, no. 4, pp. 237–250, 2014.

[39] M. Balfegò, S. Canivell, F. A. Hanzu et al., "Effects of sardine-enriched diet on metabolic control, inflammation and gut microbiota in drug-naïve patients with type 2 diabetes: a pilot randomized trial," *Lipids in Health and Disease*, vol. 15, no. 1, p. 78, 2016.

[40] S. Zhao, W. Liu, J. Wang et al., "*Akkermansia muciniphila* improves metabolic profiles by reducing inflammation in chow diet-fed mice," *Journal of Molecular Endocrinology*, vol. 58, no. 1, pp. 1–14, 2017.

[41] J. Li, S. Lin, P. M. Vanhoutte, C. W. Woo, and A. Xu, "Akkermansia muciniphila protects against atherosclerosis by preventing metabolic endotoxemia-induced inflammation in Apoe–/– mice," *Circulation*, vol. 133, no. 24, pp. 2434–2446, 2016.

[42] R. L. Greer, X. Dong, A. C. F. Moraes et al., "*Akkermansia muciniphila* mediates negative effects of IFNγ on glucose metabolism," *Nature Communications*, vol. 7, p. 13329, 2016.

[43] M. C. Dao, A. Everard, J. Aron-Wisnewsky et al., "Akkermansia muciniphila and improved metabolic health during a dietary intervention in obesity: relationship with gut microbiome richness and ecology," *Gut*, vol. 65, no. 3, pp. 426–436, 2016.

[44] M. Schneeberger, A. Everard, A. G. Gomez-Valades et al., "Akkermansia muciniphila inversely correlates with the onset of inflammation, altered adipose tissue metabolism and metabolic disorders during obesity in mice," *Scientific Reports*, vol. 5, no. 1, p. 16643, 2015.

[45] M. Yan, M. M. Song, R. X. Bai, S. Cheng, and W. M. Yan, "Effect of Roux-en-Y gastric bypass surgery on intestinal Akkermansia muciniphila," *World Journal of Gastrointestinal Surgery*, vol. 8, no. 4, pp. 301–307, 2016.

[46] L. R. Malamug, R. Karnchanasorn, R. Samoa, and K. C. Chiu,

"The role of *Helicobacter pylori* seropositivity in insulin sensitivity, beta cell function, and abnormal glucose tolerance," *Scientifica*, vol. 2014, Article ID 870165, 7 pages, 2014.

[47] T. Kozyrieva, E. Kolesnikova, and I. Shut, "Correlation of Helicobacter pylori infection with development of cardiovascular risk in patients with coronary heart disease in association with type 2 diabetes mellitus," *Georgian Medical News*, vol. 256-257, pp. 24–29, 2016.

[48] K. Tsang and S. Lam, "Extragastroduodenal conditions associated with Helicobacter pylori infection," *Hong Kong Medical Journal*, vol. 5, no. 2, pp. 169–174, 1999.

[49] W. A. Nasif, M. H. Mukhtar, M. M. Nour Eldein, and S. S. Ashgar, "Oxidative DNA damage and oxidized low density lipoprotein in type II diabetes mellitus among patients with Helicobacter pylori infection," *Diabetology & Metabolic Syndrome*, vol. 8, no. 1, p. 34, 2016.

Permissions

All chapters in this book were first published in JDR, by Hindawi Publishing Corporation; hereby published with permission under the Creative Commons Attribution License or equivalent. Every chapter published in this book has been scrutinized by our experts. Their significance has been extensively debated. The topics covered herein carry significant findings which will fuel the growth of the discipline. They may even be implemented as practical applications or may be referred to as a beginning point for another development.

The contributors of this book come from diverse backgrounds, making this book a truly international effort. This book will bring forth new frontiers with its revolutionizing research information and detailed analysis of the nascent developments around the world.

We would like to thank all the contributing authors for lending their expertise to make the book truly unique. They have played a crucial role in the development of this book. Without their invaluable contributions this book wouldn't have been possible. They have made vital efforts to compile up to date information on the varied aspects of this subject to make this book a valuable addition to the collection of many professionals and students.

This book was conceptualized with the vision of imparting up-to-date information and advanced data in this field. To ensure the same, a matchless editorial board was set up. Every individual on the board went through rigorous rounds of assessment to prove their worth. After which they invested a large part of their time researching and compiling the most relevant data for our readers.

The editorial board has been involved in producing this book since its inception. They have spent rigorous hours researching and exploring the diverse topics which have resulted in the successful publishing of this book. They have passed on their knowledge of decades through this book. To expedite this challenging task, the publisher supported the team at every step. A small team of assistant editors was also appointed to further simplify the editing procedure and attain best results for the readers.

Apart from the editorial board, the designing team has also invested a significant amount of their time in understanding the subject and creating the most relevant covers. They scrutinized every image to scout for the most suitable representation of the subject and create an appropriate cover for the book.

The publishing team has been an ardent support to the editorial, designing and production team. Their endless efforts to recruit the best for this project, has resulted in the accomplishment of this book. They are a veteran in the field of academics and their pool of knowledge is as vast as their experience in printing. Their expertise and guidance has proved useful at every step. Their uncompromising quality standards have made this book an exceptional effort. Their encouragement from time to time has been an inspiration for everyone.

The publisher and the editorial board hope that this book will prove to be a valuable piece of knowledge for researchers, students, practitioners and scholars across the globe.

List of Contributors

Selvalakshmi Rathinavelu and Crissy Guidry-Elizondo
Department of Health and Biomedical Sciences, College of Health Affairs, University of Texas Rio Grande Valley, 1201, W University Dr, Edinburg, TX 78539, USA

Jameela Banu
Department of Health and Biomedical Sciences, College of Health Affairs, University of Texas Rio Grande Valley, 1201, W University Dr, Edinburg, TX 78539, USA
Department of Biology, College of Sciences, University of Texas Rio Grande Valley, 1201, W University Dr, Edinburg, TX 78539, USA

Konstantinos Batzias, Alexios S. Antonopoulos, Evangelos Oikonomou, Gerasimos Siasos, Evanthia Bletsa, Panagiota K. Stampouloglou, Chara-Vasiliki Mistakidi, Periklis Karopoulos, Georgios Charalambous and Dimitris Tousoulis
1st Department of Cardiology, Hippokration Hospital, National and Kapodistrian University of Athens Medical School, Athens, Greece

Marina Noutsou and Anastasia Thanopoulou
Diabetes Center, 2nd Department of Internal Medicine, Medical School, National and Kapodistrian University of Athens, Hippokration General Hospital of Athens, Athens, Greece

Niki Katsiki
Second Department of Internal Medicine, Hippokration University Hospital, Aristotle University of Thessaloniki, Thessaloniki, Greece

Nicholas Tentolouris
First Department of Propaedeutic and Internal Medicine, Division of Diabetes, Laiko University Hospital, National and Kapodistrian University of Athens Medical School, Athens, Greece

Pu Wang, Yu Cheng Lu and Lan Wang
School of Life Sciences, Shanxi University, Taiyuan, Shanxi 030006, China

Yuan Fei Li
Department of Oncology, The First Clinical Hospital of Shanxi Medical University, Taiyuan, Shanxi 030006, China

Shao Chin Lee
School of Life Sciences, Shanxi University, Taiyuan, Shanxi 030006, China
Department of Bological Science, School of Life Sciences, Jiangsu Normal University, Xuzhou, Jiangsu 221000, China

Osei Sarfo-Kantanka, Eunice Oparebea Ansah and Ishmael Kyei
Komfo Anokye Teaching Hospital, Kumasi, Ghana

Fred Stephen Sarfo
Komfo Anokye Teaching Hospital, Kumasi, Ghana
Kwame Nkrumah University of Science and Technology, Kumasi, Ghana

Christian Obirikorang, Emmanuel Acheampong, Bright Amakwaa, Emmanuella Nsenbah Batu and Peter Brenya
Department of Molecular Medicine, School of Medical Sciences, Kwame Nkrumah University of Science and Technology (KNUST), Kumasi, Ghana

Yaa Obirikorang
Department of Nursing, Faculty of Health and Allied Sciences, Garden City University College (GCUC), Kenyasi, Kumasi, Ghana

Enoch Odame Anto
Department of Molecular Medicine, School of Medical Sciences, Kwame Nkrumah University of Science and Technology (KNUST), Kumasi, Ghana
School of Medical and Health Sciences, Edith Cowan University, Joondalup, WA, Australia

Emmanuel Toboh
Diagnostic Unit, Dansoman Polyclinic, Ghana Health Service, Accra, Ghana

Evans Adu Asamoah
Department of Medical Laboratory Technology, Faculty of Allied Health Sciences, KNUST, Kumasi, Ghana

Ming-Kuo Ting
Division of Endocrinology and Metabolism, Chang Gung Memorial Hospital, Keelung, Taiwan

Pei-Ju Liao
Department of Health Care Administration, Oriental Institute of Technology, New Taipei City, Taiwan

I-Wen Wu
Division of Nephrology, Chang Gung Memorial Hospital, Keelung, Taiwan

Shuo-Wei Chen
Division of Gastroenterology and Hepatology, Chang Gung Memorial Hospital, Keelung, Taiwan

Ning-I Yang
Division of Cardiology, Chang Gung Memorial Hospital, Keelung, Taiwan

Tzu-Yu Lin
Healthy Aging Research Center, Chang Gung University, Taoyuan, Taiwan

Kuang-Hung Hsu
Healthy Aging Research Center, Chang Gung University, Taoyuan, Taiwan
Laboratory for Epidemiology, Department of Health Care Management, Chang Gung University, Taoyuan, Taiwan
Department of Emergency Medicine, Chang Gung Memorial Hospital, Taoyuan, Taiwan
Department of Urology, Chang Gung Memorial Hospital, Taoyuan, Taiwan

Sandra C. Fuchs and Leila B. Moreira
Postgraduate Program in Cardiology, School of Medicine, Universidade Federal do Rio Grande do Sul (UFRGS), R. Ramiro Barcelos 2600, 90035-003 Porto Alegre, RS, Brazil

Glaucia S. Tres and Fabiana Piovesan
Postgraduate Program in Cardiology, School of Medicine, Universidade Federal do Rio Grande do Sul (UFRGS), R. Ramiro Barcelos 2600, 90035-003 Porto Alegre, RS, Brazil
Hospital São Vicente de Paulo, School of Medicine, Universidade de Passo Fundo (UPF), R. Teixeira Soares 808, 99010-080 Passo Fundo, RS, Brazil

Hugo K. Lisboa
Hospital São Vicente de Paulo, School of Medicine, Universidade de Passo Fundo (UPF), R. Teixeira Soares 808, 99010-080 Passo Fundo, RS, Brazil

Patricia Koehler-Santos and Fernanda dos S. Pereira
Unidade de Análises Moleculares e de Proteínas (UAMP), Hospital de Clinicas de Porto Alegre, Universidade Federal do Rio Grande do Sul (UFRGS), R. Ramiro Barcelos 2350, 90035-903 Porto Alegre, RS, Brazil

Suzi Camey
Postgraduate Program in Cardiology, School of Medicine, Universidade Federal do Rio Grande do Sul (UFRGS), R. Ramiro Barcelos 2600, 90035-003 Porto Alegre, RS, Brazil
Department of Statistics, Mathematics Institute, Universidade Federal do Rio Grande do Sul, R. Ramiro Barcelos 2350, 90035-903 Porto Alegre, RS, Brazil
Biostatistics Unit, GPPG, Hospital de Clinicas de Porto Alegre, Universidade Federal do Rio Grande do Sul (UFRGS), R. Ramiro Barcelos 2350, 90035-903 Porto Alegre, RS, Brazil

Qian Wang, Xu Zhang, Li Fang, Qingbo Guan and Qiu Li
Department of Endocrinology, Shandong Provincial Hospital Affiliated to Shandong University, Jinan, Shandong, China
Shandong Clinical Medical Center of Endocrinology and Metabolism, Jinan, Shandong, China
Institute of Endocrinology and Metabolism, Shandong Academy of Clinical Medicine, Jinan, Shandong, China

Ling Gao
Shandong Clinical Medical Center of Endocrinology and Metabolism, Jinan, Shandong, China
Institute of Endocrinology and Metabolism, Shandong Academy of Clinical Medicine, Jinan, Shandong, China
Scientific Center, Shandong Provincial Hospital Affiliated to Shandong University, Jinan, Shandong, China

Jennifer B. Bollyky
Livongo Health, Mountain View, CA, USA
Stanford University, Hospital & Clinics, Stanford, CA, USA

Dena Bravata and Jennifer Schneider
Livongo Health, Mountain View, CA, USA
Center for Primary Care and Outcomes Research, Stanford University, Stanford, CA, USA

Jason Yang
Biomedical Informatics, Stanford University, Stanford, CA, USA

Mark Williamson
Restore Health, Palo Alto, CA, USA

Jelena P. Seferovic, Brian Claggett, Eldrin F. Lewis, Scott D. Solomon and Marc A. Pfeffer
Cardiovascular Division, Brigham and Women's Hospital, Harvard Medical School, Boston, MA, USA

Rhonda Bentley-Lewis
Massachusetts General Hospital, Harvard Medical School, Boston, MA, USA

Rafael Diaz
Estudios Clínicos Latinoamérica, Rosario, Argentina

Hertzel C. Gerstein
McMaster University, Hamilton, ON, Canada

Lars V. Køber
Rigshospitalet Copenhagen University Hospital, Copenhagen, Denmark

Francesca C. Lawson
Sanofi U.S., Bridgewater, NJ, USA

Aldo P. Maggioni
Research Center of the Italian Association of Hospital Cardiologists, Florence, Italy

John J. V. McMurray
British Heart Foundation Cardiovascular Research Centre, University of Glasgow, Glasgow, UK

Jeffrey L. Probstfield
University of Washington Medical Center, Seattle, WA, USA

Matthew C. Riddle
Oregon Health and Science University, Portland, OR, USA

Jean-Claude Tardif
Montreal Heart Institute, Université de Montréal, Montreal, Canada

Mengyao Chao, Chunyan Wang, Xiaosheng Dong and Meng Ding
College of Physical Education, Shandong Normal University, 88 Wenhuadong Street, Jinan 250014, China

Li Zheng, Wei Zhang, Aimei Li, Yan Liu, Bin Yi and Hao Zhang
Department of Nephrology, The Third Xiangya Hospital of Central South University, 138 Tongzipo Road, Changsha, Hunan, China

Farid Nakhoul
Diabetic Nephropathy Lab, Baruch Padeh Poriya Medical Center Affiliated to the Faculty of Medicine in Galilee, 15208 Lower Galilee, Israel

You Lv, Xue Zhao, Weiying Guo, Ying Gao, Shuo Yang, Zhuo Li and Guixia Wang
Department of Endocrinology and Metabolism, The First Hospital of Jilin University, Changchun, Jilin, China

Kim Lam Soh
Department of Nursing and Rehabilitations, Faculty of Medicine and Health Sciences, University Putra Malaysia (UPM), 43400 Serdang, Selangor, Malaysia

Golnaz Azami
Department of Nursing and Rehabilitations, Faculty of Medicine and Health Sciences, University Putra Malaysia (UPM), 43400 Serdang, Selangor, Malaysia
Department of Nursing, Faculty of Nursing and Midwifery, Ilam University of Medical Sciences, Ilam 693917714, Iran

Sanaz Aazami, Mosayeb Mozafari and Hamid Taghinejad
Department of Nursing, Faculty of Nursing and Midwifery, Ilam University of Medical Sciences, Ilam 693917714, Iran

Shariff Ghazali Sazlina
Department of Family Medicine, Faculty of Medicine and Health Sciences, University Putra Malaysia (UPM), 43400 Serdang, Selangor, Malaysia

Md. Said Salmiah
Department of Community Health, Faculty of Medicine and Health Sciences, University Putra Malaysia (UPM), 43400 Serdang, Selangor, Malaysia

Ablikm Tuerdi, Xiaoyun Zeng, Li Quan, Shan Xiao and Jun Zhu
Department of Endocrinology, First Affiliated Hospital of Xinjiang Medical University, Urumqi, China

Mingchen Zhang
Department of Endocrinology, First Affiliated Hospital of Xinjiang Medical University, Urumqi, China
Postdoctoral Research Station of Public Health, School of Public Health, Xinjiang Medical University, Urumqi, China

Jiangfeng Mao
Department of Endocrinology, Peking Union Medical College Hospital, Key Laboratory of Endocrinology, Ministry of Health, Beijing, China

Hua Yao
Postdoctoral Research Station of Public Health, School of Public Health, Xinjiang Medical University, Urumqi, China
The Key Laboratory of Xinjiang Metabolic Disease, Clinical Medical Research Institute, First Affiliated Hospital of Xinjiang Medical

Caroline Jane Magri
Department of Cardiology, Mater Dei Hospital and University of Malta, Msida, Malta
Department of Cardiology, Mater Dei Hospital, Msida, Malta

Robert G. Xuereb
Department of Cardiology, Mater Dei Hospital, Msida, Malta

Dillon Mintoff
Mater Dei Hospital, Msida, Malta

Liberato Camilleri
Statistics & Operations Research, Faculty of Science, University of Malta, Msida, Malta

Joseph Galea and Stephen Fava
Mater Dei Hospital and University of Malta, Msida, Malta

Cindy Feng
School of Public Health, University of Saskatchewan, Saskatoon, SK, Canada

Nathaniel D. Osgood
Department of Computer Science, University of Saskatchewan, Saskatoon, SK, Canada

Roland F. Dyck
Department of Medicine, Canadian Centre for Health and Safety in Agriculture, University of Saskatchewan, Saskatoon, SK, Canada

T. Kroner, M. Arzt and S. Stadler
Department of Internal Medicine II, University Hospital Regensburg, Franz-Josef-Strauss-Allee 11, 93053 Regensburg, Germany

M. Rheinberger and C. A. Böger
Department of Nephrology, University Hospital Regensburg, Franz-Josef-Strauss-Allee 11, 93053 Regensburg, Germany

M. Gorski and I. M. Heid
Department of Genetic Epidemiology, University of Regensburg, Franz-Josef-Strauss-Allee 11, 93053 Regensburg, Germany

Natalie Z. M. Eichner
Department of Kinesiology, University of Virginia, Charlottesville, VA, USA

Uta Erdbrügger
Division of Nephrology, University of Virginia, Charlottesville, VA, USA

Steven K. Malin
Department of Kinesiology, University of Virginia, Charlottesville, VA, USA
Division of Endocrinology and Metabolism, University of Virginia, Charlottesville, VA, USA
Robert M. Berne Cardiovascular Research Center, University of Virginia, Charlottesville, VA, USA

Zhong-Xia Lu, Wen-Jun Xu and Yi-Tao Chen
College of Life Sciences, Zhejiang Chinese Medical University, Hangzhou 310053, China

Yang-Sheng Wu and Chang-Yu Li
College of Pharmacy, Zhejiang Chinese Medical University, Hangzhou 310053, China

Yiqiang Xie, Yali Ni and Shenggang Sang
First Affiliated Hospital of Hainan Medical University, Haikou 571199, China

Man Xiao, Shangfei Jiang, Guizhu Feng and Guankui Du
Department of Biochemistry and Molecular Biology, Hainan Medical University, Haikou 571101, China

Index

www.ingramcontent.com/pod-product-compliance
Lightning Source LLC
LaVergne TN
LVHW060606210926
848485LV00005B/1378
9781639271290